AF541323

GEOGRAPHY IN HEALTH

GEOGRAPHY IN HEALTH

Dr. Panna Lal

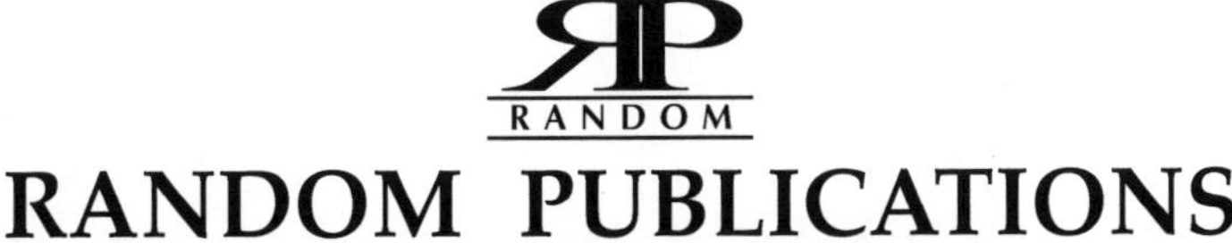

RANDOM PUBLICATIONS
NEW DELHI - 110 002 (INDIA)

Geography in Health

ISBN 978-93-51117-38-4
© Reserved

All Rights Reserved. No Part of this book may be reproduced in any manner without written permission.

Published in 2015 in India by

RANDOM PUBLICATIONS

4376-A/4B, Gali Murari Lal, Ansari Road
New Delhi-110 002
Phone: +9111-43580356, 23289044
E-mail: randomexports@gmail.com; sales@randompublications.com; info@randompublications.com

Reprinted 2024

Type Setting by: Friends Media, Delhi-110089
Digitally Printed at : Replika Press Pvt. Ltd.

Preface

Geography and health are intrinsically linked. Where we are born, live, study and work directly influences our health experiences: the air we breathe, the food we eat, the viruses we are exposed to and the health services we can access. The social, built and natural environments affect our health and well-being in ways that are directly relevant to health policy. Spatial location (the geographic context of places and the connectedness between places) plays a major role in shaping environmental risks as well as many other health effects. For example, locating health care facilities, targeting public health strategies or monitoring disease outbreaks all have a geographic context. Health geography is related to medical geography, but is much more. It should be obvious that GIS can play a major role in several areas of health geography. However, similarly, it should also be obvious that the use of technologies such as GIS must always be tempered by a critical social and cultural perspective on the issue.

The study of health geography has been influenced by (re)positioning of medical geography within the field of social geography due a shift from a medical model to a social model in healthcare, which advocates for the redefinition of health and health care away from prevention and treatment of illness only to one of promoting well-being in general. Under this model, some previous illnesses (e.g., mental ill health) are recognized as behaviour disturbances only, and other types of medicine (e.g., complementary or alternative medicine and traditional medicine) are studied by the medicine researchers, sometimes with the aid of health geographers without medical education. This shift changes the definition of care, no longer limiting it to spaces such as hospitals or doctor's offices. Also, the social model gives primacy to the intimate encounters performed at non-traditional spaces of medicine and healthcare as well as to the individuals as health consumers. This alternative methodological approach means that medical geography is broadened to incorporate philosophies such as Marxian political economy, structuralism, social interactionism, humanism, feminism and queer theory. Health geography is considered to be divided into two distinct elements. The first of which is focused on geographies of disease and ill health, involving descriptive research quantifying disease frequencies and distributions, and analytic research concerned with finding what characteristics make an individual or population susceptible to disease. This requires an understanding of epidemiology. The second stream of health geography is the geography of health care, primarily facility location, accessibility and utilization. This requires the use of spatial analysis and often borrows from Behavioural economics. Informed decision-making leads to the development of effective public health policy based on evidence. We need to understand disease risk factors and how risks such as genetics, lifestyle, environment and occupation interact with the social, built and natural environments. Understanding geography, including the arrangement of health services and the location and nature of environmental exposures, is crucial in assessing the interrelations inherent in many health-related risk exposures. Many core geographic research themes, including health inequalities and polarization, scale, globalization and urbanization, are directly related to public health.

The present book provides a comprehensive introduction to geographic approaches to studying disease and promoting health. This book is an essential introductory text for undergraduate students studying Geography, Health and Social Studies.

I thank all members of my team who have helped in the preparation of the book. My special thanks go to "Random Publications" who have published the book.

— Dr. Panna Lal

Contents

Chapter 1

Overview of Health Geography

Health geography is the application of geographical information, perspectives, and methods to the study of health, disease, and health care. The study of health geography has been influenced by (re)positioning of medical geography within the field of social geography due a shift from a medical model to a social model in healthcare, which advocates for the redefinition of health and health care away from prevention and treatment of illness only to one of promoting well-being in general. Under this model, some previous illnesses (e.g., mental ill health) are recognised as behaviour disturbances only, and other types of medicine (e.g., complementary or alternative medicine and traditional medicine) are studied by the medicine researchers, sometimes with the aid of health geographers without medical education. This shift changes the definition of care, no longer limiting it to spaces such as hospitals or doctor's offices. Also, the social model gives primacy to the intimate encounters performed at non-traditional spaces of medicine and healthcare as well as to the individuals as health consumers.

This alternative methodological approach means that medical geography is broadened to incorporate philosophies such as Marxian political economy, structuralism, social interactionism, humanism, feminism and queer theory.

History of Health Geography

The relationship between space and health dates back to Hippocrates, who stated that "airs, waters, places" all played significant roles impacting human health and history. A classic piece of research in health geography was done in 1854 as a cholera outbreak gripped a neighbourhood in London. Death tolls rang around the clock and the people feared that they were being infected by vapours coming from the ground. John Snow thought that if he could locate the source of the disease, it could be contained. He drew maps showing the homes of people who had died of cholera and the locations of water pumps. He found that one pump, the public pump on Broad Street, was central to most of the victims. He figured that infected water from the pump was the culprit. He instructed the authorities to remove the handle to the pump, making it unusable. After that the number of new cholera cases decreased.

Areas of Study

Health geography is considered to be divided into two distinct elements. The first of which is focused on geographies of disease and ill health, involving descriptive research quantifying disease frequencies and distributions, and analytic research concerned with finding what characteristics make an individual or population susceptible to disease. This requires an understanding of epidemiology. The second stream of health geography is the geography of health care, primarily facility location, accessibility and utilisation. This requires the use of spatial analysis and often borrows from Behavioural economics.

Geographies of Disease and Ill Health

Health geographers are concerned with the prevalence of different diseases along a range of scales from the local to global, and inspects the natural world, in all of its complexity, for correlations between diseases and locations. This situates health geography alongside other geographical sub-disciplines that trace human-environment relations. Health geographers use modern spatial analysis tools to map the diffusion of various diseases, as individuals spread them amongst themselves, and across wider spaces as they migrate. Health geographers also consider all types of spaces as presenting health risks, from natural disasters, to interpersonal violence, stress and other potential dangers.

Geography of Health Care Provision

Although health care is a public good, it is not equally available to all individuals. Demand for public services is continuously increasing. People need advance knowledge and fastest prediction technology, that Health Geography offers. The latest example is Telemedicine.

Medical geography, sometimes called health geography, is an area of medical research that incorporates geographic techniques into the study of health around the world and the spread of diseases. In addition, medical geography studies the impact of climate and location on an individual's health as well as the distribution of health services. Medical geography is an important field because it aims to provide an understanding of health problems and improve the health of people worldwide based on the various geographic factors influencing them.

History of Medical Geography

Medical geography has a long history. Since the time of the Greek doctor, Hippocrates (5th-4th centuries BCE), people have studied the effect of location on one's health. For example, early medicine studied the differences in diseases experienced by people living at high versus low elevation. It was easily understood that those at living low elevations near waterways would be more prone to malaria than those at higher elevations or in drier, less humid areas. Though the reasons for these variations were not fully understood at the time, the study of this spatial distribution of disease is the beginnings of medical geography.

This field of geography did not gain prominence until the mid-1800s though when cholera gripped London. As more and more people became ill, they believed they were becoming infected by vapours escaping the ground. John Snow, a doctor in London, believed that if he could isolate the source of the toxins infecting the population they and cholera could be contained.

As part of his study, Snow plotted the distribution of deaths throughout London on a map. After examining these locations, he found a cluster of unusually high deaths near a water pump on Broad Street. He then concluded that the water coming from this pump was the reason people were becoming sick and he had authorities remove the handle to the pump. Once people then stopped drinking the water, the number of cholera deaths dramatically decreased.

Snow's use of mapping to find the source of disease is the earliest and most famous example of medical geography. Since he conducted his research however, geographic techniques have found their place in a number of other medical applications.

Another example of geography aiding medicine occurred in the early 20th Century in Colorado. There, dentists noticed that children living in certain areas had fewer cavities. After plotting these locations on a map and comparing them with chemicals found in the groundwater, they concluded that the children with fewer cavities were clustered around areas that had high levels of fluoride. From there, the use of fluoride gained prominence in dentistry.

Medical Geography Today

Today, medical geography has a number of applications as well. Since the spatial distribution of disease is still a large matter of importance though, mapping plays a huge role in the field. Maps are created to show historic outbreaks of things like the 1918 influenza for example or current issues like the index of pain or Google Flu Trends across the United States. In the pain map example, factors like climate and environment can be considered to determine why high amounts of pain cluster where they do at any given time.

Other studies have also been conducted to show where the highest outbreaks of certain types of disease occur. The Centre for Disease Control and Prevention (CDC) in the United States for instance uses what they call the *Atlas of United States Mortality* to look at a wide range of health factors across the U.S. Data ranges from the spatial distribution of people at different ages to places with the best and worst air quality. Subjects such as these are important because they have implications on the population growth of an area and the instances of health problems such as asthma and lung cancer. Local governments can then consider these factors when planning their cities and/or determining the best use of city funds.

The CDC also features a website for traveller's health. Here, people can get information about the distribution of disease in countries worldwide and learn about the different vaccines needed to travel to such places. This application of medical geography is important to reducing or even stopping the spread of the world's diseases through travel.

In addition to the United States' CDC, the World Health Organisation (WHO) also features similar health data for the world with its Global Health Atlas. Here, the public, medical professionals, researchers, and other interested persons can gather data about the distribution of the world's diseases in an attempt to find patterns of transmission and possibly cures to some of the more deadly illnesses such as HIV/AIDS and various cancers.

Obstacles in Medical Geography

Although medical geography is a prominent field of study today, geographers have some obstacles to overcome when gathering data. The first problem is associated with recording a disease's location. Since people sometimes do not always go to a doctor when ill, it can be difficult to get entirely accurate data about a disease's location. The second problem is associated with the accurate diagnosis of disease. While the third deals with the timely reporting of a disease's presence. Often, doctor-patient confidentiality laws can complicate the reporting of a disease. Since, data such as this need to be as complete as possible to monitor the spread of illness effectively, the International Classification of Disease (ICD) was created to make sure that all countries use the same medical terms to classify a disease and the WHO helps monitor the global surveillance of diseases to help data get to geographers and other researchers as quickly as possible.

Through the efforts of the ICD, the WHO, other organisations, and local governments, geographers are in fact able to monitor the spread of disease fairly accurately and their work, like that of Dr. John Snow's cholera maps, are essential to reducing the spread of and understanding contagious disease. As such, medical geography has become a significant area of expertise within the discipline.

Ecological Health

Ecological health is a term that has been used in relation to both human health and the condition of the environment. In medicine, ecological health has been used to refer to multiple chemical sensitivity, which results from exposure to synthetic chemicals (pesticides, smoke, etc.) in the environment, hence the term ecological. The term has also been used in medicine with respect to management of environmental factors (taxes, health insurance surcharges) that may reduce the risk of unhealthy behaviour such as smoking. As an urban planning term, ecological health refers to the "greenness" of cities, meaning composting, recycling, and energy efficiency. With respect to broader environmental issues, ecological health has been defined as "the goal for the condition at a site that is cultivated for crops, managed for tree harvest, stocked for fish, urbanized, or otherwise intensively used." Ecological health differs from ecosystem health, the condition of ecosystems, which have particular structural and functional properties, and it differs from ecological integrity, which refers to environments with minimal human impact, although the term ecological health has also been used loosely in reference to a range of environmental issues. Human health, in its broadest sense, is recognised as having ecological foundations.

The term health is intended to evoke human environmental health concerns, which are often closely related (but as a part of medicine not ecology). As with ecocide, that term assumes that ecosystems can be said to be alive. While the term integrity or damage seems to take no position on this, it does assume that there is a definition of integrity that can be said to apply to ecosystems. The more political term ecological wisdom refers not only to recognition of a level of health, integrity or potential damage, but also, to a decision to do nothing (more) to harm that ecosystem or its dependents. An ecosystem has a good health if it is capable of self-restoration after suffering external disturbances. This is termed resilience.

Measures of broad ecological health, like measures of the more specific principle of biodiversity, tend to be specific to an ecoregion or even to an ecosystem. Measures that depend on biodiversity are valid indicators of ecological health as stability and productivity (good indicators of ecological health) are two ecological effects of biodiversity. Dependencies between species vary so much as to be difficult to express abstractly. However, there are a few universal symptoms of poor health or damage to system integrity:

- The buildup of waste material and the proliferation of simpler life forms (bacteria, insects) that thrive on it - but no consequent population growth in those species that normally prey on them;
- The loss of keystone species, often a top predator, causing smaller carnivores to proliferate, very often overstressing herbivore populations;
- A higher rate of species mortality due to disease rather than predation, climate, or food scarcity;
- The migration of whole species into or out of a region, contrary to established or historical patterns;
- The proliferation of a bioinvader or even a monoculture where previously a more biodiverse species range existed.

Some practices such as organic farming, sustainable forestry, natural landscaping, wild gardening or precision agriculture, sometimes combined into sustainable agriculture, are thought to improve or at least not to degrade ecological health, while still keeping land usable for human purposes. This is difficult to investigate as part of ecology, but is increasingly part of discourse on agricultural economics and conservation.

Ecotage is another tactic thought to be effective by some in protecting the health of ecosystems, but this is hotly disputed. In general, low confrontation and much attention to political virtues is thought to be important to maintaining ecological health, as it is far faster and simpler to destroy an ecosystem than protect it - thus wars on behalf of ecosystem integrity may simply lead to more rapid despoliation and loss due to competition.

Deforestation and the habitat destruction of deep-sea coral reef are two issues that prompt deep investigation of what makes for ecological health, and fuels a great many debates. The role of clearcuts, plantations, and trawler nets is often portrayed as negative in the extreme, held akin to the role of weapons on human life.

Disease Ecology

The interaction of the behaviour and ecology of hosts with the biology of pathogens, as it relates to the impact of diseases on populations.

Threshold Theorem

For a disease to spread, on average it must be successfully transmitted to a new host before its current host dies or recovers. This observation lies at the core of the most important idea in epidemiology: the threshold theorem. The threshold theorem states that if the density of susceptible hosts is below some critical value, then on average the transmission of a disease will not occur rapidly enough to cause the number of infected individuals to increase. In other words, the reproductive rate of a disease must be greater than 1 for there to be an epidemic, with the reproductive rate being defined as the average number of new infections created per infected individual. Human immunization programmes are based on applying the threshold theorem of epidemiology to public health; specifically, if enough individuals in a population can be vaccinated, then the density of susceptible individuals will be sufficiently lowered that epidemics are prevented.

In general, the rate of reproduction for diseases is proportional to their transmissibility and to the length of time that an individual is infectious. For this reason, extremely deadly diseases that kill their hosts too rapidly may require extremely high densities of hosts before they can spread. All diseases do not behave as simply as hypothesized by the threshold theorem, the most notable exceptions being sexually transmitted diseases. Because organisms actively seek reproduction, the rate at which a sexually transmitted disease is passed among hosts is generally much less dependent on host density.

Population Effects

Cycles in many animal populations are thought to be driven by diseases. For example, the fluctuations of larch bud moths in Europe are hypothesized to be driven by a virus that infects and kills the caterpillars of this species. Cycles of red grouse in northern England are also thought to be driven by disease, in this case by parasitic nematodes. It is only when grouse are laden with heavy worm burdens that effects are seen, and those effects take the form of reduced breeding success or higher mortality during the winter. This example highlights a common feature of diseases: their effects may be obvious only when their hosts are assaulted by other stresses as well (such as harsh winters and starvation).

The introduction of novel diseases to wild populations has created massive disruptions of natural ecosystems. For example, the introduction of rinderpest virus into African buffalo and wildebeest populations decimated them in the Serengeti. African wild ungulates have recovered in recent years only because a massive vaccination programme eliminated rinderpest from the primary reservoir for the disease, domestic cattle. But the consequences of the rinderpest epidemic among wild ungulates extended well beyond the ungulate populations. For example, human sleeping sickness increased following the rinderpest epidemic because the tsetse flies that transmit sleeping sickness suffered a shortage of game animals (the normal hosts for tsetse flies) and increasingly switched to humans to obtain meals.

It is widely appreciated that crop plants are attacked by a tremendous diversity of diseases, some of which may ruin an entire year's production. Diseases are equally prevalent among wild populations of plants, but their toll seems to be reduced because natural plant populations are so genetically variable that it is unlikely that any given pathogen strain can sweep through and kill all of the plants—there are always some resistant genotypes. But when agronomists have bred plants for uniformity, they have often depleted genetic diversity and created a situation in which a plant pathogen that evolves to attack the crop encounters plants with no resistance (all the plants are the same). For example, when leaf blight devastated the United States corn crop, 70% of that crop shared genetically identical cytoplasm, and the genetic uniformity of the host exacerbated the severity of the epidemic.

Disease Emergence

Humans are dramatically altering habitats and ecosystems. Sometimes these changes can influence disease interactions in surprising ways. Lyme disease in the eastern United States provides a good example of the interplay of human habitat modifications and diseases. Lyme disease involves a spirochete bacterium transmitted to humans by ticks. However, humans are not the normal hosts for this disease; instead, both the ticks and the bacterium are maintained primarily on deer and mouse populations. Human activities influence both deer and mice populations, and in turn tick populations, affecting potential exposure of humans to the disease. Much less certain are the impacts of anticipated global warming on diseases. There is some cause for concern about the expansion of tropical diseases into what are now temperate regions in those cases where temperature sets limits to the activity or distribution of major disease vectors.

Population Ecology

Population ecology or autoecology is a sub-field of ecology that deals with the dynamics of species populations and how these populations interact with the environment. It is the study of how the population sizes of species living together in groups change over time and space. The development of population ecology owes much to demography and actuarial life tables. Population ecology is important in conservation biology, especially in the development of population viability analysis (PVA) which makes it possible to predict the long-term probability of a species persisting in a given habitat patch, such as a national park. Although population ecology is a subfield of biology, it provides interesting problems for mathematicians and statisticians who work in population dynamics.

Fundamentals

The most fundamental law of population ecology is Thomas Malthus' exponential law of population growth.

Terms used to describe natural groups of individuals in ecological studies

Term	*Definition*
Species population	All individuals of a species.
Metapopulation	A set of spatially disjunct populations, among which there is some immigration.
Population	A group of conspecific individuals that is demographically, genetically, or spatially disjunct from other groups of individuals.
Aggregation	A spatially clustered group of individuals.
Deme	A group of individuals more genetically similar to each other than to other individuals, usually with some degree of spatial isolation as well.
Local population	A group of individuals within an investigator-delimited area smaller than the geographic range of the species and often within a population (as defined above). A local population could be a disjunct population as well.
Subpopulation	An arbitrary spatially delimited subset of individuals from within a population (as defined above).

A population will grow (or decline) exponentially as long as the environment experienced by all individuals in the population remains constant. This principle in population ecology provides the basis for formulating predictive theories and tests that follow.

Simplified population models usually start with four key variables including death, birth, immigration, and emigration. Mathematical models used to calculate changes in population demographics and evolution hold the assumption (or null hypothesis) of no external influence. Models can be more mathematically complex where "...several competing hypotheses are simultaneously confronted with the data." For example, in a closed system where immigration and emigration does not take place, the per capita rates of change in a population can be described as:

$$\frac{dN}{dT} = B - D = bN - dN = (b - d)N = rN,$$

where N is the total number of individuals in the population, B is the number of births, D is the number of deaths, b and d are the per capita rates of birth and death respectively, and r is the per capita rate of population change. This formula can be read as the rate of change in the population (dN/dT) is equal to births minus deaths (B - D).

Using these techniques, Malthus' population principle of growth was later transformed into a mathematical model known as the logistic equation:

$$\frac{dN}{dT} = aN\left(1 - \frac{N}{K}\right),$$

where N is the biomass density, a is the maximum per-capita rate of change, and K is the carrying capacity of the population. The formula can be read as follows: the rate of change in the population (dN/dT) is equal to growth (aN) that is limited by carrying capacity ($1-N/K$). From these basic mathematical principles the discipline of population ecology expands into a field of investigation that queries the demographics of real populations and tests these results against the statistical models. The field of population ecology often uses data on life history and matrix algebra to develop projection matrices on fecundity and survivorship. This information is used for managing wildlife stocks and setting harvest quotas

r/K Selection

At its most elementary level, interspecific competition involves two species utilising a similar resource. It rapidly gets more complicated, but stripping the phenomenon of all its complications, this is the basic principle: two consumers consuming the same resource.

An important concept in population ecology is the r/K selection theory. The first variable is *r* (the intrinsic rate of natural increase in population size, density independent) and the second variable is *K* (the carrying capacity of a population, density dependent). An *r*-selected species (e.g., many kinds of insects, such as aphids) is one that has high rates of fecundity, low levels of parental investment in the young, and high rates of mortality before individuals reach maturity. Evolution favours productivity in r-selected species. In contrast, a *K*-selected species (such as humans) has low rates of fecundity, high levels of parental investment in the young, and low rates of mortality as individuals mature. Evolution in *K*-selected species favours efficiency in the conversion of more resources into fewer offspring.

Metapopulation

Populations are also studied and conceptualized through the "metapopulation" concept. The metapopulation concept was introduced in 1969:

> *"as a population of populations which go extinct locally and recolonize."*

Metapopulation ecology is a simplified model of the landscape into patches of varying levels of quality. Patches are either occupied or they are not. Migrants moving among the patches are structured into metapopulations either as sources or sinks. Source patches are productive sites that generate a seasonal supply of migrants to other patch locations. Sink patches are unproductive sites that only receive migrants. In metapopulation terminology there are emigrants (individuals that leave a patch) and immigrants (individuals that move into a patch). Metapopulation models examine patch dynamics over time to answer questions about spatial and demographic ecology. An important concept in metapopulation ecology is the rescue effect, where small patches of lower quality (i.e., sinks) are maintained by a seasonal influx of new immigrants. Metapopulation structure evolves from year to year, where some patches are sinks, such as dry years, and become sources when conditions are more favourable. Ecologists utilise a mixture of computer models and field studies to explain metapopulation structure.

History

The older term, autecology, refers to roughly the same field of study as population ecology. It derives from the division of ecology into autecology—the study of individual species in relation to the environment—

and synecology—the study of groups of organisms in relation to the environment—or community ecology. Odum (1959, p. 8) considered that synecology should be divided into population ecology, community ecology, and ecosystem ecology, defining autecology as essentially "species ecology." However, for some time biologists have recognised that the more significant level of organisation of a species is a population, because at this level the species gene pool is most coherent. In fact, Odum regarded "autecology" as no longer a "present tendency" in ecology (i.e., an archaic term), although included "species ecology"—studies emphasizing life history and behaviour as adaptations to the environment of individual organisms or species—as one of four subdivisions of ecology.

Disease Transmission

In 1999, a study group on Veterinary Public Health (VPH), convened jointly by the World Health Organisation (WHO), the Food and Agriculture Organisation of the United nations (FAO), and the Office International des epizooties (OIE), and including twenty-eight experts from eighteen countries, defined veterinary public health as "the contribution to the complete physical, mental, and social well-being of humans through an understanding and application of veterinary science." The emphasis was on the human ecosystem where the contribution of veterinary science to human health has been fundamental and sustained over millennia. It is not generally appreciated that this contribution pertains not only to livestock and food production, animal traction, and transportation, which have laid the basis for most urban societies around the world. The study and management of animal diseases have also laid the basis for much of what we know about the dynamics and management of infectious human diseases, and the promotion of environmental quality.

Defined as diseases transmitted between vertebrate animals and humans, zoonotic diseases (zoonoses) include bubonic plague, Lyme disease, salmonella, and rabies. Disease-carrying animals, called reservoirs, infect humans through several pathways: when they are eaten by humans, when they bite humans, or when arthropods that have fed on them, such as mosquitoes or ticks, then feed on a human host. It has been estimated that over 60% of infectious diseases impacting humans are zoonotic in origin and zoonoses are on the rise globally, accounting for over 75% of emerging diseases.

Many important human diseases have originated in animals, and so changes in the habitats of animals that are disease vectors or reservoirs may affect human health, sometimes positively and sometimes negatively. For example, the Nipah virus is believed to have emerged after forest clearance fires in Indonesia drove carrier bats to neighbouring Malaysia, where the virus infected intensively farmed pigs, and then crossed to humans. Intensive livestock production, while providing benefits to health in terms of improved nutrition, has also created environments favourable to the emergence of diseases. Greater human contact with wild species and 'bush meat' from encroachment in forests and changes in diet also create opportunities for disease transmission. Trends ranging from forest clearance to climate-induced habitat changes also appear to have impacted certain populations of mosquitoes, ticks and midges, altering transmission patterns for diseases like malaria and lyme disease.

Until recently, zoonotic diseases have not been treated as part of ecological systems. In response to the prevalence of zoonoses, the multidisciplinary field of disease ecology has emerged. It involves the study of any ecological system that includes pathogens and incorporates the complexity of multiple interactions. The research area covers basic processes underlying the linkages between climate, ecosystems, and infectious disease, particularly the different ways that climate can influence the emergence and transmission of infectious disease agents. For example Mexican researchers adopted an ecosystem approach to better understand the complex set of factors that influenced the incidence and spread of malaria in Oaxaca. This project includes the molecular biology of the vector and the parasite, community perceptions of malaria, statistical analyses, and a geographic information-based surveillance system.

Mammals are the most common reservoirs for zoonotic diseases, with rodents leading the pack. The plague (Yersinia pestis), Lyme disease (Borrelia burgdorferi), Hantavirus pulmonary syndrome and Rocky Mountain spotted fever (Rickettsia rickettsii) all owe their spread to the presence of rodents. From an ecological perspective, rodents occupy the middle rung of the food chain. Primarily herbivores, with diets rich in plant matter, they are a food source for vertebrate predators such as foxes, and owls.

Aquatic animals that carry human parasites are also a source of disease and death. The human cost is high: The World Health Organisation (WHO 2004, 2) estimates that globally "1.8 million people die each year from diarrhoeal diseases, 200 million people are infected with schistosomiasis and more than 1 billion people suffer from soil-transmitted helminthes infections."

Unfortunately, agricultural systems, especially irrigated ones, have long been associated with manifestations of extreme human ill-health arising from water-related diseases. The major reason is that public health and disease control programmes have not been concerns of the water resources sector, which typically has focused on potential economic benefits of water bodies in terms of food production and power generation. This theme of applied ecology aims to increase knowledge of the relationship between water, human health and ecosystems; and to develop practical measures to reduce negative environmental health impacts by:

- mitigating adverse impacts due to malaria and other water-related parasitic diseases through water and land management strategies;
- managing the agricultural use of polluted water sources (including urban and industrial waste) so as to optimize food production and livelihoods benefits and minimize adverse health and environmental impacts;
- exploring the trade-offs necessary to provide for environmental water requirements in river basins, the wise use of wetland ecosystems, and the conservation of biodiversity through the application of eco-agricultural principles.

Another important issue is the dangerous integration of circumstances when animals and consumers from different ecosystems come into contact. The lack of resistance to new pathogens makes humans and animals replicating reservoirs, for viruses and bacteria to adapt and rapidly mutate. Further, the staggering numbers of animals and people in contact change one-in-a-million odds of a disease transfer into almost a daily possibility. Even under the most hygienic conditions, this pool of viruses, bacteria, and other pathogens creates optimal conditions for diseases to multiply rapidly and jump between species to exploit new potential hosts; something the most "successful" diseases do all too well. Under this scenario, two problems are created. First is the high risk of new diseases spreading into human populations. Second is that this can create a "fear factor" amongst people - their concern that wildlife is unhealthy might cause them to try to remove the threat by killing the wildlife. Shooting flying foxes was proposed in Southeast Asia when they were thought to be carrying nipa virus, even though the link has not been definitively proven and the disease is rarely found in flying foxes.

The global trade in wildlife provides disease transmission mechanisms that not only cause human disease outbreaks but also threaten livestock, international trade, rural livelihoods, native wildlife populations, and the health of ecosystems. Outbreaks resulting from wildlife trade have caused hundreds of billions of dollars of economic damage globally.

In almost all cases, eradication schemes are not cost efficient or effective means to reduce disease spread when compared to health education, sanitation, and controlling animal movement. Moreover, eradication schemes do not address the fundamental problem of our creating conditions, which maximize opportunities for disease build-up and cross-species transmission. Much research is still needed on the links between viruses in different species and human disease, and means of transmission between the two. Rather than attempting to eradicate pathogens or the wild species that may harbour them, a practical approach would include decreasing the contact rate among species, including humans, at the interface created by the wildlife trade. Since wildlife marketing functions as a system of networks with major hubs, these points provide control opportunities to maximize the effects of regulatory efforts.

Intensive production has also given rise to new disease problems, such as Bovine Spongiform Encephalopathy (Mad Cow Disease) and Avian flu. These indicate the potential for disease transmission through human food chains that are now often extended halfway across the globe. Industrialized animal production systems are now major features of human ecology. They have considerable impacts on the quality of the atmosphere, water and soil due to nutrient overloads; they impact terrestrial ecosystems directly and indirectly; in addition, disruption of marine fisheries occurs locally with pollution and runoff from production facilities and globally in terms of depletion of fish stocks where fishmeal has become a large commodity in the production of livestock feeds.

The response to the fact that several vector-borne, parasitic or zoonotic diseases have (re)-emerged and spread in Europe with major health, ecological, socio-economical and political consequences, has been the establishment of EDEN (Emerging Diseases in a changing European Environment). Most of these outbreaks are linked to global and local changes resulting from climate change, human-induced landscape changes or the activities of human populations. Europe must anticipate, prevent and control new emergences to avoid major societal and economical crises (cf. SARS in Asia, West Nile in the USA). EDEN offers a unique opportunity to prepare for uncertainties about the future of the European environment by exploring the impact of environmental.

Other aims are to identify, evaluate and catalogue European ecosystems and environmental conditions linked to global change, which can influence the spatial and temporal distribution and dynamics of human pathogenic agents.

The project will develop and co-coordinate at the European level a set of generic methods, tools and skills such as predictive emergence and spread models, early warning, surveillance and monitoring tools and scenarios, which can be used by decision makers for risk assessment, decision support for intervention and public health policies both at the EU and at the national or regional level. Part of EDEN's innovation will be to combine spatial data (earth observation data, GIS etc.) with epidemiological data.

EDEN has selected for study a range of indicator human diseases that are especially sensitive to environmental changes and will be studied within a common scientific framework (involving Landscapes, Vector and Parasite bionomics, Public Health, and Animal Reservoirs). Some of these diseases are already present in Europe (tick- and rodent-borne diseases, leishmaniasis, West Nile fever); others were present historically (malaria) and so may re-emerge, whilst others are on the fringes of Europe (Rift Valley fever) in endemic regions of West and Northern Africa.

Epidemiology

Epidemiology is the science that studies the patterns, causes, and effects of health and disease conditions in defined populations. It is the cornerstone of public health, and informs policy decisions and evidence-based practice by identifying risk factors for disease and targets for preventive healthcare. Epidemiologists help with study design, collection, and statistical analysis of data, and interpretation and dissemination of results (including peer review and occasional systematic review). Epidemiology has helped develop methodology used in clinical research, public health studies, and, to a lesser extent, basic research in the biological sciences.

Major areas of epidemiological study include disease etiology, transmission, outbreak investigation, disease surveillance and screening, biomonitoring, and comparisons of treatment effects such as in clinical trials. Epidemiologists rely on other scientific disciplines like biology to better understand disease processes, statistics to make efficient use of the data and draw appropriate conclusions, social sciences to better understand proximate and distal causes, and engineering for exposure assessment.

Etymology

Epidemiology, literally meaning "the study of what is upon the people", is derived from Greek *epi*, meaning "upon, among", *demos*, meaning "people, district", and *logos*, meaning "study, word, discourse", suggesting that it applies only to human populations. However, the term is widely used in studies of zoological populations (veterinary epidemiology), although the term "epizoology" is available, and it has also been applied to studies of plant populations (botanical or plant disease epidemiology).

The distinction between "epidemic" and "endemic" was first drawn by Hippocrates, to distinguish between diseases that are "visited upon" a population (epidemic) from those that "reside within" a population (endemic). The term "epidemiology" appears to have first been used to describe the study of epidemics in 1802 by the Spanish physician Villalba in *Epidemiología Española*. Epidemiologists also study the interaction of diseases in a population, a condition known as a syndemic.

The term epidemiology is now widely applied to cover the description and causation of not only epidemic disease, but of disease in general, and even many non-disease health-related conditions, such as high blood pressure and obesity. Therefore, this epidemiology is based upon how the pattern of the disease cause changes in the function of everyone.

History

"History of epidemiology" redirects here. The Greek physician Hippocrates, known as the father of medicine, sought a logic to sickness; he is the first person known to have examined the relationships between the occurrence of disease and environmental influences. Hippocrates believed sickness of the human body to be caused by an imbalance of the four Humors (air, fire, water and earth "atoms"). The cure to the sickness was to remove or add the humor in question to balance the body. This belief led to the application of bloodletting and dieting in medicine. He coined the terms *endemic* (for diseases usually found in some places but not in others) and *epidemic* (for diseases that are seen at some times but not others).

In ancient India, Ayurveda considered disease to be a manifestation of imbalance in 3 bodily humors, called Doshas. Around this theory, systems of diagnosis were based.

One of the earliest theories on the origin of disease was that it was primarily the fault of human luxury. This was expressed by philosophers such as Plato and Rousseau, and social critics like Jonathan Swift.

In the middle of the 16th century, a doctor from Verona named Girolamo Fracastoro was the first to propose a theory that these very small, unseeable, particles that cause disease were alive. They were considered to be able to spread by air, multiply by themselves and to be destroyable by fire. In this way he refuted Galen's miasma theory (poison gas in sick people). In 1543 he wrote a book *De contagione et contagiosis morbis*, in which he was the first to promote personal and environmental hygiene to prevent disease. The development of a sufficiently powerful microscope by Anton van Leeuwenhoek in 1675 provided visual evidence of living particles consistent with a germ theory of disease.

Another pioneer, Thomas Sydenham (1624–1689), was the first to distinguish the fevers of Londoners in the later 1600s. His theories on cures of fevers met with much resistance from traditional physicians at the time. He was not able to find the initial cause of the smallpox fever he researched and treated.

John Graunt, a haberdasher and amateur statistician, published *Natural and Political Observations ... upon the Bills of Mortality* in 1662. In it, he analysed the mortality rolls in London before the Great Plague, presented one of the first life tables, and report time trends for many diseases, new and old. He provided statistical evidence for many theories on disease, and also refuted some widespread ideas on them.

Modern Era

John Snow is famous for his investigations into the causes of the 19th century cholera epidemics, and is also known as the father of (modern) epidemiology. He began with noticing the significantly higher death rates in two areas supplied by Southwark Company. His identification of the Broad Street pump as the cause of the Soho epidemic is considered the classic example of epidemiology. Snow used chlorine in an attempt to clean the water and removed the handle; this ended the outbreak. This has been perceived as a major event in the history of public health and regarded as the founding event of the science of epidemiology, having helped shape public health policies around the world. However, Snow's research and preventive measures to avoid further outbreaks were not fully accepted or put into practice until after his death.

Other pioneers include Danish physician Peter Anton Schleisner, who in 1849 related his work on the prevention of the epidemic of neonatal tetanus on the Vestmanna Islands in Iceland. Another important pioneer was Hungarian physician Ignaz Semmelweis, who in 1847 brought down infant mortality at a Vienna hospital by instituting a disinfection procedure. His findings were published in 1850, but his work was ill received by his colleagues, who discontinued the procedure. Disinfection did not become widely practiced until British surgeon Joseph Lister 'discovered' antiseptics in 1865 in light of the work of Louis Pasteur.

In the early 20th century, mathematical methods were introduced into epidemiology by Ronald Ross, Janet Lane-Claypon, Anderson Gray McKendrick and others.

Another breakthrough was the 1954 publication of the results of a British Doctors Study, led by Richard Doll and Austin Bradford Hill, which lent very strong statistical support to the suspicion that tobacco smoking was linked to lung cancer.

In the late 20th century, with advancement of biomedical sciences, a number of molecular markers in blood, other biospecimens and environment were identified as predictors of development or risk of a certain disease. Epidemiology research to examine the relationship between these biomarkers analysed at the molecular level and disease was broadly named "molecular epidemiology". Specifically, "genetic epidemiology" has been used for epidemiology of germline genetic variation and disease. Genetic variation is typically determined using DNA from peripheral blood leukocytes. Since the 2000s, genome-wide association studies (GWAS) have been commonly performed to identify genetic risk factors for many diseases and health conditions.

While most molecular epidemiology studies are still using conventional disease diagnosis and classification system, it is increasingly recognised that disease evolution represents inherently heterogeneous process differing from person to person. Conceptually, each individual has a unique disease process different from any other individual ("the unique disease principle"), considering uniqueness of the exposome (a totality of endogenous and exogenous / environmental exposures) and its unique influence on molecular pathologic process in each individual. Studies to examine the relationship between an exposure and molecular pathologic signature of disease (particularly, cancer) became increasingly common throughout the 2000s. However, the use of molecular pathology in epidemiology posed unique challenges including lack of research guidelines and standardized statistical methodologies, and paucity of interdisciplinary experts and training programmes. Furthermore, the concept of disease heterogeneity appears to conflict with the long-standing premise in epidemiology that individuals with the same disease name have similar etiologies and disease processes. To resolve these issues and advance population health science in the era of molecular precision medicine, "molecular pathology" and "epidemiology" was integrated to create a new interdisciplinary field of "molecular pathological epidemiology" (MPE), defined as "epidemiology of molecular pathology and heterogeneity of disease".

In MPE, investigators analyse the relationships between; (A) environmental, dietary, lifestyle and genetic factors; (B) alterations in cellular or extracellular molecules; and (C) evolution and progression of disease. A better understanding of heterogeneity of disease pathogenesis will further contribute to elucidate etiologies of disease. The MPE approach can be applied to not only neoplastic diseases but also non-neoplastic diseases. The concept and paradigm of MPE have become widespread in the 2010s.

The Profession

To date, few universities offer epidemiology as a course of study at the undergraduate level. Many epidemiologists are physicians, or hold graduate degrees such as a Master of Public Health (MPH), Master of Science of Epidemiology (MSc.). Doctorates include the Doctor of Public Health (DrPH), Doctor of Pharmacy (PharmD), Doctor of Philosophy (PhD), Doctor of Science (ScD), Doctor of Social Work (DSW), Doctor of Clinical Practice (DClinP), Doctor of Podiatric Medicine (DPM), Doctor of Veterinary Medicine (DVM), Doctor of Nursing Practice (DNP), Doctor of Physical Therapy (DPT), or for clinically trained physicians, Doctor of Medicine (MD) and Doctor of Osteopathic Medicine (DO). In the United Kingdom, the title of 'doctor' is by long custom used to refer to general medical practitioners, whose professional degrees are usually those of Bachelor of Medicine and Surgery (MBBS or MBChB).

As public health/health protection practitioners, epidemiologists work in a number of different settings. Some epidemiologists work 'in the field'; i.e., in the community, commonly in a public health/health protection service and are often at the forefront of investigating and combating disease outbreaks.

Others work for non-profit organisations, universities, hospitals and larger government entities such as the Centres for Disease Control and Prevention (CDC), the Health Protection Agency, the World Health Organisation (WHO), or the Public Health Agency of Canada. Epidemiologists can also work in for-profit organisations such as pharmaceutical and medical device companies in groups such as market research or clinical development.

The Practice

Epidemiologists employ a range of study designs from the observational to experimental and generally categorized as descriptive, analytic (aiming to further examine known associations or hypothesized relationships), and experimental (a term often equated with clinical or community trials of treatments and other interventions). In observational studies, nature is allowed to "take its course", as epidemiologists observe from the sidelines.

Conversely, in experimental studies, the epidemiologist is the one in control of all of the factors entering a certain case study. Epidemiological studies are aimed, where possible, at revealing unbiased relationships between exposures such as alcohol or smoking, biological agents, stress, or chemicals to mortality or morbidity. The identification of causal relationships between these exposures and outcomes is an important aspect of epidemiology. Modern epidemiologists use informatics as a tool.

Observational studies have two components: descriptive, or analytical. Descriptive observations pertain to the "who, what, where and when of health-related state occurrence". However, analytical observations deal more with the 'how' of a health-related event.

Experimental epidemiology contains three case types: randomized control trial (often used for new medicine or drug testing), field trial (conducted on those at a high risk of conducting a disease), and community trial (research on social originating diseases).

Unfortunately, many epidemiology studies conducted cause false or misinterpreted information to circulate the public. According to a class taught by professor Madhukar Pai MD, PhD at McGill, "...optimism bias is pervasive, most studies biased or inconclusive or false, most discovered true associations are inflated, fear and panic inducing rather than helpful; media-induced panic, cannot detect small effects; big effects are not to be found anymore".

The term 'epidemiologic triad' is used to describe the intersection of *Host*, *Agent*, and *Environment* in analyzing an outbreak.

As Causal Inference

Although epidemiology is sometimes viewed as a collection of statistical tools used to elucidate the associations of exposures to health outcomes, a deeper understanding of this science is that of discovering *causal* relationships.

"Correlation does not imply causation" is a common theme for much of the epidemiological literature. For epidemiologists, the key is in the term inference. Epidemiologists use gathered data and a broad range of biomedical and psychosocial theories in an iterative way to generate or expand theory, to test hypotheses, and to make educated, informed assertions about which relationships are causal, and about exactly how they are causal. Epidemiologists Rothman and Greenland emphasize that the "one cause – one effect" understanding is a simplistic misbelief. Most outcomes, whether disease or death, are caused by a chain or web consisting of many component causes. Causes can be distinguished as necessary, sufficient or probabilistic conditions. If a necessary condition can be identified and controlled (e.g., antibodies to a disease agent), the harmful outcome can be avoided.

Bradford Hill Criteria

In 1965 Austin Bradford Hill proposed a series of considerations to help assess evidence of causation, which have come to be commonly known as the "Bradford Hill criteria". In contrast to the explicit intentions of their author, Hill's considerations are now sometimes taught as a checklist to be implemented for assessing causality. Hill himself said "None of my nine viewpoints can bring indisputable evidence for or against the cause-and-effect hypothesis and none can be required *sine qua non.*"

1. Strength: A small association does not mean that there is not a causal effect, though the larger the association, the more likely that it is causal.
2. Consistency: Consistent findings observed by different persons in different places with different samples strengthens the likelihood of an effect.
3. Specificity: Causation is likely if a very specific population at a specific site and disease with no other likely explanation. The more specific an association between a factor and an effect is, the bigger the probability of a causal relationship.
4. Temporality: The effect has to occur after the cause (and if there is an expected delay between the cause and expected effect, then the effect must occur after that delay).
5. Biological gradient: Greater exposure should generally lead to greater incidence of the effect. However, in some cases, the mere presence of the factor can trigger the effect. In other cases, an inverse proportion is observed: greater exposure leads to lower incidence.

6. Plausibility: A plausible mechanism between cause and effect is helpful (but Hill noted that knowledge of the mechanism is limited by current knowledge).
7. Coherence: Coherence between epidemiological and laboratory findings increases the likelihood of an effect. However, Hill noted that "... lack of such [laboratory] evidence cannot nullify the epidemiological effect on associations".
8. Experiment: "Occasionally it is possible to appeal to experimental evidence".
9. Analogy: The effect of similar factors may be considered.

Legal Interpretation

Epidemiological studies can only go to prove that an agent could have caused, but not that it did cause, an effect in any particular case:

> *"Epidemiology is concerned with the incidence of disease in populations and does not address the question of the cause of an individual's disease. This question, sometimes referred to as specific causation, is beyond the domain of the science of epidemiology. Epidemiology has its limits at the point where an inference is made that the relationship between an agent and a disease is causal (general causation) and where the magnitude of excess risk attributed to the agent has been determined; that is, epidemiology addresses whether an agent can cause a disease, not whether an agent did cause a specific plaintiff's disease."*

In United States law, epidemiology alone cannot prove that a causal association does not exist in general. Conversely, it can be (and is in some circumstances) taken by US courts, in an individual case, to justify an inference that a causal association does exist, based upon a balance of probability.

The subdiscipline of forensic epidemiology is directed at the investigation of specific causation of disease or injury in individuals or groups of individuals in instances in which causation is disputed or is unclear, for presentation in legal settings.

Advocacy

As a public health discipline, epidemiologic evidence is often used to advocate both personal measures like diet change and corporate measures like removal of junk food advertising, with study findings disseminated to the general public to help people to make informed decisions about their health. Often the uncertainties about these findings are not communicated well; news articles often prominently report the latest result of one study with little mention of its limitations, caveats, or context.

Epidemiological tools have proved effective in establishing major causes of diseases like cholera and lung cancer, but experience difficulty in regards to more subtle health issues where causation is more complex. Notably, conclusions drawn from observational studies may be reconsidered as later data from randomized controlled trials becomes available, as was the case with the association between the use of hormone replacement therapy and cardiac risk.

Chapter 2

Population-based Health Management

Epidemiological practice and the results of epidemiological analysis make a significant contribution to emerging population-based health management frameworks.

Population-based health management encompasses the ability to:

- Assess the health states and health needs of a target population;
- Implement and evaluate interventions that are designed to improve the health of that population; and
- Efficiently and effectively provide care for members of that population in a way that is consistent with the community's cultural, policy and health resource values.

Modern population-based health management is complex, requiring a multiple set of skills (medical, political, technological, mathematical etc.) of which epidemiological practice and analysis is a core component, that is unified with management science to provide efficient and effective health care and health guidance to a population. This task requires the forward looking ability of modern risk management approaches that transform health risk factors, incidence, prevalence and mortality statistics (derived from epidemiological analysis) into management metrics that not only guide how a health system responds to current population health issues, but also how a health system can be managed to better respond to future potential population health issues.

Examples of organisations that use population-based health management that leverage the work and results of epidemiological practice include Canadian Strategy for Cancer Control, Health Canada Tobacco Control Programmes, Rick Hansen Foundation, Canadian Tobacco Control Research Initiative.

Each of these organisations use a population-based health management framework called Life at Risk that combines epidemiological quantitative analysis with demographics, health agency operational research and economics to perform:

- *Population Life Impacts Simulations*: Measurement of the future potential impact of disease upon the population with respect to new disease cases, prevalence, premature death as well as potential years of life lost from disability and death;
- *Labour Force Life Impacts Simulations*: Measurement of the future potential impact of disease upon the labour force with respect to new disease cases, prevalence, premature death and potential years of life lost from disability and death;
- *Economic Impacts of Disease Simulations*: Measurement of the future potential impact of disease upon private sector disposable income impacts (wages, corporate profits, private health care costs) and public sector disposable income impacts (personal income tax, corporate income tax, consumption taxes, publicly funded health care costs).

Types of Studies

Case Series

Case-series may refer to the qualitative study of the experience of a single patient, or small group of patients with a similar diagnosis, or to a statistical technique comparing periods during which patients are exposed to some factor with the potential to produce illness with periods when they are unexposed.

The former type of study is purely descriptive and cannot be used to make inferences about the general population of patients with that disease. These types of studies, in which an astute clinician identifies an unusual feature of a disease or a patient's history, may lead to formulation of a new hypothesis. Using the data from the series, analytic studies could be done to investigate possible causal factors. These can include case control studies or prospective studies. A case control study would involve matching comparable controls without the disease to the cases in the series. A prospective study would involve following the case series over time to evaluate the disease's natural history.

The latter type, more formally described as self-controlled case-series studies, divide individual patient follow-up time into exposed and unexposed periods and use fixed-effects Poisson regression processes to compare the incidence rate of a given outcome between exposed and unexposed periods. This technique has been extensively used in the study of adverse reactions to vaccination, and has been shown in some circumstances to provide statistical power comparable to that available in cohort studies.

Case Control Studies

Case control studies select subjects based on their disease status. It is a retrospective study. A group of individuals that are disease positive (the "case" group) is compared with a group of disease negative individuals (the "control" group). The control group should ideally come from the same population that gave rise to the cases.

The case control study looks back through time at potential exposures that both groups (cases and controls) may have encountered. A 2×2 table is constructed, displaying exposed cases (A), exposed controls (B), unexposed cases (C) and unexposed controls (D). The statistic generated to measure association is the odds ratio (OR), which is the ratio of the odds of exposure in the cases (A/C) to the odds of exposure in the controls (B/D), i.e. OR = (AD/BC).

	Cases	***Controls***
Exposed	A	B
Unexposed	C	D

If the OR is clearly greater than 1, then the conclusion is "those with the disease are more likely to have been exposed," whereas if it is close to 1 then the exposure and disease are not likely associated. If the OR is far less than one, then this suggests that the exposure is a protective factor in the causation of the disease.

Case control studies are usually faster and more cost effective than cohort studies, but are sensitive to bias (such as recall bias and selection bias). The main challenge is to identify the appropriate control group; the distribution of exposure among the control group should be representative of the distribution in the population that gave rise to the cases. This can be achieved by drawing a random sample from the original population at risk. This has as a consequence that the control group can contain people with the disease under study when the disease has a high attack rate in a population.

A major drawback for case control studies is that, in order to be considered to be statistically significant, the minimum number of cases required at the 95% confidence interval is related to the odds ratio by the equation:

total cases = (a+c) = (1.96)^2× (1+N)×(1 ÷ln(OR))^2 ×((OR+2√OR +1)÷√OR) ≈ 15.5×(1+N)×(1÷ln(OR))^2

where N = the ratio of cases to controls. As the odds ratio approached 1, approaches 0; rendering case control studies all but useless for low odds ratios. For instance, for an odds ratio of 1.5 and cases = controls, the table shown above would look like this:

.....	*Cases*	*Controls*
Exposed	103	84
Unexposed	84	103

For an odds ratio of 1.1:

.....	*Cases*	*Controls*
Exposed	1732	1652
Unexposed	1652	1732

Cohort Studies

Cohort studies select subjects based on their exposure status. The study subjects should be at risk of the outcome under investigation at the beginning of the cohort study; this usually means that they should be disease free when the cohort study starts. The cohort is followed through time to assess their later outcome status. An example of a cohort study would be the investigation of a cohort of smokers and non-smokers over time to estimate the incidence of lung cancer. The same 2×2 table is constructed as with the case control study. However, the point estimate generated is the relative risk (RR), which is the probability of disease for a person in the exposed group, $P_e = A / (A + B)$ over the probability of disease for a person in the unexposed group, $P_u = C / (C + D)$, i.e. $RR = P_e / P_u$.

.....	*Case*	*Non-case*	*Total*
Exposed	*A*	*B*	*(A + B)*
Unexposed	*C*	*D*	*(C + D)*

As with the OR, a RR greater than 1 shows association, where the conclusion can be read "those with the exposure were more likely to develop disease."

Prospective studies have many benefits over case control studies. The RR is a more powerful effect measure than the OR, as the OR is just an estimation of the RR, since true incidence cannot be calculated in a case control study where subjects are selected based on disease status. Temporality can be established in a prospective study, and confounders are more easily controlled for. However, they are more costly, and there is a greater chance of losing subjects to follow-up based on the long time period over which the cohort is followed.

Cohort studies also are limited by the same equation for number of cases as for cohort studies, but, if the base incidence rate in the study population is very low, the number of cases required is reduced by ½.

Validity: Precision and Bias

Different fields in epidemiology have different levels of validity. One way to assess the validity of findings is the ratio of false-positives (claimed effects that are not correct) to false-negatives (studies which fail to support a true effect). To take the field of genetic epidemiology, candidate-gene studies produced over 100 false-positive findings for each false-negative. By contrast genome-wide association appear close to the reverse, with only one false positive for every 100 or more false-negatives. This ratio has improved over time in genetic epidemiology as the field has adopted stringent criteria. By contrast other epidemiological fields have not required such rigorous reporting and are much less reliable as a result.

Random Error

Random error is the result of fluctuations around a true value because of sampling variability. Random error is just that: random. It can occur during data collection, coding, transfer, or analysis. Examples of random error include: poorly worded questions, a misunderstanding in interpreting an individual answer from a particular respondent, or a typographical error during coding. Random error affects measurement in a transient, inconsistent manner and it is impossible to correct for random error. There is random error in all sampling procedures. This is called sampling error. Precision in epidemiological variables is a measure of random error. Precision is also inversely related to random error, so that to reduce random error is to increase precision. Confidence intervals are computed to demonstrate the precision of relative risk estimates. The narrower the confidence interval, the more precise the relative risk estimate. There are two basic ways to reduce random error in an epidemiological study. The first is to increase the sample size of the study. In other words, add more subjects to your study. The second is to reduce the variability in measurement in the study. This might be accomplished by using a more precise measuring device or by increasing the number of measurements.

Note, that if sample size or number of measurements are increased, or a more precise measuring tool is purchased, the costs of the study are usually increased. There is usually an uneasy balance between the need for adequate precision and the practical issue of study cost.

Systematic Error

A systematic error or bias occurs when there is a difference between the true value (in the population) and the observed value (in the study) from any cause other than sampling variability. An example of systematic error is if, unknown to you, the pulse oximeter you are using is set incorrectly and adds two points to the true value each time a measurement is taken. The measuring device could be precise but not accurate. Because the error happens in every instance, it is systematic. Conclusions you draw based on that data will still be incorrect. But the error can be reproduced in the future (e.g., by using the same mis-set instrument).

A mistake in coding that affects *all* responses for that particular question is another example of a systematic error.

The validity of a study is dependent on the degree of systematic error. Validity is usually separated into two components:

- Internal validity is dependent on the amount of error in measurements, including exposure, disease, and the associations between these variables. Good internal validity implies a lack of error in measurement and suggests that inferences may be drawn at least as they pertain to the subjects under study.
- External validity pertains to the process of generalizing the findings of the study to the population from which the sample was drawn (or even beyond that population to a more universal statement). This requires an understanding of which conditions are relevant (or irrelevant) to the generalization. Internal validity is clearly a prerequisite for external validity.

Three Types of Bias

Selection Bias: Selection bias is one of three types of bias that can threaten the validity of a study. Selection bias occurs when study subjects are selected or become part of the study as a result of a third, unmeasured variable which is associated with both the exposure and outcome of interest. For instance, it has repeatedly been noted that cigarette smokers and non smokers tend to differ in their study participation rates. (Sackett D cites the example of Seltzer et al., in which 85% of non smokers and 67% of smokers returned mailed questionnaires.) It is important to note that such a difference in response will not lead to bias if it is not also associated with a systematic difference in outcome between the two response groups.

Information Bias: Information bias is bias arising from systematic error in the assessment of a variable. An example of this is recall bias. A typical example is again provided by Sackett in his discussion of a study examining the effect of specific exposures on fetal health: "in questioning mothers whose recent pregnancies had ended in fetal death or malformation (cases) and a matched group of mothers whose pregnancies ended normally (controls) it was found that 28% of the former, but only 20% of the latter, reported exposure to drugs which could not be substantiated either in earlier prospective interviews or in other health records". In this example, recall bias probably occurred as a result of women who had had miscarriages having an apparent tendency to better recall and therefore report previous exposures.

Confounding

Confounding has traditionally been defined as bias arising from the co-occurrence or mixing of effects of extraneous factors, referred to as confounders, with the main effect(s) of interest. A more recent definition of confounding invokes the notion of *counterfactual* effects. According to this view, when one observes an outcome of interest, say Y=1 (as opposed to Y=0), in a given population A which is entirely exposed (i.e. exposure $X = 1$ for every unit of the population) the risk of this event will be R_{A1}. The counterfactual or unobserved risk R_{A0} corresponds to the risk which would have been observed if these same individuals had been unexposed (i.e. $X = 0$ for every unit of the population). The true effect of exposure therefore is: $R_{A1} - R_{A0}$ (if one is interested in risk differences) or R_{A1}/R_{A0} (if one is interested in relative risk). Since the counterfactual risk R_{A0} is unobservable we approximate it using a second population B and we actually measure the following relations: R_{A1} - R_{B0} or R_{A1}/R_{B0}. In this situation, confounding occurs when $R_{A0} \neq R_{B0}$. (NB: Example assumes binary outcome and exposure variables.)

Some epidemiologists prefer to think of confounding separately from common categorizations of bias since, unlike selection and information bias, confounding stems from real causal effects.

Geographic Mobility

Geographic mobility is the measure of how populations move over time. Geographic mobility, population mobility, or more simply mobility is also a statistic that measures migration within a population. Commonly used in demography and human geography, it may also be used to describe the movement of animals between populations. These moves can be as large scale as international migrations or as small as regional commuting arrangements.

Geographic mobility has a large impact on many sociological factors in a community and is a current topic of academic research. It varies between different regions depending on both formal policies and established social norms, and has different effects and responses in different societies. Population mobility has implications ranging from administrative changes in government and impacts on local economic growth to housing markets and demand for regional services.

Measurement

Geographic mobility data is available from census and public government records in the United States, The European Union, The People's Republic of China and many other countries.

In the United States

Mobility estimates in the Current Population Survey (CPS), produced by the United States Census Bureau, define mobility status on the basis of a comparison between the place of residence of each individual to the time of the March survey and the place of residence one year earlier. Non-movers are all people who were living in the same house at the end of the migration period and the beginning of the migration period. Movers are all people who were living in a different house at the end of the period rather than at the beginning. They are further classified as to whether they were living in the same or different county, state, region, or were movers from abroad. Movers are also categorized by whether they moved within or between central cities, suburbs, and non-metropolitan areas of the United States.

The CPS includes information on reasons for a move. These include work-related factors, such as a job transfer, job loss or looking for work, and wanting to be closer to work. Housing factors include wanting to own a home, rather than rent, seeking a better home or better neighbourhoods, or wanting cheaper housing. Additional mobility factors include attending college, changes in marital status, retirement, or health-related moves.

In the European Union

The Eurobarometer survey measures mobility in a similar manner to the US census. Direct comparison of the two is difficult due to social constraints of travelling between countries in the European Union not encountered with interstate travel within the United States. Differences include language barriers, cultural resistance, and the added hurdle of international labour laws.

In China

Several scholarly surveys have been conducted to measure geographic mobility in China, but no single comprehensive census is available. Since the year 2000 the National Bureau of Statistics of China has added migrant worker estimates to their annual household survey. The Chinese Development Research Centre of the State Council also undertook a study in 2010 characterizing the scope of migration for work and relevant statistics of that population. The survey measured demographics such as age, education level, job type, income, expenses, housing, and leisure activities.

Other Measures

Population turnover is a related statistic that measures gross moves in relation to the size of the population, for example movement of residents into and out of a geographic location between census counts.

Influencing Factors

Economic Reasons: Most theoretical models attribute the desire to relocate to the impact of wages and employment on personal expected earnings. The prospect of gainful employment in another region leads to movement to capitalize on new opportunities and/or resources unavailable in the original community. Perceptions, gaps in prospective incomes, availability of accurate information, and geographic distance all play a part in the decision to migrate. Studies have shown that unemployment rates statistically correlate to measured migrations in the EU (a relatively mobile society). Further, there is evidence that comparable statistical results can be obtained using labour availability interchangeably with population migration data.

Surveys show potential movers also face anxiety about the prospects of actually finding a suitable job in their new location. The capacity to migrate depends on current income or access to credit to support the move, and is always up to chance. Economists have shown that the decline in home values in the US in the late 2000s diminished state-to-state migration, with roughly 110,000 to 150,000 fewer individuals migrating across state lines in any given year. Socialized unemployment insurance programmes help to increase individual liquidity and lessen the burden of search costs and movement risk. Research has shown that overall the presence of social insurance does not have a strong effect on the rate of personal movement because while it lowers relative movement costs, it also increases the opportunity costs of movement.

Current international laws present challenges to ideal geographic mobility. Migrants must have a physical means (legal or illegal) over which to travel to a new country. An increase in individual income was shown to increase access to long distance transportation and enable individuals more freedom of travel. Seeking a job in another country often requires sponsorship, visas, or may not even be possible in a given situation. Government support is in no way guaranteed for international geographic mobility. Existing language and cultural barriers also severely hamper geographic mobility on both regional and national levels.

Personal Preferences

Personal preference factors besides economic logic can exert a strong influence on an individual's geographic mobility. Concerns such as climate, the strength of regional housing markets, cultural comfort, family, and local social capital all play into the decision to move or not. Individualization of the job market in industrializing countries has led to an increased preference among workers to follow market opportunities. Media driven self-awareness and highly individualistic symbolism exported from the western world have allowed people to imagine themselves living completely different lifestyles. Western media glamorizes the image of the self-sufficient youth, showing examples of both men and women who lead strong, individualistic, empowered lifestyles. Globalization has destabilized previously immutable social institutions, shifting cultural value away from old traditions to new more individualist and market friendly ideas. This combined with a privatization and individualization of labour has in many ways made fluidity more than norm than structure.

The availability of geographic mobility can also directly affect an individual's self-empowerment. Large numbers of women in South Korea, Japan, and China are taking advantage of newly available travel opportunities: experiencing life overseas and touring or studying. In South Korea progressive educational reforms have led to large numbers of women receiving higher level degrees, but structural inequality in the job market makes it difficult for them to get middle or upper class jobs. 93% of women graduate from high school and 63% from college, but only 46.7% of college grads are employed. Further, those employed women suffer from a 76% wage differential compared to like qualified men. Japan has similar structural issues where half of the employed women in the country only work part-time. Geographic relocation presents social opportunities to both seek a more favourable job climate and a social order more accepting of educated women. The prospect of greater control over their own lives and careers draws many of these young women to build their futures away from their immediate surroundings: 80% of Japanese people studying abroad are women.

Social Forces

Social forces can also foster individual geographic mobility. Support from the community can increase the probability of relocation- it has been shown that the chances of a migration in India improve when groups of houses from same sub-caste all decide to move together. Worldly exposure also increase one's tendency to be mobile. Public health studies measured higher geographic mobility among female sex workers who: drank, had experienced violence, had worked for more than 4 years, and had a regular non-paying partner than those who did not.

Demographically, research shows that one's level of education tends to correlate to higher mobility, especially among university graduates. Youth and a lack of a family or children correlate to increased mobility too, with the peak in mobility occurring in the mid-late 20s for populations surveyed in Europe.

Economic Effects

Labour Supply: Geographical mobility of labour allows the labour supply to respond to regional disparities, limiting economic inefficiencies. Low labour mobility quickly leads to inequality between static economic regions and a misappropriation of labour resources. Geographic mobility can help alleviate asymmetric shocks between regions with diversified economies, like in the European Union. A mobile population allows a region to shed workers when jobs are scarce and gives those workers the opportunity seek employment elsewhere where opportunities might be better. While an increase in geographic mobility increases overall economic efficiency, the increased competition for jobs on the local level in otherwise prosperous regions could lead to higher unemployment than before the migration.

Female labour supply rates actually have larger statistical effect on mobility than male rates. Traditionally male jobs in the developing world have much more inelastic demand than female ones, so the variations in the female rate lead to more drastic changes in employment that more strongly affect mobility.

Resource Allocation

Labour mobility theoretically leads to a more balanced and economically efficient distribution of jobs and resources overall. Individual employees can better match their skills to potential jobs on the open job market. They can seek out ideal jobs instead of artificially limiting themselves to their geographic areas. The opportunity to study abroad is a major vehicle of entry to western countries for Asian women. Moving to the West to study is a common career move for Asian women in their 20s, allowing them to abandon the traditional marriage track and pursue economic ventures outside the home.

On the other hand, mobility can also have negative consequences on a region facing widespread emigration. Brain drain and labour resource diminishment make it more difficult for troubled regions to recover after an economic stumble. Additional people migrating into a region can also place extra stress on existing social infrastructure for services like healthcare, welfare, and unemployment.

Remittances

Geographic mobility allows for remittances from distant family members back to support local needs. Loans and transfers can flow back from migrated members of a community to sustain those who remain behind. Remittances are one of the primary benefits of migration to the country of origin, not only substantially enhancing local family income but also spilling over into benefits of increased capital flow in the entire local economy. Remittances play a large role in sustaining the economies of many developing nations, for example bringing over US$1bn into the Philippines every month and eclipsing the entire tourism profit of Morocco.

Female Mobility

Empowerment: With heightened self-awareness, educated women hope to grasp opportunities from moving, leading to increased female individualization and empowerment. Given access to travel, international education provides one of few avenues for women in China to live non-traditional personally emancipated lives. In Japan geographic mobility offers an opportunity to gain real job experience and advance a career too. Japanese society places a great social pressure on women to get married, but many young women feel the need to "escape" and can find their independent selves in another setting.

Many migrants do choose to continue to benefit and rely on older home ties though. These women cannot change behaviour too much from social norms or risk being cut off. Studies show that household choices in India are affected by distance from the ancestral home, especially within the caste system. There are also other new risks for women in new locations. Female sex workers have statistically higher sexually transmitted diseases and HIV rates when more mobile. There is also potential for male backlash in a new setting. Domestic violence can be sparked by power struggles when newly empowered women regain some control traditionally held by men.

Participation

Female labour participation is vital to improving regional disparities in a competitive world and will increase in value over time. Women's participation and creative energy is vital for the success of economies on a global scale. Female labour participation can act as a substitute for more generalized labour mobility too. In the European Union women provide a dynamic substitute for male labour with fluctuations in the economy. This allows for more geographic stability while maintaining the variability of a flexible labour economy. When families do migrate, woman often get employed first and become the breadwinner for house. Even if this only lasts for a duration of time, the experience is empowering and helps shape social dynamics within the home.

Often a relocation is primarily motivated by lack of any better opportunities in their prior situation though. Many of the women go through the trial of moving and starting over due to economic and social circumstances outside of her control. Research also seems to indicate that women and minorities migrating into a new area often act as economic substitutes for local minorities rather than paving their own new ground. Female income effects from migration will only kick in if there are sufficient differences between males and females too, so long term changes will likely not happen quickly.

Transportation Access

Women have traditionally had more limited access to improved means of personal transportation and thus had more limited local mobility. Women surveyed in England were less likely overall than men to have drivers licenses and took longer to get to key destinations. Women often seek work closer to home compared to men, taking jobs in a more geographically confined area and relying more on non-automobile transportation. Access to personal transportation could improve women's choice of feasible destinations and decrease average trip time.

Effects on Children, Family, & Education

Increased geographic mobility can offer new opportunities to previously isolated groups. In India, increasing mobility allows families the chance to strengthen family ties by sending children to traditional homes or expand educational opportunities with options to attend urban schools. Additional economic freedom bolstered by additional capital from remittances can allow children to stay in school longer without having to worry about supporting the core family.

Increased geographic mobility and long distance moves do place strains on the household. The loss of established strong ties decreases social support and can lower productivity. Geographic isolation from previous relationships increases personal dependence on the nuclear family unit and can lead to power unbalances within the household.

Migration for work allows the migrants themselves to develop new skills and receive new technical training abroad. Migrants surveyed in Australia and the US have lower rates of continual training than their native born peers as a whole, but are likely to continue gaining technical skills after establishing an initial technical aptitude. The appeal of new educational opportunities to migrants also loses appeal with age; older movers see less of an incentive to spend time to improve upon their existing skills.

Increased global mobility has helped to destabilize the prospects of young people looking for reliable work and led to a greater assumption of risk on behalf of young people. Coping strategies push them to put off long term commitments, decreasing the formation of families and lowering birth rates. Labour market volatility increases the dangers of settling down since incomes are cannot be relied upon long term. Women in the workplace also face more disincentives to having children since they could be more easily replaced if forced to leave their job temporarily.

Effects on Culture

Cultural Exchange: Increased geographic mobility increases the depth and quality of cultural exchange between communities. Travel and cooperation bring people together across cultural bounds and facilitate the trade of customs and ideas.

New community members bring unique talents and skills that can improve overall services and bring additional opportunity to an area. Additional population "churn" can also increase diversity and lower tensions that would arise otherwise with large concentrations of particular demographic groups.

On the other hand, accelerated cultural exchange can dilute existing customs and cause social friction between competing immigrating populations too. Residents in communities with a large percentage of highly mobile occupants also worry about long term social cohesion. Rapid turnover can lead to cultural isolation and sometimes prevents neighbours from building close cohesive relationships.

Social Networks

Increasing long range personal mobility tends to lead to geographic expansion of an individual's support network. Long distance connections require more time to visit and minimizes the occurrence of unplanned social interaction.

Increased mobility can decrease an individual's attachment to a local community and weaken local support networks. People often turn to information technology to maintain connections across distance, strengthening distance relationships and allowing people to pursue career opportunities despite geographic distance from a partner.

Migrant Health

There are an estimated 1 billion migrants in the world today of whom 214 million international migrants and 740 million internal migrants. The collective health needs and implications of this sizeable population are considerable. Migration flows comprise a wide range of populations, such as workers, refugees, students, undocumented migrants and others, with each different health determinants, needs and levels of vulnerability.

In a globalized world defined by profound disparities, skill shortages, demographic imbalances, climate change as well as economic and political crises, natural as well as man-made disasters, migration is omnipresent. Migration is also essential for some societies to compensate for demographic trends and skill shortages and to assist home communities with remittances.

Epidemiological Transition

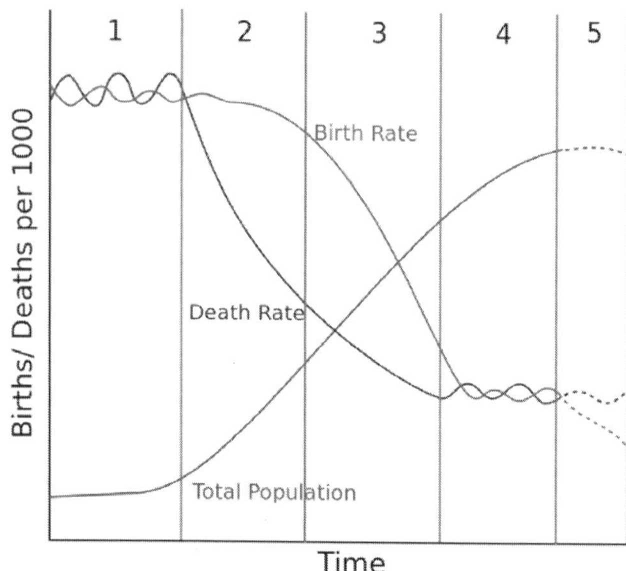

Figure: *Diagram showing sharp birth rate and death rate decreases between Time 1 and Time 4, the congruent increase in population caused by delayed birth rate decreases, and the subsequent re-levelling of population growth by Time 5.*

In demography and medical geography, epidemiological transition is a phase of development witnessed by a sudden and stark increase in population growth rates brought about by medical innovation in disease or sickness therapy and treatment, followed by a re-levelling of population growth from subsequent declines in fertility rates. "Epidemiological transition" accounts for the replacement of infectious diseases by chronic diseases over time due to expanded public health and sanitation. This theory was originally posited by Abdel Omran in 1971.

Theory

Omran divided the epidemiological transition of mortality into three phases, in the last of which chronic diseases replace infection as the primary cause of death. These phases are:

1. *The Age of Pestilence and Famine*: Where mortality is high and fluctuating, precluding sustained population growth, with low and variable life expectancy, vacillating between 20 and 40 years.
2. *The Age of Receding Pandemics*: Where mortality progressively declines, with the rate of decline accelerating as epidemic peaks decrease in frequency. Average life expectancy increases

steadily from about 30 to 50 years. Population growth is sustained and begins to be exponential.

3. *The Age of Degenerative and Man-Made Diseases*: Mortality continues to decline and eventually approaches stability at a relatively low level.

The epidemiological transition occurs as a country undergoes the process of modernisation from developing nation to developed nation status. The developments of modern healthcare, and medicine like antibiotics, drastically reduces infant mortality rates and extends average life expectancy which, coupled with subsequent declines in fertility rates, reflects a transition to chronic and degenerative diseases as more important causes of death.

History

In general human history, Omran's first phase occurs when human population sustains cyclic, low-growth, and mostly linear, up-and-down patterns associated with wars, famine, epidemic outbreaks, as well as small golden ages, and localized periods of "prosperity". In early pre-agricultural history, infant mortality rates were high and average life expectancy low. Today, life expectancy in third world countries remains relatively low, as in many Sub-Saharan African nations where it typically doesn't exceed 60 years of age.

The second phase involves advancements in medicine and the development of a healthcare system. One treatment breakthrough of note was the discovery of penicillin in the mid 20th century which led to widespread and dramatic declines in death rates from previously serious diseases such as syphilis. Population growth rates surged in the 1950s, 1960s and 1970s, to 1.8% per year and higher, with the world gaining 2 billion people between 1950 and the 1980s alone.

Omran's third phase occurs when human birth rates drastically decline from highly positive replacement numbers to stable replacement rates. In several European nations replacement rates have even become negative. As this transition generally represents the net effect of individual choices on family size (and the ability to implement those choices), it is more complicated. Omran gives three possible factors tending to encourage reduced fertility rates:

1. *Biophysiologic factors*, associated with reduced infant mortality and the expectation of longer life in parents,
2. *Socioeconomic factors*, associated with childhood survival and the economic perceptions of large family size, and

3. *Psychologic or emotional factors*, where society as a whole changes its rationale and opinion on family size and parental energies are redirected to qualitative aspects of child-raising.

This transition may also be associated with the sociological adaptations associated with demographic movements to urban areas, and a shift from agriculture and labour based production output to technological and service-sector-based economies.

Regardless, Chronic and degenerative diseases, and accidents and injuries, became more important causes of death. This shift in demographic and disease profiles is currently under way in most developing nations, however every country is unique in its transition speed based on a myriad of geographical and socio-political factors.

Controversy

Many question whether or not epidemiological transition really took place during the twentieth century. The transition during this time describes the replacement of infectious diseases by chronic diseases. This replacement of diseases has been identified to be caused by multiple factors such as antibiotics and increased overall public sanitation. Even though these factors undeniably affected society in ways such as increased life-span, many believe that the increase from infectious disease to chronic disease may be an illusion. It is debated that there was an actual increase in chronic diseases. Instead it is argued that due to new techniques of diagnosing and managing diseases that previously had been undiagnosed and untreated, it gave the appearance of an emergence of new chronic illnesses. Multiple factors made chronic diseases more visible to health care professionals such as increased use of hospitals as treatment centres and improved statistical evaluation. This led to the question, "Was an epidemiological transition really taking place in the twentieth century?"

Demographic Transition

Demographic transition (DT) refers to the transition from high birth and death rates to low birth and death rates as a country develops from a pre-industrial to an industrialized economic system. This is typically demonstrated through a demographic transition model (DTM). The theory is based on an interpretation of demographic history developed in 1929 by the American demographer Warren Thompson (1887–1973). Thompson observed changes, or transitions, in birth and death rates in industrialized societies over the previous 200 years. Most developed countries are in stage 3 or 4 of the model; the majority of developing countries have reached stage 2 or stage 3. The major (relative) exceptions are some poor countries, mainly in sub-Saharan Africa and some Middle Eastern countries, which are poor or affected by government policy or civil strife, notably Pakistan, Palestinian Territories, Yemen and Afghanistan.

Although this model predicts ever decreasing fertility rates, recent data show that beyond a certain level of development fertility rates increase again.

A correlation matching the demographic transition has been established; however, it is not certain whether industrialization and higher incomes lead to lower population or if lower populations lead to industrialization and higher incomes. In countries that are now developed this demographic transition began in the 18th century and continues today. In less developed countries, this demographic transition started later and is still at an earlier stage.

Summary of the Theory

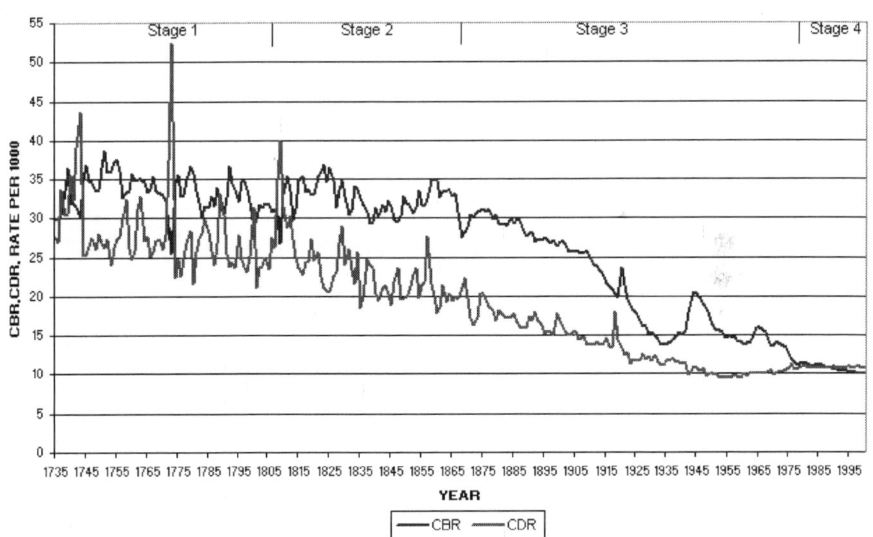

Figure: *Demographic change in Sweden from 1735 to 2000. Crude death rate (CDR), blue line: (crude) birth rate (CBR)*

The transition involves four stages, or possibly five.

- In stage one, pre-industrial society, death rates and birth rates are high and roughly in balance. All human populations are believed to have had this balance until the late 18th century, when this balance ended in Western Europe. In fact, growth rates were less than 0.05% at least since the Agricultural Revolution over 10,000 years ago. Birth and death rates both tend to be very high in this stage. Because both rates are approximately in balance, population growth is typically very slow in stage one.

- In stage two, that of a developing country, the death rates drop rapidly due to improvements in food supply and sanitation, which increase life spans and reduce disease. The improvements specific to food supply typically include selective breeding and crop rotation and farming techniques. Other improvements generally include access to technology, basic healthcare, and education. For example, numerous improvements in public health reduce mortality, especially childhood mortality. Prior to the mid-20th century, these improvements in public health were primarily in the areas of food handling, water supply, sewage, and personal hygiene. One of the variables often cited is the increase in female literacy combined with public health education programmes which emerged in the late 19th and early 20th centuries. In Europe, the death rate decline started in the late 18th century in northwestern Europe and spread to the south and east over approximately the next 100 years. Without a corresponding fall in birth rates this produces an imbalance, and the countries in this stage experience a large increase in population.
- In stage three, birth rates fall due to access to contraception, increases in wages, urbanization, a reduction in subsistence agriculture, an increase in the status and education of women, a reduction in the value of children's work, an increase in parental investment in the education of children and other social changes. Population growth begins to level off. The birth rate decline in developed countries started in the late 19th century in northern Europe. While improvements in contraception do play a role in birth rate decline, it should be noted that contraceptives were not generally available nor widely used in the 19th century and as a result likely did not play a significant role in the decline then. It is important to note that birth rate decline is caused also by a transition in values; not just because of the availability of contraceptives.
- During stage four there are both low birth rates and low death rates. Birth rates may drop to well below replacement level as has happened in countries like Germany, Italy, and Japan,

leading to a shrinking population, a threat to many industries that rely on population growth. As the large group born during stage two ages, it creates an economic burden on the shrinking working population. Death rates may remain consistently low or increase slightly due to increases in lifestyle diseases due to low exercise levels and high obesity and an aging population in developed countries. By the late 20th century, birth rates and death rates in developed countries levelled off at lower rates.

As with all models, this is an idealized picture of population change in these countries. The model is a generalization that applies to these countries as a group and may not accurately describe all individual cases. The extent to which it applies to less-developed societies today remains to be seen. Many countries such as China, Brazil and Thailand have passed through the Demographic Transition Model (DTM) very quickly due to fast social and economic change. Some countries, particularly African countries, appear to be stalled in the second stage due to stagnant development and the effect of AIDS.

Stage One

In pre-industrial society, death rates and birth rates were both high and fluctuated rapidly according to natural events, such as drought and disease, to produce a relatively constant and young population. Family planning and contraception were virtually nonexistent; therefore, birth rates were essentially only limited by the ability of women to bear children. Emigration depressed death rates in some special cases (for example, Europe and particularly the Eastern United States during the 19th century), but, overall, death rates tended to match birth rates, often exceeding 40 per 1000 per year. Children contributed to the economy of the household from an early age by carrying water, firewood, and messages, caring for younger siblings, sweeping, washing dishes, preparing food, and working in the fields. Raising a child cost little more than feeding him or her; there were no education or entertainment expenses. Thus, the total cost of raising children barely exceeded their contribution to the household. In addition, as they became adults they become a major input to the family business, mainly farming, and were the primary form of insurance for adults in old age. In India, an adult son was all that prevented a widow from falling into destitution. While death rates remained high there was no question as to the need for children, even if the means to prevent them had existed.

During this stage, the society evolves in accordance with Malthusian paradigm, with population essentially determined by the food supply. Any fluctuations in food supply (either positive, for example, due to technology improvements, or negative, due to droughts and pest invasions) tend to translate directly into population fluctuations. Famines resulting in significant mortality are frequent. Overall, the population dynamics during stage one is highly reminiscent of that commonly observed in animals.

Stage Two

This stage leads to a fall in death rates and an increase in population. The changes leading to this stage in Europe were initiated in the Agricultural Revolution of the 18th century and were initially quite slow. In the 20th century, the falls in death rates in developing countries tended to be substantially faster. Countries in this stage include Yemen, Afghanistan, the Palestinian territories, Bhutan and Laos and much of Sub-Saharan Africa (but do not include South Africa, Zimbabwe, Botswana, Swaziland, Lesotho, Namibia, Kenya and Ghana, which have begun to move into stage 3).

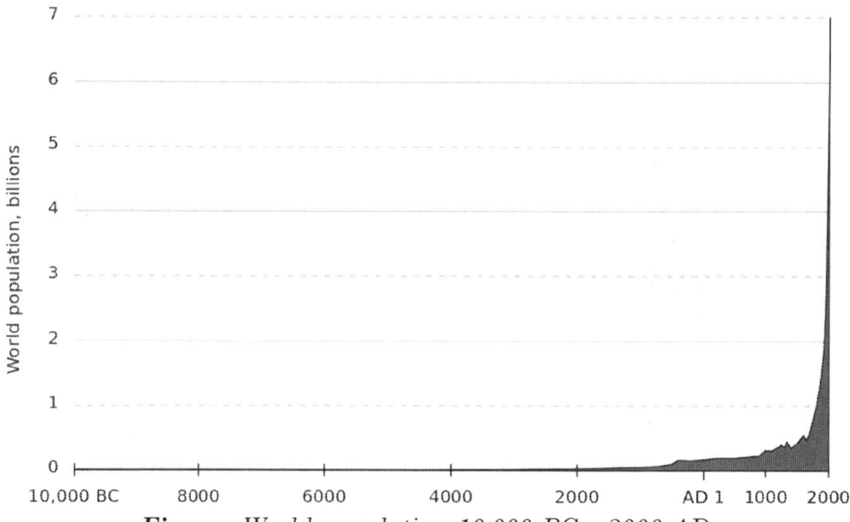

Figure: *World population 10,000 BC - 2000 AD*

The decline in the death rate is due initially to two factors:

- First, improvements in the food supply brought about by higher yields in agricultural practices and better transportation prevent death due to starvation and lack of water. Agricultural improvements included crop rotation, selective breeding, and seed drill technology.

- Second, significant improvements in public health reduce mortality, particularly in childhood. These are not so many medical breakthroughs (Europe passed through stage two before the advances of the mid-20th century, although there was significant medical progress in the 19th century, such as the development of vaccination) as they are improvements in water supply, sewerage, food handling, and general personal hygiene following from growing scientific knowledge of the causes of disease and the improved education and social status of mothers.

A consequence of the decline in mortality in Stage Two is an increasingly rapid rise in population growth (a "population explosion") as the gap between deaths and births grows wider. Note that this growth is not due to an increase in fertility (or birth rates) but to a decline in deaths. This change in population occurred in north-western Europe during the 19th century due to the Industrial Revolution. During the second half of the 20th century less-developed countries entered Stage Two, creating the worldwide population explosion that has demographers concerned today. In this stage of DT, countries are vulnerable to become failed states in the absence of progressive governments.

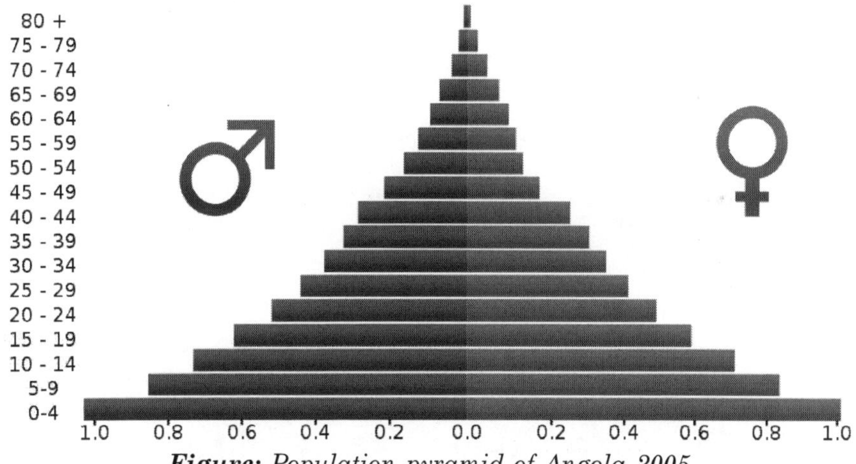

Figure: *Population pyramid of Angola 2005*

Another characteristic of Stage Two of the demographic transition is a change in the age structure of the population. In Stage One, the majority of deaths are concentrated in the first 5–10 years of life. Therefore, more than anything else, the decline in death rates in Stage Two entails the increasing survival of children and a growing population. Hence, the age structure of the population becomes increasingly youthful and more of these children enter the reproductive cycle of their lives while maintaining the high fertility rates of their parents. The bottom of the "age pyramid" widens first, accelerating population growth. The age structure of such a population is illustrated by using an example from the Third World today.

Stage Three

Stage Three moves the population towards stability through a decline in the birth rate. Several factors contribute to this eventual decline, although some of them remain speculative:

- In rural areas continued decline in childhood death means that at some point parents realise they need not require so many children to be born to ensure a comfortable old age. As childhood death continues to fall and incomes increase parents can become increasingly confident that fewer children will suffice to help in family business and care for them in old age.
- Increasing urbanization changes the traditional values placed upon fertility and the value of children in rural society. Urban living also raises the cost of dependent children to a family. A recent theory suggests that urbanization also contributes to reducing the birth rate because it disrupts optimal mating patterns. A 2008 study in Iceland found that the most fecund marriages are between distant cousins. Genetic incompatibilities inherent in more distant outbreeding makes reproduction harder.
- In both rural and urban areas, the cost of children to parents is exacerbated by the introduction of compulsory education acts and the increased need to educate children so they can take up a respected position in society. Children are increasingly prohibited under law from working outside the household and make an increasingly limited contribution to the household, as school children are increasingly exempted from the expectation of making a significant contribution to domestic work. Even in equatorial Africa, children now need to be clothed, and may even require school uniforms. Parents begin to consider it a duty to buy children books and toys. Partly due to education and access to family planning, people begin to reassess their need for children and their ability to raise them.
- Increasing female literacy and employment lowers the uncritical acceptance of childbearing and motherhood as measures of the status of women. Working women have less time to raise children; this is particularly an issue where fathers traditionally make little or no contribution to child-raising, such as southern Europe or Japan. Valuation of women beyond childbearing and motherhood becomes important.

- Improvements in contraceptive technology are now a major factor. Fertility decline is caused as much by changes in values about children and sex as by the availability of contraceptives and knowledge of how to use them.

The resulting changes in the age structure of the population include a reduction in the youth dependency ratio and eventually population aging. The population structure becomes less triangular and more like an elongated balloon. During the period between the decline in youth dependency and rise in old age dependency there is a demographic window of opportunity that can potentially produce economic growth through an increase in the ratio of working age to dependent population; the demographic dividend.

However, unless factors such as those listed above are allowed to work, a society's birth rates may not drop to a low level in due time, which means that the society cannot proceed to Stage Four and is locked in what is called a demographic trap.

Countries that have experienced a fertility decline of over 40% from their pre-transition levels include: Costa Rica, El Salvador, Panama, Jamaica, Mexico, Colombia, Ecuador, Guyana, Philippines, Indonesia, Malaysia, Sri Lanka, Turkey, Azerbaijan, Turkmenistan, Uzbekistan, Egypt, Tunisia, Algeria, Morocco, Lebanon, South Africa, India, Saudi Arabia, and many Pacific islands.

Countries that have experienced a fertility decline of 25-40% include: Honduras, Guatemala, Nicaragua, Paraguay, Bolivia, Vietnam, Myanmar, Bangladesh, Tajikistan, Jordan, Qatar, Albania, United Arab Emirates, Zimbabwe, and Botswana. Countries that have experienced a fertility decline of 10-25% include: Haiti, Papua New Guinea, Nepal, Pakistan, Syria, Iraq, Libya, Sudan, Kenya, Ghana and Senegal.

Stage Four

This occurs where birth and death rates are both low, leading to a total population which is high and stable. Death rates are low for a number of reasons, primarily lower rates of diseases and higher production of food. The birth rate is low because people have more opportunities to choose if they want children; this is made possible by improvements in contraception or women gaining more independence and work opportunities. Some theorists consider there are only 4 stages and that the population of a country will remain at this level. The DTM is only a suggestion about the future population levels of a country, not a prediction. Countries that are at this stage (Total Fertility Rate of less than 2.5 in 1997) include: United States, Canada, Argentina, Australia, New Zealand, most of Europe, Bahamas, Puerto Rico, Trinidad and Tobago, Brazil, Sri Lanka, South Korea, Singapore, Iran, China, Turkey, Thailand and Mauritius.

Stage Five and/or Six

The original Demographic Transition model has just four stages, but additional stages have been proposed. Both more-fertile and less-fertile futures have been claimed as a Stage Five.

Some countries have sub-replacement fertility (that is, below 2.1 children per woman). Replacement fertility is typically 2.1 because this replaces the two parents and adds population to compensate for deaths (i.e. members of the population who die without reproducing) with the additional 0.1. Many European and East Asian countries now have higher death rates than birth rates. Population aging and population decline may eventually occur, assuming that the fertility rate does not change and sustained mass immigration does not occur.

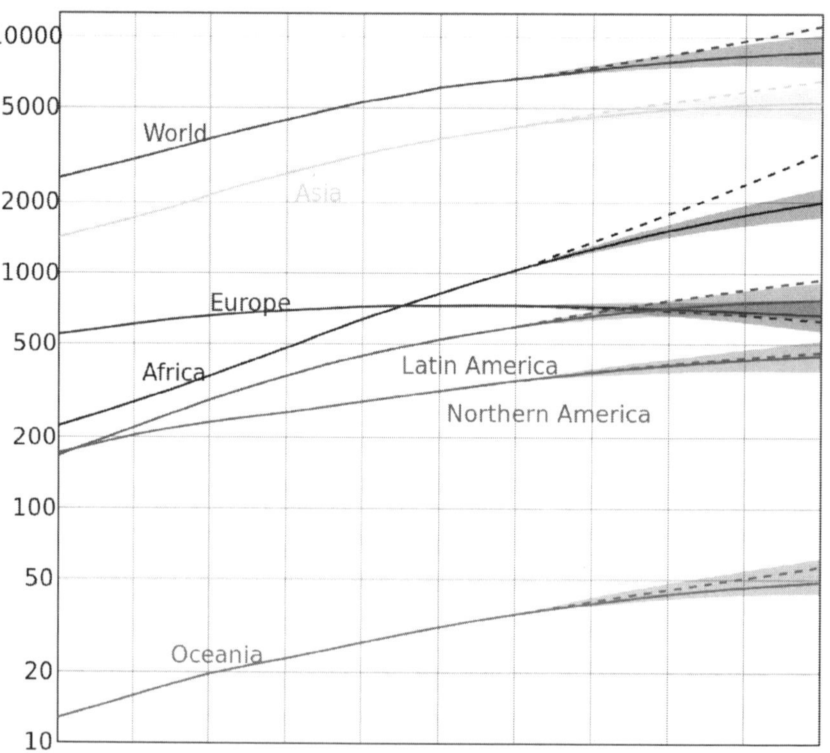

Figure: *United Nation's population projections by location. Note the vertical axis is logarithmic and represents millions of people.*

In an article in the August 2009 issue of *Nature*, Myrskyla, Kohler and Billari show that the previously negative relationship between national wealth (as measured by the Human Development Index (HDI)) and birth rates has become J-shaped. Development promotes fertility decline at low and medium HDI levels, but advanced HDI promotes a rebound in fertility. In many countries with very high levels of development fertility rates are now approaching two children per woman — although there are exceptions, notably Germany, Italy, Japan.

In the current century, most developed countries have increased fertility. From the point of view of evolutionary biology, richer people having fewer children is unexpected, as natural selection would be expected to favour individuals who are willing and able to convert plentiful resources into plentiful fertile descendants.

Effects on Age Structure

The decline in death rate and birth rate that occurs during the demographic transition leads to a radical transformation of the age structure. When the death rate declines during the second stage of the transition, the result is primarily an increase in the child population. The reason is that when the death rate is high (stage one), the infant mortality rate is very high, often above 200 deaths per 1000 children born. When the death rate falls or improves, this, in general, results in a significantly lower infant mortality rate and, hence, increased child survival. Over time, as cohorts increased by higher survival rates get older, there will also be an increase in the number of older children, teenagers, and young adults. This implies that there is an increase in the fertile population which, with constant fertility rates, will lead to an increase in the number of children born. This will further increase the growth of the child population. The second stage of the demographic transition, therefore, implies a rise in child dependency.

Historical Studies

Britain: Between 1750 and 1975 England experienced the transition from high levels of both mortality and fertility, to low levels. A major factor was the sharp decline in the death rate for infectious diseases, which has fallen from about 11 per 1,000 to less than 1 per 1,000. By contrast, the death rate from other causes was 12 per 1,000 in 1850 and has not declined markedly. The agricultural revolution and the development of transport, initiated by the construction of canals, led to greater availability of food and coal, and enabled the Industrial Revolution to improve the standard of living. Scientific discoveries and medical breakthroughs did not, in general, contribute importantly to the early major decline in infectious disease mortality, and the decline in fertility occurred before efficient contraception became available.

Ireland: In the 1980s and early 1990s, the Irish demographic status converged to the European norm. Mortality rose above the European Community average, and in 1991 Irish fertility fell to replacement level. The peculiarities of Ireland's past demography and its recent rapid changes challenge established theory. The recent changes have mirrored inward changes in Irish society, with respect to family planning, women in the work force, the sharply declining power of the Catholic Church, and the emigration factor.

France: France displays real divergences from the standard model of Western demographic evolution. The uniqueness of the French case arises from its specific demographic history, its historic cultural values, and its internal regional dynamics. France's demographic transition was unusual in that the mortality and the natality decreased at the same time, thus there was no demographic boom in the 19th century.

France's demographic profile is similar to its European neighbours and to developed countries in general, yet it seems to be staving off the population decline of Western countries. With 62.9 million inhabitants in 2006, it is the second most populous country in the European Union, and it displays a certain demographic dynamism, with a growth rate of 2.4% between 2000 and 2005, above the European average. More than two-thirds of that growth can be ascribed to a natural increase resulting from high fertility and birthrates. In contrast, France is one of the developed nations whose migratory balance is rather weak, which is an original feature at the European level. Several interrelated reasons account for such singularities, in particular the impact of pro-family policies accompanied by greater unmarried households and out-of-wedlock births. These general demographic trends parallel equally important changes in regional demographics. Since 1982 the same significant tendencies have occurred throughout mainland France: demographic stagnation in the least-populated rural regions and industrial regions in the northwest, with strong growth in the southwest and along the Atlantic coast, plus dynamism in metropolitan areas. Shifts in population between regions account for most of the differences in growth. The varying demographic evolution regions can be analysed though the filter of several parameters, including residential facilities, economic growth, and urban dynamism, which yield several distinct regional profiles. The distribution of the French population therefore seems increasingly defined not only by interregional mobility but also by the residential preferences of individual households. These challenges, linked to configurations of population and the dynamics of distribution, inevitably raise the issue of town and country planning. The most recent census figures show that an outpouring of the urban population means that fewer rural areas are continuing to register a negative migratory flow - two-thirds of rural communities have shown some since 2000. The spatial demographic expansion of large cities amplifies the process of peri-urbanization yet is also accompanied by movement of selective residential flow, social selection, and socio-spatial segregation based on income.

Asia: McNicoll (2006) examines the common features behind the striking changes in health and fertility in East and Southeast Asia in the 1960s–1990s, focusing on seven countries: Taiwan and South Korea ("tiger" economies), Thailand, Malaysia, and Indonesia ("second wave" countries), and China and Vietnam ("market-Leninist" economies). Demographic change can be seen as a byproduct of social and economic development together with, in some cases, strong governmental pressures. The transition sequence entailed the establishment of an effective, typically authoritarian, system of local administration, providing a framework for promotion and service delivery in health, education, and family planning. Subsequent economic liberalization offered new opportunities for upward mobility — and risks of backsliding —, accompanied by the erosion of social capital and the breakdown or privatization of service programmes.

India: As of year 2013, India is in later half of third stage demographic transition with 1.23 billion population. It is nearly 40 years behind in demographic transition process compared to EU countries, Japan, etc. The present demographic transition stage of India along with its higher population base will yield rich demographic dividend in future decades.

Korea: Cha (2007) analyses a panel data set to explore how industrial revolution, demographic transition, and human capital accumulation interacted in Korea from 1916–38. Income growth and public investment in health caused mortality to fall, which suppressed fertility and promoted education. Industrialization, skill premium, and closing gender wage gap further induced parents to opt for child quality. Expanding demand for education was accommodated by an active public school building programme. The interwar agricultural depression aggravated traditional income inequality, raising fertility and impeding the spread of mass schooling. Landlordism collapsed in the wake of de-colonization, and the consequent reduction in inequality accelerated human and physical capital accumulation, hence leading to growth in South Korea.

Africa: Campbell has studied the demography of 19th-century Madagascar in the light of demographic transition theory. Both supporters and critics of the theory hold to an intrinsic opposition between human and "natural" factors, such as climate, famine, and disease, influencing demography. They also suppose a sharp chronological divide between the precolonial and colonial eras, arguing that whereas "natural" demographic influences were of greater importance in the former period, human factors predominated thereafter. Campbell argues that in 19th-century Madagascar the human factor, in the form of the Merina state, was the predominant demographic influence. However, the impact of the state was felt through natural forces, and it varied over time. In the late 18th and early 19th centuries Merina state policies stimulated agricultural production, which helped to create a larger and healthier population and laid the foundation for Merina military and economic expansion within Madagascar. From 1820, the cost of such expansionism led the state to increase its exploitation of forced labour at the expense of agricultural production and thus transformed it into a negative demographic force. Infertility and infant mortality, which were probably more significant influences on overall population levels than the adult mortality rate, increased from 1820 due to disease, malnutrition, and stress, all of which stemmed from state forced labour policies. Available estimates indicate little if any population growth for Madagascar between 1820 and 1895. The demographic "crisis" in Africa, ascribed by critics of the demographic transition theory to the colonial era, stemmed in Madagascar from the policies of the imperial Merina regime, which in this sense formed a link to the French regime of the colonial era. Campbell thus questions the underlying assumptions governing the debate about historical demography in Africa and suggests that the demographic impact of political forces be re-evaluated in terms of their changing interaction with "natural" demographic influences.

Russia: In the 1980s and 1990s Russia underwent a unique demographic transition; observers call it a "demographic catastrophe": the number of deaths exceeded the number of births, life expectancy fell sharply (especially for males) and the number of suicides increased. From 1992 through 2011, the number of deaths exceeded the number of births.

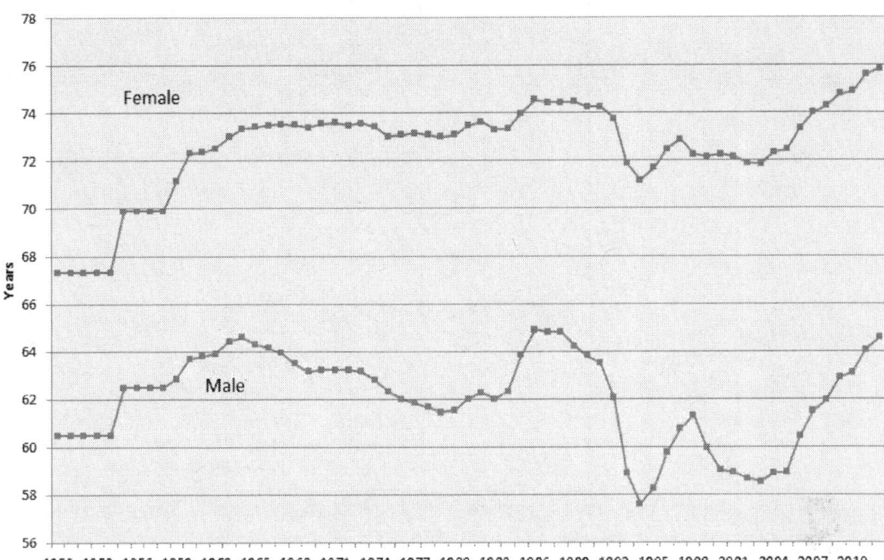

Figure: *Russian male and female life expectancy since **1950.***

United States

Greenwood and Seshadri (2002) show that from 1800 to 1940 there was a demographic shift from a mostly rural US population with high fertility, with an average of seven children born per white woman, to a minority (43%) rural population with low fertility, with an average of two births per white woman.

This shift resulted from technological progress. A sixfold increase in real wages made children more expensive in terms of forgone opportunities to work and increases in agricultural productivity reduced rural demand for labour, a substantial portion of which traditionally had been performed by children in farm families.

A simplification of the DTM theory proposes an initial decline in mortality followed by a later drop in fertility. The changing demographics of the U.S. in the last two centuries did not parallel this model. Beginning around 1800, there was a sharp fertility decline; at this time, an average woman usually produced seven births per lifetime, but by 1900 this number had dropped to nearly four. A mortality decline was not observed in the U.S. until almost 1900—a hundred years following the drop in fertility.

However, this late decline occurred from a very low initial level. It's been estimated that the crude death rate in 17th century rural New England was already as low as 20 deaths per 1000 residents per year (levels of up to 40 per 1000 being typical during stages one and two). The phenomenon is explained by the pattern of colonization of the United States: high death rates unavoidably had to match high birth rates in densely populated Europe, whereas in the United States, westward expansion of the frontier into sparsely populated interior allowed ample room to absorb all the excess people, resulting in exponential population growth (from less than 4 million people in 1790, to 23 million in 1850, to 76 million in 1900.)

Today, the U.S. is recognised as having both low fertility and mortality rates. Specifically, birth rates stand at 14 per 1000 per year and death rates at 8 per 1000 per year.

Critical Evaluation

It has to be remembered that the DTM is only a model and cannot necessarily predict the future. It does however give an indication of what the future birth and death rates may be for an underdeveloped country, together with the total population size. Most particularly, of course, the DTM makes no comment on change in population due to migration. It is not applicable for high levels of development, as it has been shown that after a HDI of 0.9 the fertility increases again.

Non-applicability to Less-developed Countries

DTM has a questionable applicability to less economically developed countries (LEDCs), where wealth and information access are limited. For example, the DTM has been validated primarily in Europe, Japan and North America where demographic data exists over centuries, whereas high quality demographic data for most LEDCs did not become widely available until the mid-20th century. DTM does not account for recent phenomena such as AIDS; in these areas HIV has become the leading source of mortality. Some trends in waterborne bacterial infant mortality are also disturbing in countries like Malawi, Sudan and Nigeria; for example, progress in the DTM clearly arrested and reversed between 1975 and 2005. The DTM did not include government interventions (population control e.g. one child policy of China).

Economic development not sufficient cause to affect demographic change

DTM assumes that population changes are induced by industrial changes and increased wealth, without taking into account the role of social change in determining birth rates, e.g., the education of women. In recent decades more work has been done on developing the social mechanisms behind it.

DTM assumes that the birth rate is independent of the death rate. Nevertheless, demographers maintain that there is no historical evidence for society-wide fertility rates rising significantly after high mortality events. Notably, some historic populations have taken many years to replace lives after events such as the Black Death.

Some have claimed that DTM does not explain the early fertility declines in much of Asia in the second half of the 20th century or the delays in fertility decline in parts of the Middle East. Nevertheless, the demographer John C. Caldwell has suggested that the reason for the rapid decline in fertility in some developing countries compared to Western Europe, the United States of America, Canada, Australia and New Zealand is mainly due to government programmes and a massive investment in education both by governments and parents.

Spatial Epidemiology

Spatial epidemiology is a subfield of health geography focused on the study of the spatial distribution of health outcomes.

Specifically, spatial epidemiology is concerned with the description and examination of disease and its geographic variations. This is done in consideration of "demographic, environmental, behavioural, socioeconomic, genetic, and infections risk factors ".

Types of Studies

Disease Mapping:

- Disease maps are visual representations of intricate geographic data that provide a quick overview of said information. Mainly used for explanatory purposes, disease maps can be presented to survey high-risk areas and to help policy and resource allocation in said areas.

Geographic Correlation Studies:

- Geographic correlation studies attempt to study the geographical factors and their effects on geographically differentiated health outcomes. Measured on an ecologic scale, these factors include environmental variables (quality of surrounding space), socioeconomic and demographic statistics (income and race), or even lifestyle choices (nutrition or diet) of the population groups under study. This approach has the convenience of being able to employ already available data from various surveying sources.

Clustering, Disease Clusters, and Surveillance:

- Disease clusters, or spatial groupings of proximity and characteristically related epidemics. While the term itself is relatively poorly defined, it generally "implies an excess of cases above some background rate bounded in time and space." Although clustering is not the most precise method for spatial analysis, it can and has proved useful for health-related surveillance and monitoring.

Because the statistical models used to draw up such research are complex, the data analysis and the interpretation of results should be carried out by qualified statisticians. Sometimes, the proliferation of errors in disease mapping has led to inefficient decision-making, implementation of inappropriate health policies and negative impact on the advancement of scientific knowledge.

Future Challenges

Data Availability and Quality:

- Since spatial epidemiology is almost entirely based on the analysis of data and its various visual representations, data collection methods must be routine, accurate, and publicly available. With the advent of specialised and accurate health equipment and global information networks, these methods can be relatively and easily improved. Compiling and standardizing data can also be done efficiently and usefully given the right tools and processes.

Data Protection and Confidentiality:

- In our current time, legislation in the United States regarding individual human rights are gaining increasing support, especially in regards to the confidentiality of personal health data and consent over its use in medical investigations. Safe and secure data is a crucial aspect of successful epidemiologic research.

Exposure Assessment and Mapping:

- Typically always seen as an analytical weakness, the quality of exposure data, or reported accuracy of the spatial reach of epidemics, is especially important in spatial epidemiology. With the more mainstream use of geographic information systems, the capabilities of spatial interpolation and mapping have been tremendously improved, yet these still greatly depend on the precision and legitimacy of the source data commissioned.

Cluster (Epidemiology)

A cluster refers to a grouping of health-related events that are related temporally and in proximity. Typically, when clusters are recognised, they are reported to public health departments in the local area. The 1854 cholera outbreak which occurred in London is a classical example of a cluster. If clusters are of sufficient size and importance, they may be re-evaluated as outbreaks.

Chapter 3

Public Health

Public health is "the science and art of preventing disease, prolonging life and promoting health through the organised efforts and informed choices of society, organisations, public and private, communities and individuals." It is concerned with threats to health based on population health analysis. The population in question can be as small as a handful of people, or as large as all the inhabitants of several continents (for instance, in the case of a pandemic). The dimensions of health can encompass "a state of complete physical, mental and social well-being and not merely the absence of disease or infirmity", as defined by the United Nations' World Health Organisation. Public health incorporates the interdisciplinary approaches of epidemiology, biostatistics and health services. Environmental health, community health, behavioural health, health economics, public policy, insurance medicine and occupational safety and health are other important subfields.

The focus of public health intervention is to improve health and quality of life through the prevention and treatment of disease and other physical and mental health conditions, through surveillance of cases and health indicators, and through the promotion of healthy behaviours. Promotion of hand washing and breastfeeding, delivery of vaccinations, and distribution of condoms to control the spread of sexually transmitted diseases are examples of common public health measures.

Modern public health practice requires multidisciplinary teams of public health workers and professionals including physicians specialising in public health/community medicine/infectious disease, psychologists epidemiologists, biostatisticians, medical assistants or Assistant Medical Officers, public health nurses, midwives, medical microbiologists, environmental health officers / public health inspectors, pharmacists, dental hygienists, dietitians and nutritionists, veterinarians, public health engineers, public health lawyers, sociologists, community development workers, communications experts, bioethicists, and others.

Objectives

The focus of a public health intervention is to prevent and manage diseases, injuries and other health conditions through surveillance of cases and the promotion of healthy behaviours, communities and environments. Many diseases are preventable through simple, non-medical methods. For example, research has shown that the simple act of hand washing with soap can prevent many contagious diseases. In other cases, treating a disease or controlling a pathogen can be vital to preventing its spread to others, such as during an outbreak of infectious disease, or contamination of food or water supplies. Public health communications programmes, vaccination programmes, and distribution of condoms are examples of common public health measures. Measures such as these have contributed greatly to the health of populations and increases in life expectancy.

Public health plays an important role in disease prevention efforts in both the developing world and in developed countries, through local health systems and non-governmental organisations. The World Health Organisation (WHO) is the international agency that coordinates and acts on global public health issues. Most countries have their own government public health agencies, sometimes known as ministries of health, to respond to domestic health issues. For example in the United States, the front line of public health initiatives are state and local health departments. The United States Public Health Service (PHS), led by the Surgeon General of the United States, and the Centres for Disease Control and Prevention, headquartered in Atlanta, are involved with several international health activities, in addition to their national duties. In Canada, the Public Health Agency of Canada is the national agency responsible for public health, emergency preparedness and response, and infectious and chronic disease control and prevention. The Public health system in India is managed by the Ministry of Health & Family Welfare of the government of India with state owned health care facilities.

There is a great disparity in access to health care and public health initiatives between developed nations and developing nations. In the developing world, public health infrastructures are still forming. There may not be enough trained health workers or monetary resources to provide even a basic level of medical care and disease prevention. As a result, a large majority of disease and mortality in the developing world results from and contributes to extreme poverty. For example, many African governments spend less than US$10 per person per year on health care, while, in the United States, the federal government spent approximately US$4,500 per capital in 2000. However, expenditures on health care should not be confused with spending on public health. Public health measures may not generally be considered "health care" in the strictest sense. For example, mandating the use of seat belts in cars can save countless lives and contribute to the health of a population, but typically money spent enforcing this rule would not count as money spent on health care.

History

Early History

Public health has early roots in antiquity. From the beginnings of human civilization, it was recognised that polluted water and lack of proper waste disposal spread communicable diseases (theory of miasma). Early religions attempted to regulate behaviour that specifically related to health, from types of food eaten, to regulating certain indulgent behaviours, such as drinking alcohol or sexual relations. Leaders were responsible for the health of their subjects to ensure social stability, prosperity, and maintain order.

By Roman times, it was well understood that proper diversion of human waste was a necessary tenet of public health in urban areas. The ancient Chinese medical doctors developed the practice of variolation following a smallpox epidemic around 1000 BC. An individual without the disease could gain some measure of immunity against it by inhaling the dried crusts that formed around lesions of infected individuals. Also, children were protected by inoculating a scratch on their forearms with the pus from a lesion.

During the 14th century Black Death in Europe, it was believed that removing bodies of the dead would further prevent the spread of the bacterial infection. This did little to stem the plague, however, which was most likely spread by rodent-borne fleas. Burning parts of cities resulted in much greater benefit, since it destroyed the rodent infestations . The development of quarantine in the medieval period helped mitigate the effects of other infectious diseases.

In 1485 the Republic of Venice established a Permanent Court of supervisors of health with special attention to the prevention of the spread of epidemics in the territory from abroad. The three supervisors were initially appointed by the Venetian Senate. In 1537 it was assumed by the Grand Council, and in 1556 added two judges, with the task of control, on behalf of the Republic, the efforts of the supervisors.

However, according to Michel Foucault, the plague model of governmentality was later controverted by the cholera model. A Cholera pandemic devastated Europe between 1829 and 1851, and was first fought by the use of what Foucault called "social medicine", which focused on flux, circulation of air, location of cemeteries, etc. All those concerns, born of the miasma theory of disease, were mixed with urbanistic concerns for the management of populations, which Foucault designated as the concept of "biopower". The German conceptualized this in the *Polizeiwissenschaft* ("Police science").

Modern Public Health

The 18th century saw rapid growth in voluntary hospitals in England. The latter part of the century brought the establishment of the basic pattern of improvements in public health over the next two centuries: a social evil was identified, private philanthropists brought attention to it, and changing public opinion led to government action.

The practice of vaccination became prevalent in the 1800s, following the pioneering work of Edward Jenner in treating smallpox. James Lind's discovery of the causes of scurvy amongst sailors and its mitigation via the introduction of fruit on lengthy voyages was published in 1754 and led to the adoption of this idea by the Royal Navy. Efforts were also made to promulgate health matters to the broader public; in 1752 the British physician Sir John Pringle published *Observations on the Diseases of the Army in Camp and Garrison*, in which he advocated for the importance of adequate ventilation in the military barracks and the provision of latrines for the soldiers.

With the onset of the Industrial Revolution, living standards amongst the working population began to worsen, with cramped and unsanitary urban conditions. In the first four decades of the 19th century alone, London's population doubled and even greater growth rates were recorded in the new industrial towns, such as Leeds and Manchester. This rapid urbanisation exacerbated the spread of disease in the large conurbations that built up around the workhouses and factories. These settlements were cramped and primitive with no organised sanitation. Disease was inevitable and its incubation in these areas was encouraged by the poor lifestyle of the inhabitants. Unavailable housing led to the rapid growth of slums and the per capita death rate began to rise alarmingly, almost doubling in Birmingham and Liverpool. Thomas Malthus warned of the dangers of overpopulation in 1798. His ideas, as well as those of Jeremy Bentham, became very influential in government circles in the early years of the 19th century.

Public Health Legislation

The first attempts at sanitary reform and the establishment of public health institutions were made in the 1840s. Thomas Southwood Smith, physician at the London Fever Hospital, began to write papers on the importance of public health, and was one of the first physicians brought in to give evidence before the Poor Law Commission in the 1830s, along with Neil Arnott and James Phillips Kay. Smith advised the government on the importance of quarantine and sanitary improvement for limiting the spread of infectious diseases such as cholera and yellow fever.

The Poor Law Commission reported in 1838 that "the expenditures necessary to the adoption and maintenance of measures of prevention would ultimately amount to less than the cost of the disease now constantly engendered". It recommended the implementation of large scale government engineering projects to alleviate the conditions that allowed for the propagation of disease. The Health of Towns Association was formed in Exeter on 11 December 1844, and vigorously campaigned for the development of public health in the United Kingdom. Its formation followed the 1843 establishment of the Health of Towns Commission, chaired by Sir Edwin Chadwick, which produced a series of reports on poor and insanitary conditions in British cities.

These national and local movements led to the Public Health Act, finally passed in 1848. It aimed to improve the sanitary condition of towns and populous places in England and Wales by placing the supply of water, sewerage, drainage, cleansing and paving under a single local body with the General Board of Health as a central authority. The Act was passed by the Liberal government of Lord John Russell, in response to the urging of Edwin Chadwick. Chadwick's seminal report on *The Sanitary Condition of the Labouring Population* was published in 1842 and was followed up with a supplementary report a year later.

Vaccination for various diseases was made compulsory in the United Kingdom in 1851, and by 1871 legislation required a comprehensive system of registration run by appointed vaccination officers.

Further interventions were made by a series of subsequent Public Health Acts, notably the 1875 Act. Reforms included latrinization, the building of sewers, the regular collection of garbage followed by incineration or disposal in a landfill, the provision of clean water and the draining of standing water to prevent the breeding of mosquitoes. So began the inception of the modern public health.

In the U.S., the first public health organisation based on a state health department and local boards of health was founded in New York City in 1866.

Epidemiology

The science of epidemiology was founded by John Snow's identification of a polluted public water well as the source of an 1854 cholera outbreak in London. Dr. Snow believed in the germ theory of disease as opposed to the prevailing miasma theory. He first publicized his theory in an essay, *On the Mode of Communication of Cholera*, in 1849, followed by a more detailed treatise in 1855 incorporating the results of his investigation of the role of the water supply in the Soho epidemic of 1854.

By talking to local residents (with the help of Reverend Henry Whitehead), he identified the source of the outbreak as the public water pump on Broad Street (now Broadwick Street). Although Snow's chemical and microscope examination of a water sample from the Broad Street pump did not conclusively prove its danger, his studies of the pattern of the disease were convincing enough to persuade the local council to disable the well pump by removing its handle.

Snow later used a dot map to illustrate the cluster of cholera cases around the pump. He also used statistics to illustrate the connection between the quality of the water source and cholera cases. He showed that the Southwark and Vauxhall Waterworks Company was taking water from sewage-polluted sections of the Thames and delivering the water to homes, leading to an increased incidence of cholera. Snow's study was a major event in the history of public health and geography. It is regarded as the founding event of the science of epidemiology.

Disease Control

With the pioneering work in bacteriology of French chemist Louis Pasteur and German scientist Robert Koch, methods for isolating the bacteria responsible for a given disease and vaccines for remedy were developed at the turn of the 20th century. British physician Ronald Ross identified the mosquito as the carrier of malaria and laid the foundations for combating the disease. Joseph Lister revolutionized surgery by the introduction of antiseptic surgery to eliminate infection. French epidemiologist Paul-Louis Simond proved that plague was carried by fleas on the back of rats, and the Americans Walter Reed and James Carroll demonstrated that mosquitoes carry the virus responsible for yellow fever.

With onset of the epidemiological transition and as the prevalence of infectious diseases decreased through the 20th century, public health began to put more focus on chronic diseases such as cancer and heart disease. Previous efforts in many developed countries had already led to dramatic reductions in the infant mortality rate using preventative methods. In Britain, the infant mortality rate fell from over 15% in 1870 to 7% by 1930.

In the United States, public health worker Dr. Sara Josephine Baker established many programmes to help the poor in New York City keep their infants healthy, leading teams of nurses into the crowded neighbourhoods of Hell's Kitchen and teaching mothers how to dress, feed, and bathe their babies.

Dramatic increases in average life span in the late 19th century and 20th century, is widely credited to public health achievements, such as vaccination programmes and control of many infectious diseases including polio, diphtheria, yellow fever and smallpox; effective health and safety policies such as road traffic safety and occupational safety; improved family planning; tobacco control measures; and programmes designed to decrease non-communicable diseases by acting on known risk factors such as a person's background, lifestyle and environment.

Another major public health improvement was the decline in the "urban penalty" brought about by improvements in sanitation. These improvements included chlorination of drinking water, filtration and sewage treatment which led to the decline in deaths caused by infectious waterborne diseases such as cholera and intestinal diseases.

Recent

Large parts of the developing world remained plagued by largely preventable or treatable infectious diseases and poor maternal and child health, exacerbated by malnutrition and poverty. The WHO reports that a lack of exclusive breastfeeding during the first six months of life contributes to over a million avoidable child deaths each year. Intermittent preventive therapy aimed at treating and preventing malaria episodes among pregnant women and young children is one public health measure in endemic countries.

Each day brings new front-page headlines about public health: emerging infectious diseases such as SARS, rapidly making its way from China to Canada, the United States and other geographically distant countries; reducing inequities in health care access through publicly funded health insurance programmes; the HIV/AIDS pandemic and its spread from certain high-risk groups to the general population in many countries, such as in South Africa; the increase of childhood obesity and the concomitant increase in type II diabetes among children; the social, economic and health effects of adolescent pregnancy; and the public health challenges related to natural disasters such as the 2004 Indian Ocean tsunami, 2005's Hurricane Katrina in the United States and the 2010 Haiti earthquake.

Since the 1980s, the growing field of population health has broadened the focus of public health from individual behaviours and risk factors to population-level issues such as inequality, poverty, and education. Modern public health is often concerned with addressing determinants of health across a population. There is a recognition that our health is affected by many factors including where we live, genetics, our income, our educational status and our social relationships; these are known as "social determinants of health." A social gradient in health runs through society. The poorest generally suffer the worst health, but even the middle classes will generally have worse health outcomes than those of a higher social stratum. The new public health advocates for population-based policies that improve health in an equitable manner.

Public Health 2.0

Public Health 2.0 is a movement within public health that aims to make the field more accessible to the general public and more user-driven. The term is used in three senses. In the first sense, "Public Health 2.0" is similar to "Health 2.0" and describes the ways in which traditional public health practitioners and institutions are reaching out (or could reach out) to the public through social media and health blogs.

In the second sense, "Public Health 2.0" describes public health research that uses data gathered from social networking sites, search engine queries, cell phones, or other technologies. In the third sense, "Public Health 2.0" is used to describe public health activities that are completely user-driven. An example is the collection and sharing of information about environmental radiation levels after the March 2011 tsunami in Japan. In all cases, Public Health 2.0 draws on ideas from Web 2.0, such as crowdsourcing, information sharing, and user-centred design.

Education and Training

Education and training of public health professionals is available throughout the world in Medical Schools, Veterinary Schools, Schools of Nursing, Schools of Public Health, and Schools of Public Affairs.

The training typically requires a university degree with a focus on core disciplines of biostatistics, epidemiology, health services administration, health policy, health education, behavioural science and environmental health. The National Commission for Health Education Credentialing (NCHEC) offers a national certification, Certified Health Education Specialist, C.H.E.S., for those who meet the eligibility requirements.

Schools of Public Health

In the United States, the Welch-Rose Report of 1915 has been viewed as the basis for the critical movement in the history of the institutional schism between public health and medicine because it led to the establishment of schools of public health supported by the Rockefeller Foundation. The report was authored by William Welch, founding dean of the Johns Hopkins Bloomberg School of Public Health, and Wycliffe Rose of the Rockefeller Foundation. The report focused more on research than practical education. Some have blamed the Rockefeller Foundation's 1916 decision to support the establishment of schools of public health for creating the schism between public health and medicine and legitimizing the rift between medicine's laboratory investigation of the mechanisms of disease and public health's nonclinical concern with environmental and social influences on health and wellness.

Even though schools of public health had already been established in Canada, Europe and North Africa, the United States had still maintained the traditional system of housing faculties of public health within their medical institutions. A $25,000 donation from businessman Samuel Zemurray instituted the School of Public Health and Tropical Medicine at Tulane University in 1912 conferring its first doctor of public health degree in 1914. The Johns Hopkins School of Hygiene and Public Health became the an independent, degree-granting institution for research and training in public health, and the largest public health training facility in the United States, when it was founded in 1916. By 1922, schools of public health were established at Columbia, Harvard and Yale on the Hopkins model. By 1999 there were twenty nine schools of public health in the US, enrolling around fifteen thousand students.

Over the years, the types of students and training provided have also changed. In the beginning, students who enrolled in public health schools typically had already obtained a medical degree; public health school training was largely a second degree for medical professionals. However, in 1978, 69% of American students enrolled in public health schools had only a bachelor's degree.

Degrees in Public Health

Schools of public health offer a variety of degrees which generally fall into two categories: professional or academic. The two major postgraduate degrees are the Master of Public Health (M.P.H.) or the Master of Science in Public Health (MSPH). Doctoral studies in this field include Doctor of Public Health (DrPH) and Doctor of Philosophy (Ph.D.) in a subspeciality of greater Public Health disciplines. DrPH is regarded as a professional leadership degree and Ph.D. as more of an academic degree.

Professional degrees are oriented towards practice in public health settings. The Master of Public Health, Doctor of Public Health, Doctor of Health Science (DHSc) and the Master of Health Care Administration are examples of degrees which are geared towards people who want careers as practitioners of public health in health departments, managed care and community-based organisations, hospitals and consulting firms among others. Master of Public Health degrees broadly fall into two categories, those that put more emphasis on an understanding of epidemiology and statistics as the scientific basis of public health practice and those that include a more eclectic range of methodologies. A Master of Science of Public Health is similar to an MPH but is considered an academic degree (as opposed to a professional degree) and places more emphasis on quantitative methods and research. The same distinction can be made between the DrPH and the DHSc. The DrPH is considered a professional degree and the DHSc is an academic degree.

Academic degrees are more oriented towards those with interests in the scientific basis of public health and preventive medicine who wish to pursue careers in research, university teaching in graduate programmes, policy analysis and development, and other high-level public health positions. Examples of academic degrees are the Master of Science, Doctor of Philosophy, Doctor of Science (ScD), and Doctor of Health Science (DHSc). The doctoral programmes are distinct from the MPH and other professional programmes by the addition of advanced coursework and the nature and scope of a dissertation research project.

In the United States, the Association of Schools of Public Health represents Council on Education for Public Health (CEPH) accredited schools of public health. Delta Omega is the honour society for graduate studies in public health. The society was founded in 1924 at the Johns Hopkins School of Hygiene and Public Health. Currently, there are approximately 68 chapters throughout the United States and Puerto Rico.

Public Health Programmes

Today, most governments recognise the importance of public health programmes in reducing the incidence of disease, disability, and the effects of aging and other physical and mental health conditions, although public health generally receives significantly less government funding compared with medicine. In recent years, public health programmes providing vaccinations have made strides in promoting health, including the eradication of smallpox, a disease that plagued humanity for thousands of years.

The World Health Organisation (WHO) identifies core functions of public health programmes including:

- providing leadership on matters critical to health and engaging in partnerships where joint action is needed;
- shaping a research agenda and stimulating the generation, translation and dissemination of valuable knowledge;
- setting norms and standards and promoting and monitoring their implementation;
- articulating ethical and evidence-based policy options;
- monitoring the health situation and assessing health trends.

In particular, public health surveillance programmes can:

- serve as an early warning system for impending public health emergencies;
- document the impact of an intervention, or track progress towards specified goals; and
- monitor and clarify the epidemiology of health problems, allow priorities to be set, and inform health policy and strategies.
- diagnose, investigate, and monitor health problems and health hazards of the community

Public health surveillance has led to the identification and prioritization of many public health issues facing the world today, including HIV/AIDS, diabetes, waterborne diseases, zoonotic diseases, and antibiotic resistance leading to the re-emergence of infectious diseases such as tuberculosis. Antibiotic resistance, also known as drug resistance, was the theme of World Health Day 2011. Although the prioritization of pressing public health issues is important, Laurie Garrett argues that there are following consequences. When foreign aid is funnelled into disease-specific programmes, the importance of public health in general is disregarded. This public health problem of stovepiping is thought to create a lack of funds to combat other existing diseases in a given country.

For example, the WHO reports that at least 220 million people worldwide suffer from diabetes. Its incidence is increasing rapidly, and it is projected that the number of diabetes deaths will double by the year 2030. In a June 2010 editorial in the medical journal *The Lancet*, the authors opined that "The fact that type 2 diabetes, a largely preventable disorder, has reached epidemic proportion is a public health humiliation." The risk of type 2 diabetes is closely linked with the growing problem of obesity. The WHO's latest estimates highlighted that globally approximately 1.5 billion adults were overweight in 2008, and nearly 43 million children under the age of five were overweight in 2010. The United States is the leading country with 30.6% of its population being obese. Mexico follows behind with 24.2% and the United Kingdom with 23%. Once considered a problem in high-income countries, it is now on the rise in low-income countries, especially in urban settings. Many public health programmes are increasingly dedicating attention and resources to the issue of obesity, with objectives to address the underlying causes including healthy diet and physical exercise.

Some programmes and policies associated with public health promotion and prevention can be controversial. One such example is programmes focusing on the prevention of HIV transmission through safe sex campaigns and needle-exchange programmes. Another is the control of tobacco smoking. Changing smoking behaviour requires long-term strategies, unlike the fight against communicable diseases, which usually takes a shorter period for effects to be observed. Many nations have implemented major initiatives to cut smoking, such as increased taxation and bans on smoking in some or all public places. Proponents argue by presenting evidence that smoking is one of the major killers, and that therefore governments have a duty to reduce the death rate, both through limiting passive (second-hand) smoking and by providing fewer opportunities for people to smoke. Opponents say that this undermines individual freedom and personal responsibility, and worry that the state may be emboldened to remove more and more choice in the name of better population health overall.

Simultaneously, while communicable diseases have historically ranged uppermost as a global health priority, non-communicable diseases and the underlying behaviour-related risk factors have been at the bottom. This is changing however, as illustrated by the United Nations hosting its first General Assembly Special Summit on the issue of non-communicable diseases in September 2011.

Many health problems are due to maladaptive personal behaviours. From an evolutionary psychology perspective, over consumption of novel substances that are harmful is due to the activation of an evolved reward system for substances such as drugs, tobacco, alcohol, refined salt, fat, and carbohydrates. New technologies such as modern transportation also cause reduced physical activity. Research has found that behaviour is more effectively changed by taking evolutionary motivations into consideration instead of only presenting information about health effects. Thus, the increased use of soap and hand-washing to prevent diarrhea is much more effectively promoted if its lack of use is associated with the emotion of disgust. Disgust is an evolved system for avoiding contact with substances that spread infectious diseases. Examples might include films that show how fecal matter contaminates food. The marketing industry has long known the importance of associating products with high status and attractiveness to others. Conversely, it has been argued that emphasizing the harmful and undesirable effects of tobacco smoking on other persons and imposing smoking bans in public places have been particularly effective in reducing tobacco smoking.

Applications in Health Care

As well as seeking to improve population health through the implementation of specific population-level interventions, public health contributes to medical care by identifying and assessing population needs for health care services, including:

- Assessing current services and evaluating whether they are meeting the objectives of the health care system
- Ascertaining requirements as expressed by health professionals, the public and other stakeholders
- Identifying the most appropriate interventions
- Considering the effect on resources for proposed interventions and assessing their cost-effectiveness
- Supporting decision making in health care and planning health services including any necessary changes.
- Informing, educating, and empowering people about health issues

Implementing Effective Improvement Strategies

To improve public health, one important strategy is to promote modern medicine and scientific neutrality to drive the public health policy and campaign, which is recommended by Armanda Solorzana, through a case study of the Rockefeller Foundation's hookworm campaign in Mexico in the 1920s. Soloranza argues that public health policy can't concern only politics or economics. Political concerns can lead government officials to hide the real numbers of people affected by disease in their regions, such as upcoming elections. Therefore, scientific neutrality in making public health policy is critical; it can ensure treatment needs are met regardless of political and economic conditions.

The history of public health care clearly shows the global effort to improve health care for all. However, in modern-day medicine, real, measurable change has not been clearly seen, and critics argue that this lack of improvement is due to ineffective methods that are being implemented. As argued by Paul E. Farmer, structural interventions could possibly have a large impact, and yet there are numerous problems as to why this strategy has yet to be incorporated into the health system. One of the main reasons that he suggests could be the fact that physicians are not properly trained to carry out structural interventions, meaning that the ground level health care professionals cannot implement these improvements. While structural interventions can not be the only area for improvement, the lack of coordination between socioeconomic factors and health care for the poor could be counterproductive, and end up causing greater inequity between the health care services received by the rich and by the poor. Unless health care is no longer treated as a commodity, global public health can ultimately not be achieved. This being the case, without changing the way in which health care is delivered to those who have less access to it, the universal goal of public health care cannot be achieved.

Social Model of Disability

The social model of disability is a reaction to the dominant medical model of disability which in itself is a functional analysis of the body as machine to be fixed in order to conform with normative values. The social model of disability identifies systemic barriers, negative attitudes and exclusion by society (purposely or inadvertently) that mean society is the main contributory factor in disabling people. While physical, sensory, intellectual, or psychological variations may cause individual functional limitation or impairments, these do not have to lead to disability unless society fails to take account of and include people regardless of their individual differences. The origins of the approach can be traced to the 1960s; the specific term emerged from the United Kingdom in the 1980s.

History

In 1975, the UK organisation Union of the Physically Impaired Against Segregation (UPIAS) claimed: "In our view it is society which disables physically impaired people. Disability is something imposed on top of our impairments by the way we are unnecessarily isolated and excluded from full participation in society."

In 1983, the disabled academic Mike Oliver coined the phrase "social model of disability" in reference to these ideological developments. Oliver focused on the idea of an individual model (of which the medical was a part) versus a social model, derived from the distinction originally made between impairment and disability by the UPIAS.

The "social model" was extended and developed by academics and activists in the UK, US and other countries, and extended to include all disabled people, including those who have learning difficulties / learning disabilities / or who are mentally handicapped, or people with emotional, mental health or behavioural problems.

Oliver did not intend the "social model of disability" to be an all encompassing theory of disability, rather a starting point in reframing how society views disability.

Components and Usage

A fundamental aspect of the social model concerns equality. The struggle for equality is often compared to the struggles of other socially marginalized groups. Equal rights are said to give empowerment and the "ability" to make decisions and the opportunity to live life to the fullest. A related phrase often used by disability rights campaigners, as with other social activism, is "Nothing About Us Without Us."

The social model of disability focuses on changes required in society. These might be in terms of:

- Attitudes, for example a more positive attitude towards certain mental traits or behaviours, or not underestimating the potential quality of life of those with impairments,
- Social support, for example help dealing with barriers; resources, aids or positive discrimination to overcome them, for example providing a buddy to explain work culture for an employee with autism,
- Information, for example using suitable formats (e.g. braille) or levels (e.g. simplicity of language) or coverage (e.g. explaining issues others may take for granted),
- Physical structures, for example buildings with sloped access and elevators, or
- Flexible work hours for people with circadian rhythm sleep disorders or, for example, for people who experience anxiety/ panic attacks in rush hour traffic.

The social model of disability implies that attempts to change, "fix" or "cure" individuals, especially when used against the wishes of the patient, can be discriminatory and prejudiced. This attitude, which may be seen as stemming from a medical model and a subjective value system, can harm the self-esteem and social inclusion of those constantly subjected to it (e.g. being told they are not as good or valuable, in an overall and core sense, as others). Some communities have actively resisted "treatments", while, for example, defending a unique culture or set of abilities. In the deaf community, sign language is valued even if most people do not know it and some parents argue against cochlear implants for deaf infants who cannot consent to them. People diagnosed with an autism spectrum disorder may argue against efforts to change them to be more like others. They argue instead for acceptance of neurodiversity and accommodation to different needs and goals. Some people diagnosed with a mental disorder argue that they are just different and don't necessarily conform. The biopsychosocial model of disease/disability is a holistic attempt by practitioners to address this.

The social model implies that practices such as eugenics are founded on social values and a prejudiced understanding of the potential and value of those labelled disabled. "Over 200,000 disabled people were the first victims of the holocaust."

A 1986 article stated: "It is important that we do not allow ourselves to be dismissed as if we all come under this one great metaphysical category 'the disabled'. The effect of this is a depersonalization, a sweeping dismissal of our individuality, and a denial of our right to be seen as people with our own uniqueness, rather than as the anonymous constituents of a category or group. These words that lump us all together -'the disabled', 'spina bifida', 'tetraplegic', 'muscular dystrophy', - are nothing more than terminological rubbish bins into which all the important things about us as people get thrown away."

The social model of disability is based on a distinction between the terms "impairment" and "disability." Impairment is used to refer to the actual attributes (or lack of attributes), the abnormality, of a person, whether in terms of limbs, organs or mechanisms, including psychological. Disability is used to refer to the restrictions caused by society when it does not give equivalent attention and accommodation to the needs of individuals with impairments.

The social model also relates to economics. It proposes that people can be disabled by a lack of resources to meet their needs. It addresses issues such as the under-estimation of the potential of people to contribute to society and add economic value to society, if given equal rights and equally suitable facilities and opportunities as others. In Autumn 2001, the UK Office for National Statistics identified that approximately one fifth of the working age population were disabled - 7.1 million disabled people as opposed to 29.8 million able people - and in this analysis also provided insight into some of the reasons why disabled people were unwilling to enter the labour market, such as that the reduction in disability benefits in entering the labour market would not make it worthwhile to enter into employment. A three pronged approach was suggested: "incentives to work via the tax and benefit system, for example through the Disabled Person's Tax Credit; helping people back into work, for example via the New Deal for Disabled People; and tackling discrimination in the workplace via anti-discrimination policy. Underpinning this are the Disability Discrimination Act (DDA) 1995 and the Disability Rights Commission."

Law and Public Policy

In the United Kingdom, the Disability Discrimination Act defines disability using the medical model - disabled people are defined as people with certain conditions, or certain limitations on their ability to carry out "normal day-to-day activities." But the requirement of employers and service providers to make "reasonable adjustments" to their policies or practices, or physical aspects of their premises, follows the social model. By making adjustments, employers and service providers are removing the barriers that disable - according to the social model, they are effectively removing the person's disability. In 2006, amendments to the act called for local authorities and others to actively promote disability equality. This enforcement came in the shape of the Disability Equality Duty in December 2006. In 2010, The Disability Discrimination Act (1995) was amalgamated into the Equality Act 2010 along with other pertinent discrimination legislation. It extends the law on discrimination to indirect discrimination. For example if a carer of a person with a disability is discriminated against, this is now also unlawful. From October 2010 when it came into effect it is now unlawful for employers to ask questions about illness or disability at interview for a job or for a referee to comment on such in a reference, except where there is a need to make reasonable adjustments for an interview to proceed. Following an offer of a job, an employer can then lawfully ask such questions.

In the United States, the Americans with Disabilities Act of 1990 (ADA), revision of 2008 effective in January 2009, is a wide-ranging civil rights law that prohibits discrimination based on disability. It affords similar protections against discrimination to Americans with disabilities as the Civil Rights Act of 1964, which made discrimination based on race, religion, sex, national origin, and other characteristics illegal. Certain specific conditions are excluded, such as alcoholism and transsexualism.

In Australia, the federal Disability Discrimination Act 1992 contains a broad medical definition that incorporates all forms of medically diagnosable disease or dysfunction, real or imputed, temporary or permanent, and past or present. The Australian Act is loosely based on the US ADA.

In 2007, the European Court of Justice in the Chacon Navas v Eurest Colectividades SA court case, defined disability narrowly according to a medical definition that excluded temporary illness, when considering the Directive establishing a general framework for equal treatment in employment and occupation (Council Directive 2000/78/ EC). The directive did not provide for any definition of disability, despite discourse in policy documents previously in the EU about endorsing the social model of disability. This allowed the Court of Justice to take a narrow medical definition.

Nutrition Transition

Nutrition transition is the shift in dietary consumption and energy expenditure that coincides with economic, demographic, and epidemiological changes. Specifically the term is used for the recent transition of developing countries from traditional diets high in cereal and fibre to more Western pattern diets high in sugars, fat, and animal-source food.

Historical Framework

The nutrition transition model was first proposed in 1993 by Barry Popkin, and is the most cited framework in literature regarding the nutrition transition, although it has been subject to some criticism for being overly simplified. Popkin posits that two other historic transitions affect and are affected by nutritional transition. The first is the demographic transition, whereby a pattern of high fertility and high mortality transforms to one of low fertility and low mortality. Secondly, an epidemiological transition occurs, wherein a shift from a pattern of high prevalence of infectious diseases associated with malnutrition, and with periodic famine and poor environmental sanitation, to a pattern of high prevalence of chronic and degenerative diseases associated with urban-industrial lifestyles is shown. These concurrent and dynamically influenced transitions share an emphasis on the ways in which populations move from one pattern to the next. Popkin used five broad patterns to help summarize the nutrition transition model. While these patterns largely appear chronological, it is important to note that they are not restricted to certain periods of human history and still characterize certain geographic and socioeconomic subpopulations. The first pattern is that of collecting food, a characterization of hunter-gatherers, whose diets were high in carbohydrates and low in fat, especially unsaturated fat. The second pattern is defined by famine, a marked scarcity and reduced variation of the food supply. The third pattern is one of receding famine. Fruits, vegetables, and animal protein consumption increases, and starchy staples become less important in the diet. The fourth pattern is one of degenerative diseases onset by a diet high in total fat, cholesterol, sugar, and other refined carbohydrates and low in polyunsaturated fatty acids and fibre. This pattern is often accompanied by an increasingly sedentary lifestyle. The fifth pattern, and most recently emerging pattern, is characterized by a behavioural change reflective of a desire to prevent or delay degenerative diseases. Recent and rapid changes seen in developing countries from the second and third pattern to the fourth is the common focus of nutrition transition research and desire for policy that would emphasize a healthier overall diet characterizes the shift from the fourth to the fifth pattern.

Relation to Economic Development

The nutrition transition has much of its roots in economic factors related to the development of a nation or subpopulations within a nation. It was once believed that current nutrition transition was endemic only to industrialized nations like the United States, but increasing research has indicated that not only is nutrition transition occurring most rapidly in low- and middle-income developing countries, the stress of its effects stands to burden the poorest populations of these countries the most as well. This shift is attributable to many causes. Globalization has played a large role in altering the access and availability of foods in formerly undeveloped nations. Demographic shifts from rural to urban areas are central to this as well as the liberalization of food markets, global food marketing, and the emergence of transnational food companies in developing countries. All these forces of globalization are creating lifestyle changes that contribute to the nutrition transition. Technological advancements are making previously arduous labour less difficult and thus altering energy expenditure that would have helped offset the caloric increases in the diet. Daily tasks and leisure are also affected by technological advancements and contributing to greater rates of inactivity. The aforementioned increases in calorie are due to increased consumption of edible oils, animal-source foods, caloric sweeteners, accompanied by reduced consumption of grains and fruits and vegetables. These changes play into human biological preferences seen across the world. Socioeconomic factors also play an important role as do cultural values tied to appearance and status.

Globalization and Economic Factors

The current nutrition transition seen in the emerging markets of Asia, Latin America, the Middle East, North Africa, and urban areas of sub-Saharan Africa is largely a product of globalization. International food trade, investment, commercialization and marketing are drastically impacting the availability of and access to energy-dense, but nutrient-deficient foods causing the aforementioned shift from traditional diet. Another byproduct of globalization has been a marked demographic transition in these countries from rural areas to urban ones. Urban populations are more susceptible to current trends in nutrition transition because of the improved transportation, commercial food distribution and marketing, less labour-intensive-occupations, and changes in household eating habits and structure. The liberalization of food markets has had a drastic effect on consumption patterns across the globe. Liberalization and commercialization of domestic agricultural markets are opening up food trading since this is needed to compete in the world market. This had led to changes in the types of food produced, and increases in amounts of food imported into developing countries, which affects the relative availability and prices of different foods. Food demand is being shaped by increases in income and urbanization. As these rapidly developing nations continue to accrue high incomes per capita, their food spending is increasing as well. They elect to use these higher incomes on more calorically-dense foods that are sweeter and higher in fats. For example, in China, for the same extra dollar of income, an average Chinese person is purchasing higher calorie food today than that person would have done for the same extra yuan in 1990. Rapid urbanization has also shaped food demand globally. The demographic transition from rural areas to urban populations is a well documented byproduct of globalization and technological advancements. This is because agro-food systems have replaced local subsistence farming in many rural areas. The supply of food is directly sculpted by increasing demand in these areas with growing income. Urbanization is increasing access to new foods and therefore altering the supply chain. This is why transnational food companies have grown so rapidly over the past few decades. These companies are making processed and fast foods much cheaper and more widely available through the growth of transnational supermarkets and chain restaurants. Food is not only easier to obtain in urban areas; it is also cheaper and less time-consuming to acquire which creates an imbalance between energy intake and output. Their advertising and promotional strategies have a strong affect on consumer choices and desire. Foreign direct investment is also stimulating processed food sales in these supermarkets by lowering prices and creating incentives for advertising and promotion. A large proportion of this advertising is for energy-dense processed foods and is being directed at children and youth. Technological and transportation advancements are reducing the barriers that once limited global food trade. These techniques are critical to facilitating the production and distribution needed in a global market. Better preservation techniques are helping to reduce waste which contributes to lower prices for consumers. Technology is creating higher yields which also reduce prices.

Lifestyle Changes

The forces of globalization are strongly influencing many lifestyle changes in developing countries. Major changes in economic structures from agrarian economies to industrialized economies are reducing physical activity levels in occupations around the world. Even in agricultural work, gas-powered technologies are helping reduce the energy expenditure needed to perform pertinent farming tasks. These reduced activity levels are not just seen in the workplace, but in homes as well. Daily tasks that were once laborious engagements are now much easier with the help of technological advancements, with examples being appliances such as washing machines, refrigerators, and stoves. Also, recent leaps in the efficiency of food production (canning, refrigeration, freezing, and packaging being a few of the most notable) and improvements in cookware, such as the introduction of improved metal stoves which use fossil fuels and microwave ovens, have helped reduce domestic efforts greatly.

Leisure is being greatly impacted as well. Activities such as playing sports outside are being replaced with television watching and computer games. Decreasing physical leisure activities can also be contributed to urbanization wherein access to fields needed to play such games as soccer are not available due to such dense populations and their subsequent demand for land. Other important lifestyle changes fuelling the nutrition transition relate to the composition of diets. These dietary shifts have been mentioned previously several times but deserve greater scrutiny. Diets rich in legumes, other vegetables, and coarse grains are disappearing in all regions and countries. Taking their place are diets characterized by fat-rich edible and vegetable oils, cheap animal-source foods high in fat and protein, and artificially sweetened foods high in sugar and refined carbohydrates. Consumption of caloric beverages such as soda represented 21% of all calorie intake in Mexico from 1996 to 2002. Processes of globalization that have influenced food markets have made these products much cheaper, flavourful, and easier to produce which has in turn driven up their demand. So while globalization and the accompanying economic development has created higher levels of food security for developing countries, the ongoing trend of eating in a more Western fashion has caused increased rates of adverse health and childhood obesity.

Biopsychosocial Forces

The desires for these new diets and lifestyles are very understandable from a biological and psychosocial perspective. For example, humans have an innate preference for sweets dating back to hunter-gatherer populations. These sweets signaled a good source of energy for hunter-gatherers that were not food secure. This same concept also relates to human predisposition for energy-dense fatty foods. These foods were needed to sustain long journeys and provided a safety net for times of famine. Humans also desire to eliminate physical exertion. This can explain the shift to more sedentary lifestyles from occupational, domestic, and leisurely activities that were previously much more physical taxing. Socioeconomic and cultural influences also contribute to lifestyle changes associated with nutrition transition. The transfer of tastes by means of tourism and open food trade has introduced developing nations to foods previously enjoyed only by industrialized countries. Global food advertising and promotion has only further cemented these dietary changes. Additionally some cultures view obese body types in high regard as they relate them to power, beauty and affluence. Several studies suggest that socioeconomic status contributes greatly to nutrition transition wherein there is a lack of healthy food alternatives completely or a lack of affordable healthy food alternatives.

Health and Economic Outcomes

While increased food security is a major benefit of global nutrition transition, there are a myriad of coinciding negative health and economic consequences. Rates of obesity are soaring across the world and recent trends suggest that incidences of overnutrition in coming decades will overtake that of undernutrition in the developing world.

As well there will be a marked epidemiological shift from infectious disease to degenerative, non-communicable disease, NCDs in these countries. As it stands now these countries face a unique paradox in having to deal with both over- and undernutrition, a dual burden of malnutrition, that will inevitably be accompanied by both infectious and noncommunicable diseases, a dual burden of disease. The economic impact will be enormous as well. In addition to reduced productivity, the health systems of these countries stand to face a tremendous burden.

Health Outcomes

The foremost health outcome of the global nutrition transition will be an increased prevalence of obesity across the world. Obesity prevalence in developing countries increased from 2.3% in 1988 to 19.6% in 1998. Incidences are highest among women and children, indicating health inequities across global populations. Obesity is strongly linked to degenerative, NCDs such as coronary heart disease, diabetes, stroke, and hypertension. WHO estimates place NCDs as the principal global cause of morbidity and mortality, and global prevalence of chronic diseases is projected to increase substantially over the next 2 decades in developing countries. Between 1990 and 2020, mortality from cardiovascular diseases, CVDs, in developing countries is expected to increase 120% for women and 137% for men compared to 29 and 49% respectively in industrialized countries. In many of the countries facing epidemics of overnutrition, there is still widespread undernutrition.

Dual Burden of Disease

Deemed as a developmental challenge of epidemic proportions, the double burden of disease (DBD) is an emerging global health challenge, that exists predominately in low-to-middle income countries. More specifically, the DBD refers to the dual burden of communicable and non-communicable diseases(NCD). Today, over 90 per cent of the world's disease burden occurs in developing regions, and most are attributed to communicable diseases. Communicable diseases are infectious diseases that "can be passed between people through proximity, social contact or intimate contact." Common diseases in this category include whooping cough or tuberculosis, HIV/AIDs, malaria, influenza (the flu), and mumps. As low-to-middle income countries continue to develop, the types of diseases that affecting populations within these countries shifts primarily from infectious diseases, such as diarrhea and pneumonia, to primarily non-communicable diseases, such as cardiovascular disease, cancer and obesity. This shift is increasingly being referred to as the risk transition. Thus, as globalization and the proliferation of pre-packaged foods continues, traditional diets and lifestyles are changing in many developing countries. As such, it is becoming increasingly common to see low-to-middle income countries battle with century old issues such as food insecurity and under nutrition, in addition to emerging health epidemics such as chronic heart disease, hypertension, stroke, and diabetes. Diseases once characteristic of industrialized nations, are increasingly becoming health challenges of epidemic proportions in many low-to-middle income countries.

Economic Impact

The economic impact of these rising rates and dual burdens of disease looks to be tremendous. Disability, decreased quality of life, greater use of health care facilities, and increased absenteeism are strong associated with obesity. With inadequate resources, poorly construed health systems, and a general lack of expertise to address the burden of infective diseases, the disease burden for low-to-middle countries is exacerbated by the rising rate of non-communicable diseases. This is often attributed to the fact that these countries by nature have ill-health systems that possess inadequate resources to detect and prevent many non-communicable diseases." Social constructs within these countries often amplify the risk of the double burden, as inequality, gender, and other social determinants often have a role to play in disparate access and allocation of health services and resources. If current trends are maintained, the World Health Organisation predicts that low-and-middle income countries will be unable to support the burden of disease within the foreseeable future.

Implications for Policy

Because of the nature of the dual burden of disease, most experts endorse a holistic approach to tackling the heath complications these nations will face rather than just focusing on reducing overnutrition. Public policy must be re-engineered across a number of areas because of the interdisciplinary nature of this problem. These suggested areas include agriculture, manufacturing, retail, education, culture, trade, and economics. Prevention is the most cost-effective method but few successful models exist. Strategies should focus on especially at-risk populations such as women, youth, and the poor. School-based approaches and community initiatives have shown encouraging results. Government interventions that place Pigovian taxes on unhealthy foods such as soft drinks and fast food, are controversial, but could manipulate the market in a way that would encourage healthier eating. Other ways to manipulate the market include providing subsidies for healthier, unprocessed foods that would make them cheaper and more affordable for poorer populations. Political debate arises over whether obesity is an outcome of individual behaviour or a consequence of an increasingly obesogenic environment. In order to reduce obesity and its subsequent health and economic consequences, policy will need to be targeted at both the individual and the environment.

Case Studies

Case studies for individual nations are plentiful. The BRICS countries are specifically studied in great depth because of their rapidly transitioning economies, but more slowly developing nations are well studied too.

Industrialized Nations

Case studies in the United States and United Kingdom are particularly bountiful.

Developing Countries

Reports based in Latin America, Asia, the Middle East, North Africa, and developed areas of sub-Saharan Africa are easy to find.

Aboriginal Populations

Worldwide, Aboriginal populations have experienced radical changes in diet. Traditional diets and food intakes have been replaced by diets consisting of foods high in fat, sugar and salt. This change in diet is related to the life-style changes during the last century: for example, Hunter-gatherer communities became more settled, and traditional food gathering methods changed. The nutrition transition has been linked to increased rates of non-communicable diseases amongst Aboriginal populations. Industrialization introduced a less complicated way to access food; a protein rich diet was replaced by white bread, processed food and sugary beverages. A study conducted in northern Ontario proved that on-reserve food contributed to lower calorie and higher Ω-3 PUFA intake, which stabled the glucose level and prevents people from developing diabetes. Traditional food of First Nations included burbot filet (or muscle) and moose liver. Food consumption provided essential fats (i.e., fatty acids) and proteins that played a key medicinal role in the prevention and reduction of obesity and obesity-related diseases.

Population Health

Population health has been defined as "the health outcomes of a group of individuals, including the distribution of such outcomes within the group". It is an approach to health that aims to improve the health of an entire human population. This concept does not refer to animal or plant populations. A priority considered important in achieving this aim is to reduce health inequities or disparities among different population groups due to, among other factors, the social determinants of health, SDOH.

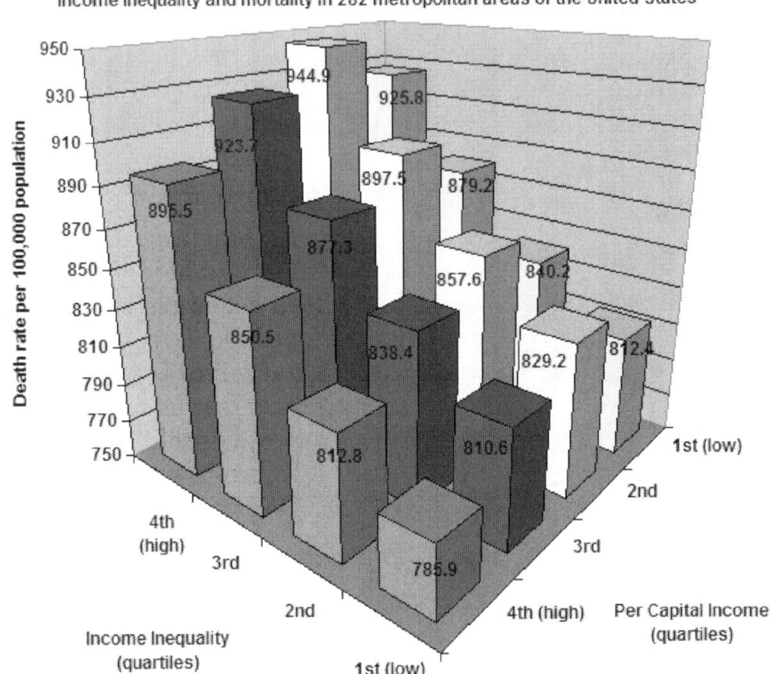

Figure: *Income inequality and mortality in 282 metropolitan areas of the United States. Mortality is correlated with both income and inequality.*

The SDOH include all the factors: social, environmental, cultural and physical the different populations are born into, grow up and function with throughout their lifetimes which potentially have a measurable impact on the health of human populations. The Population Health concept represents a change in the focus from the individual-level, characteristic of most mainstream medicine. It also seeks to complement the classic efforts of public health agencies by addressing a broader range of factors shown to impact the health of different populations. The World Health Organisation's Commission on Social Determinants of Health, reported in 2008, that the SDOH factors were responsible for the bulk of diseases and injuries and these were the major causes of health inequities in all countries. In the US, SDOH were estimated to account for 70% of avoidable mortality.

From a population health perspective, health has been defined not simply as a state free from disease but as "the capacity of people to adapt to, respond to, or control life's challenges and changes". The World Health Organisation (WHO) defined health in its broader sense in 1946 as "a state of complete physical, mental, and social well-being and not merely the absence of disease or infirmity."

Healthy People 2020

Healthy People 2020 is a web site sponsored by the US Department of Health and Human Services, representing the cumulative effort of 34 years of interest by the Surgeon General's office and others. It identifies 42 topics considered Social determinants of health and approximately 1200 specific goals considered to improve population health. It provides links to the current research available for selected topics and identifies and supports the need for community involvement considered essential to address these problems realistically.

The Human Role of Economic Inequality

Recently, human role has been encouraged by the influence of population growth there has been increasing interest from epidemiologists on the subject of economic inequality and its relation to the health of populations. There is a very robust correlation between socioeconomic status and health. This correlation suggests that it is not only the poor who tend to be sick when everyone else is healthy, heart disease, ulcers, type 2 diabetes, rheumatoid arthritis, certain types of cancer, and premature aging. Despite the reality of the SES Gradient, there is debate as to its cause. A number of researchers.

Other researchers such as Richard G. Wilkinson, J. Lynch, and G.A. Kaplan have found that socioeconomic status strongly affects health even when controlling for economic resources and access to health care. Most famous for linking social status with health are the Whitehall studies—a series of studies conducted on civil servants in London. The studies found that, despite the fact that all civil servants in England have the same access to health care, there was a strong correlation between social status and health. The studies found that this relationship stayed strong even when controlling for health-affecting habits such as exercise, smoking and drinking. Furthermore, it has been noted that no amount of medical attention will help decrease the likelihood of someone getting type 1 diabetes or rheumatoid arthritis—yet both are more common among populations with lower socioeconomic status. Lastly, it has been found that amongst the wealthiest quarter of countries on earth (a set stretching from

Luxembourg to Slovakia) there is no relation between a country's wealth and general population health—suggesting that past a certain level, absolute levels of wealth have little impact on population health, but relative levels within a country do. The concept of psychosocial stress attempts to explain how psychosocial phenomenon such as status and social stratification can lead to the many diseases associated with the SES gradient. Higher levels of economic inequality tend to intensify social hierarchies and generally degrades the quality of social relations—leading to greater levels of stress and stress related diseases. Richard Wilkinson found this to be true not only for the poorest members of society, but also for the wealthiest. Economic inequality is bad for everyone's health. Inequality does not only affect the health of human populations. David H. Abbott at the Wisconsin National Primate Research Centre found that among many primate species, less egalitarian social structures correlated with higher levels of stress hormones among socially subordinate individuals. Research by Robert Sapolsky of Stanford University provides similar findings.

Research

There is well-documented variation in health outcomes and health care utilisation & costs by geographic variation in the U.S., down to the level of Hospital Referral Regions (defined as a regional health care market, which may cross state boundaries, of which there are 306 in the U.S.). There is ongoing debate as to the relative contributions of race, gender, poverty, education level and place to these variations. The Office of Epidemiology of the Maternal and Child Health Bureau recommends using an analytic approach (Fixed Effects or hybrid Fixed Effects) to research on health disparities to reduce the confounding effects of neighbourhood (geographic) variables on the outcomes.

The Importance of Family Planning Programmes

Family planning programmes (including contraceptives, sexuality education, and promotion of safe sex) play a major role in population health. Family planning is one of the most highly cost-effective interventions in medicine. Family planning saves lives and money by reducing unintended pregnancy and the transmission of sexually transmitted infections. For example, the United States Agency for International Development lists as benefits of its international family planning programme:

- "Protecting the health of women by reducing high-risk pregnancies"
- "Protecting the health of children by allowing sufficient time between pregnancies"

- "Fighting HIV/AIDS through providing information, counselling, and access to male and female condoms"
- "Reducing abortions"
- "Supporting women's rights and opportunities for education, employment, and full participation in society"
- "Protecting the environment by stabilizing population growth"

Population Health Management (PHM)

One method to improve population health is population health management (PHM), which has been defined as "the technical field of endeavour which utilises a variety of individual, organisational and cultural interventions to help improve the morbidity patterns (i.e., the illness and injury burden) and the health care use behaviour of defined populations". PHM is distinguished from disease management by including more chronic conditions and diseases, by use of "a single point of contact and coordination", and by "predictive modelling across multiple clinical conditions". PHM is considered broader than disease management in that it also includes "intensive care management for individuals at the highest level of risk" and "personal health management... for those at lower levels of predicted health risk". Many PHM-related articles are published in *Population Health Management*, the official journal of DMAA: The Care Continuum Alliance.

The following road map has been suggested for helping healthcare organisations navigate the path towards implementing effective population health management:

- Establish precise patient registries
- Determine patient-provider attribution
- Define precise numerators in the patient registries
- Monitor and measure clinical and cost metrics
- Adhere to basic clinical practice guidelines
- Engage in risk-management outreach
- Acquire external data
- Communicate with patients
- Educate patients and engage with them
- Establish and adhere to complex clinical practice guidelines
- Coordinate effectively between care team and patient
- Track specific outcomes

Chapter 4

Community Health

Community health, a field of public health, is a discipline which concerns itself with the study and improvement of the health characteristics of biological communities. While the term community can be broadly defined, community health tends to focus on geographical areas rather than people with shared characteristics.

The health characteristics of a community are often examined using geographic information system (GIS) software and public health datasets. Some projects, such as InfoShare or GEOPROJ combine GIS with existing datasets, allowing the general public to examine the characteristics of any given community in participating countries.

Because 'health III' (broadly defined as well-being) is influenced by a wide array of socio-demographic characteristics, relevant variables range from the proportion of residents of a given age group to the overall life expectancy of the neighbourhood/community. Medical interventions aimed at improving the health of a community range from improving access to medical care to public health communications campaigns. Recent research efforts have focused on how the built environment and socio-economic status affect health.

Community health may be studied within three broad categories:

- Primary healthcare which refers to interventions that focus on the individual or family such as hand-washing, immunization, circumcision
- Secondary healthcare refers to those activities which focus on the environment such as draining puddles of water near the house, clearing bushes and spraying insecticides to control vectors like mosquitoes.

- Tertiary healthcare on the other hand refers to those interventions that take place in a hospital setting such as intravenous rehydration or surgery.

The success of community health programmes relies upon the transfer of information from health professionals to the general public using one-to-one or one to many communication (mass communication). The latest shift is towards health marketing.

Non-communicable Disease

A non-communicable disease, or NCD, is a medical condition or disease which by definition is non-infectious and non-transmissible among people. NCDs may be chronic diseases of long duration and slow progression, or they may result in more rapid death such as some types of sudden stroke. They include autoimmune diseases, heart disease, stroke, most cancers, asthma, diabetes, chronic kidney disease, osteoporosis, Alzheimer's disease, cataracts, and more. While sometimes (incorrectly) referred to as synonymous with "chronic diseases", NCDs are distinguished only by their non-infectious cause, not necessarily by their duration. Some chronic diseases of long duration, such as HIV/AIDS, are caused by transmittable infections. Chronic diseases require chronic care management as do all diseases that are slow to develop and of long duration.

The World Health Organisation (WHO) reports NCDs to be by far the leading cause of death in the world, representing over 60% of all deaths. Out of the 36 million people who died from NCDs in 2005, half were under age 70 and half were women. Of the 57 million global deaths in 2008, 36 million were due to NCDs. That is approximately 63% of total deaths worldwide. Risk factors such as a person's background, lifestyle and environment are known to increase the likelihood of certain NCDs. Every year, at least 5 million people die because of tobacco use and about 2.8 million die from being overweight. High cholesterol accounts for roughly 2.6 million deaths and 7.5 million die because of high blood pressure.

Causes and Risk Factors

Risk factors such as a person's background; lifestyle and environment are known to increase the likelihood of certain non-communicable diseases. They include age, gender, genetics, exposure to air pollution, and behaviours such as smoking, unhealthy diet and physical inactivity which can lead to hypertension and obesity, in turn leading to increased risk of many NCDs. Most NCDs are considered preventable because they are caused by modifiable risk factors.

The WHO's *World Health Report 2002* identified five important risk factors for non-communicable disease in the top ten leading risks to health. These are raised blood pressure, raised cholesterol, tobacco use, alcohol consumption, and overweight. The other factors associated with higher risk of NCDs include a person's economic and social conditions, also known as the "[social determinants of health]."

It has been estimated that if the primary risk factors were eliminated, 80% of the cases of heart disease, stroke and type 2 diabetes and 40% of cancers could be prevented. Interventions targeting the main risk factors could have a significant impact on reducing the burden of disease worldwide. Efforts focused on better diet and increased physical activity have been shown to control the prevalence of NCDs

Environmental Diseases

NCDs include many environmental diseases covering a broad category of avoidable and unavoidable human health conditions caused by external factors, such as sunlight, nutrition, pollution, and lifestyle choices. The diseases of affluence are non-infectious diseases with environmental causes. Examples include:

- Many types of cardiovascular disease (CVD)
- Chronic obstructive pulmonary disease (COPD) caused by smoking tobacco
- Diabetes mellitus type 2
- Lower back pain caused by too little exercise
- Malnutrition caused by too little food, or eating the wrong kinds of food (e.g. scurvy from lack of Vitamin C)
- Skin cancer caused by radiation from the sun
- Obesity

Inherited Diseases

Genetic disorders are caused by errors in genetic information that produce diseases in the affected people. The origin of these genetic errors can be:

- Spontaneous errors or mutations to the genome:
- A change in chromosome numbers, such as Down syndrome.
- A defect in a gene caused by mutation, such as Cystic fibrosis.
- An increase in the amount of genetic information, such as Chimerism or Heterochromia.

Cystic fibrosis is an example of an inherited disease that is caused by a mutation on a gene. The faulty gene impairs the normal movement of sodium chloride in and out of cells, which causes the mucus-secreting organs to produce abnormally thick mucus. The gene is recessive, meaning that a person must have two copies of the faulty gene for them to develop the disease. Cystic fibrosis affects the respiratory, digestive and reproductive systems, as well as the sweat glands. The mucus secreted is very thick and blocks passageways in the lungs and digestive tracts. This mucus causes problems with breathing and with the digestion and absorption of nutrients.

- Inherited genetic errors from parents:
- Dominant genetic diseases, such as Huntingtons, require the inheritance of one erroneous gene to be expressed.
- Recessive genetic diseases, such as Tay–Sachs, require the inheritance of two erroneous genes to be expressed.

NCDs and Global Health

Referred to as a "lifestyle" disease, because the majority of these diseases are preventable illnesses, the most common causes for non-communicable diseases (NCD) include tobacco use (smoking), alcohol abuse, poor diets (high consumption of sugar, salt, saturated fats, and trans fatty acids) and physical inactivity. Currently, NCD kills 36 million people a year, a number that by some estimates is expected to rise by 17–24% within the next decade.

Historically, many NCDs were associated with economic development and were so-called a "diseases of the rich". The burden of non communicable diseases in developing countries has increased however, with an estimated 80% of the four main types of NCDs — cardiovascular diseases, cancers, chronic respiratory diseases and diabetes — now occurring in low- and middle-income countries. Action Plan for the Global Strategy for the Prevention and Control of Noncommunicable Diseases and with two-thirds of people who are affected by diabetes now residing in developing nations, NCD can no longer be considered just a problem affecting affluent estimation of the economic impact of chronic noncommunicable diseases in selected countries. New WHO report: deaths from noncommunicable diseases on the rise, with developing world hit hardes. As previously stated, in 2008 alone, NCD's were the cause of 63% of deaths worldwide; a number that is expected to rise considerably in the near future if measures are not taken.

If present growth trends are maintained, by 2020, NCDs will attribute to 7 out of every 10 deaths in developing countries, killing 52 million people annually worldwide by 2030. With statistics such as these, it comes as no surprise that international entities such as the World Health Organisation & World Bank Human Development Network have identified the prevention and control of NCDs as an increasingly important discussion item on the global health agenda.

Thus, should policy makers and communities mobilize "and make prevention and targeted treatment of such diseases a priority," sustainable measures can be implemented to stagnate (and eventually even reverse) this emerging global health threat. Potential measures currently being discussed by the (World Health Organisation)-Food and Agriculture Organisation includes reducing the levels of salt in foods, limiting inappropriate marketing of unhealthy foods and non-alcoholic beverages to children, imposing controls on harmful alcohol use, raising taxes on tobacco, and curbing legislation to curb smoking in public places.

NCDs and the United Nations

The World Health Organisation is the specialised agency of the United Nations (UN) that acts as coordinating authority on international public health issues, including NCDs. In May 2008, the 193 Member States of the WHO approved a six-year plan to address non-communicable diseases, especially the rapidly increasing burden in low- and middle-income countries. The plan calls for raising the priority given to NCDs in international development work'.

During the 64th session of the United Nations General Assembly in 2010, a resolution was passed to call for a high-level meeting of the General Assembly on the prevention and treatment NCDs with the participation of heads of state and government. The resolution also encouraged UN Member States to address the issue of non-communicable diseases at the 2010 Review Summit for the Millennium Development Goals.

Global Non-communicable Disease Network

In order to better coordinate efforts around the globe, in 2009 the WHO announced the launch of the *Global Non-communicable Disease Network* (NCDnet). NCDnet will consist of leading health organisations and experts from around the world in order to fight against diseases such as cancer, cardiovascular disease, and diabetes. Ala Alwan, assistant director-general for Non-communicable Diseases and Mental Health at the WHO, said: "integrating the prevention of non-communicable diseases and injuries into the national and global development agendas is not only achievable but also a priority for developing countries."

NCD Alliance

The NCD Alliance is a global partnership founded in May 2009 by four international federations representing cardiovascular disease, diabetes, cancer, and chronic respiratory disease. The NCD Alliance brings together roughly 900 national member associations to fight non-communicable disease. Long term aims of the Alliance include:

1. NCD/disease national plans for all
2. A tobacco free world
3. Improved lifestyles
4. Strengthened health systems
5. Global access to affordable and good quality medicines and technologies
6. Human rights for people with NCDs.

Economics of NCDs

Previously, chronic NCDs were considered a problem limited mostly to high income countries, while infectious diseases seemed to affect low income countries. The burden of disease attributed to NCDs has been estimated at 85% in industrialized nations, 70% in middle income nations, and nearly 50% in countries with the lowest national incomes. In 2008, chronic NCDs accounted for more than 60% (over 35 million) of the 57 million deaths worldwide. Given the global population distribution, almost 80% of deaths due to chronic NCDs worldwide now occur in low and middle income countries, while only 20% occur in higher income countries.

National economies are reportedly suffering significant losses because of premature deaths or inability to work resulting from heart disease, stroke and diabetes. For instance, China is expected to lose roughly $558 billion in national income between 2005 and 2015 due to early deaths. In 2005, heart disease, stroke and diabetes caused an estimated loss in international dollars of national income of 9 billion in India and 3 billion in Brazil.

Absenteeism and Presenteeism

The burden of chronic NCDs including mental health conditions is felt in workplaces around the world, notably due to elevated levels of absenteeism, or absence from work because of illness, and presenteeism, or productivity lost from staff coming to work and performing below normal standards due to poor health. For example, the United Kingdom experienced a loss of about 175 million days in

2006 to absence from illness among a working population of 37.7 million people. The estimated cost of absences due to illness was over 20 billion pounds in the same year. The cost due to presenteeism is likely even larger, although methods of analysing the economic impacts of presenteeism are still being developed. Methods for analysing the distinct workplace impacts of NCDs versus other types of health conditions are also still being developed.

Key NCDs

Cancer: For the vast majority of cancers, risk factors are environmental or lifestyle-related, thus cancers are mostly preventable NCD. Greater than 30% of cancer is preventable via avoiding risk factors including: tobacco, being overweight or obesity, low fruit and vegetable intake, physical inactivity, alcohol, sexually transmitted infections, and air pollution. Infectious agents are responsible for some cancers, for instance almost all cervical cancers are caused by human papillomavirus infection.

Cardiovascular Disease

The first studies on cardiovascular health were performed in 1949 by Jerry Morris using occupational health data and were published in 1958. The causes, prevention, and/or treatment of all forms of cardiovascular disease remain active fields of biomedical research, with hundreds of scientific studies being published on a weekly basis. A trend has emerged, particularly in the early 2000s, in which numerous studies have revealed a link between fast food and an increase in heart disease. These studies include those conducted by the Ryan Mackey Memorial Research Institute, Harvard University and the Sydney Centre for Cardiovascular Health. Many major fast food chains, particularly McDonald's, have protested the methods used in these studies and have responded with healthier menu options.

A fairly recent emphasis is on the link between low-grade inflammation that hallmarks atherosclerosis and its possible interventions. C-reactive protein (CRP) is a common inflammatory marker that has been found to be present in increased levels in patients at risk for cardiovascular disease. Also osteoprotegerin which involved with regulation of a key inflammatory transcription factor called NF-êB has been found to be a risk factor of cardiovascular disease and mortality.

Diabetes

Type 2 Diabetes Mellitus is a chronic condition which is largely preventable and manageable but difficult to cure. Management concentrates on keeping blood sugar levels as close to normal ("euglycemia") as possible without presenting undue patient danger. This can usually be with close dietary management, exercise, and use of appropriate medications (insulin only in the case of type 1 diabetes mellitus. Oral medications may be used in the case of type 2 diabetes, as well as insulin).

Patient education, understanding, and participation is vital since the complications of diabetes are far less common and less severe in people who have well-managed blood sugar levels. Wider health problems may accelerate the deleterious effects of diabetes. These include smoking, elevated cholesterol levels, obesity, high blood pressure, and lack of regular exercise.

Chronic Kidney Disease

Although chronic kidney disease (CKD) is not currently identified as one of WHO's main targets for global NCD control, there is compelling evidence that CKD is not only common, harmful and treatable but also a major contributing factor to the incidence and outcomes of at least three of the diseases targeted by WHO (diabetes, hypertension and CVD). CKD strongly predisposes to hypertension and CVD; diabetes, hypertension and CVD are all major causes of CKD; and major risk factors for diabetes, hypertension and CVD (such as obesity and smoking) also cause or exacerbate CKD. In addition, among people with diabetes, hypertension, or CVD, the subset who also have CKD are at highest risk of adverse outcomes and high health care costs. Thus, CKD, diabetes and cardiovascular disease are closely associated conditions that often coexist; share common risk factors and treatments; and would benefit from a coordinated global approach to prevention and control.

Paleopathology

Paleopathology, also spelled palaeopathology, is the study of ancient diseases. It is useful in understanding the history of diseases, and uses this understanding to predict its course in the future.

History of Paleopathology

From the Renaissance to the mid nineteenth century, there was increasing reference to ancient disease, initially within prehistoric animals although later the importance of studying the antiquity of human disease began to be emphasised. The true genesis of the field of human palaeopathology is generally considered to occur between the mid nineteenth century and World War I when a number of pioneering physicians and anthropologists, such as Marc Armand Ruffer, clarified the medical nature of ancient skeletal pathologies. This included a review of human paleopathology published by H.U.

Williams in 1929 and a book published by Pales in 1930 on paleopathology and comparative pathology. This work was consolidated between the world wars with methods such as radiology, histology and serology being applied more frequently, improving diagnosis and accuracy with the introduction of statistical analysis. It was at this point that palaeopathology can truly be considered to have become a scientific discipline.

After World War II palaeopathology began to be viewed in a different way: as an important tool for the understanding of past populations, and it was at this stage that the discipline began to be related to epidemiology and demography.

New techniques in molecular biology also began to add new information to what was already known about ancient disease, as it became possible to retrieve DNA from samples that were centuries old.

Human Paleopathology

Human Osteopathology is classified into several general groups:

- Arthropathy
- Infection
- Oral pathology
- Trauma
- Tumor

Whilst traumatic injuries such as broken and malformed bones can be easy to spot, evidence of other conditions, for example infectious diseases such as tuberculosis and syphilis, can also be found in bones. Arthropathies, that is joint diseases such as osteoarthritis and gout, are also not uncommon.

The first exhaustive reference of human paleopathology evidence in skeletal tissue was published in 1976 by Ortner & Putschar. In identifying pathologies, physical anthropologists rely heavily on good archaeological documentation regarding location, age of site and other environmental factors. These provide the foundation on which further analysis is built and are required for accurate populations studies. From there, the paleopathology researcher determines a number of key biological indicators on the specimen including age and sex. These provide a foundation for further analysis of bone material and evaluation of lesions or other anomalies identified.

Archaeologists increasingly use paleopathology as an important main tool for understanding the lives of ancient peoples. For example, cranial deformation is evident in the skulls of the Maya, where a straight line between nose and forehead may have been preferred over an angle or slope. There is also evidence for trepanation, or drilling holes in the cranium, either singly or several times in a single individual. Partially or completely healed trepanations indicate that this procedure was often survived.

Infectious Diseases in the Archaeological Record

Several diseases are present in the archaeological record. Through archaeological evaluation these diseases can be identified and sometimes can explain the cause of death for certain individuals. Aside from looking at sex, age, etc. of a skeleton, a paleopathologist may analyse the condition of the bones to determine what sort of diseases the individual may have. The goal of a forensic anthropologist looking at the Paleopathology of certain diseases is to determine if the disease they are researching are still present over time, with the occurrence of certain events, or if this disease still exists today and why this disease may not exist today. Some disease that are found based on changes in bone include

- Tuberculosis
- Leprosy
- Syphilis

Apart from bones, molecular biology has also been used as a tool of paleopathology over the last few decades, as DNA can be recovered from human remains that are hundreds of years old. Since techniques such as PCR are highly sensitive to contamination, meticulous laboratory set-ups and protocols such as "suicide" PCR are necessary to ensure that false positive results from other materials in the laboratory do not occur.

For example, the long-held assumption that bubonic plague was the cause of the Justinian plague and the Black Death has been strongly supported by finding Yersinia pestis DNA in mass graves; whereas another proposed cause, anthrax, was not found

Tuberculosis

Some diseases are difficult to evaluate in the archaeology, however, tuberculosis can be found and dates as far back as the Neolithic period. Tuberculosis is presumed to have been transmitted from domesticated cattle to humans through ingestion of contaminated meats and the drinking of contaminated milk. It is also possible to contract tuberculosis through contact with infected persons. When an infected person coughs, they eject infected mucus from their body which can possibly infect those close by. There are several types of tuberculosis, the kind that affect cold-blooded animals, the kind that affects birds and the bovine type that causes disease in humans. Because bovine tuberculosis is often found in children, it may be that the disease is spread through the consumption of contaminated milk.

Tuberculosis manifests itself in the archaeological record through DNA extraction from the skeletal remains of people. Tuberculosis rarely manifests itself in the skeleton of individuals and when it does, it is usually only in advanced stages of the disease. The tuberculosis bacteria stays in the growth centres and spongy areas of the bone. This disease has a very long period of maturation, or the time it takes the disease to reach its full destructive potential. Because of the long period of development in the body, tuberculosis damages the body and then the body has time to repair itself. The evidence of the disease in bones can be seen in the destruction and healing of the bone structures especially in joints. Tuberculosis therefore appears in the archaeology record in the knee and hip joints and also the spine.

It was thought that there was no tuberculosis infection in North America before the arrival of Europeans but recent findings from the 80's and 90's have overturned that idea. Through extraction of DNA within the bone tuberculosis was not only found, but also dated to have been present in the Americas since 800 BC. Tuberculosis is a disease that thrives in dense populations. So the implications of finding tuberculosis in pre-Columbian society indicates that there was a large thriving community at the time. The earliest evidence of tuberculosis has been found in Italy dating to the 4th millennium BC. Evidence of tuberculosis has also been found in mummies from ancient Egypt dating to the same period. There is however, a lack of medical texts from ancient European and Mediterranean regions describing diseases that are identifiable as Tuberculosis but the bones show that there was a disease of this type.

Syphilis

Syphilis is a disease classified in a category of Treponemal disease. This group includes diseases like pinta, yaws, endemic syphilis and venereal syphilis. These diseases have symptoms that include inflammatory changes in tissues throughout the body. Initially the infected person may notice an area of inflammation at the site where the bacteria entered the body. Then the individual can expect more widespread soft tissue changes and lastly the diseases start to affect the bones. However, Only 10-20 percent of people infected with venereal syphilis show bone changes. Venereal syphilis has more severe symptoms than the other types of treponemal disease. Nervous system and circulatory disruption are unique to venereal syphilis and are not seen in yaws, endemic syphilis or pinta.

Bone changes can be seen in the archaeological record through lesions on the surface on the bone. In venereal syphilis the bone change is characterized by damage to the knees and joints. The damaged joints could be the source of infection or they could be damaged because of disruption in the nervous systems and ability to feel. In the beginning stages of the disease, the bone forms small lesions on the skull and tibiae. These lesions are caused mostly by inflammation of the marrow. In the final stages of the disease the bones start to be destroyed. Lesions that are formed tend to look similar to "worm holes" in the bone and are seen in the skull as well as large bones in the body. Most of the bone that is destroyed is due to secondary infections.

Syphilis has been seen in the Americas and Europe alike but there is debate as to what the origin of the disease is. Columbus and his sailors were said to have brought it to the Americas, however, Europeans blame Columbus for bringing the disease to Europe. There has not been any evidence of bone lesions associated with the disease that Columbus and the Europeans describe. The debate on the origins of venereal syphilis has been the subject of scientific discussions for hundreds of years and has recently been discussed and debated. At the first International Congress on the Evolution and Paleoepidemiology the subject was examined and debated by scholars from all over the world. There was no conclusive decision made as to the origin of venereal syphilis. There is however, more archaeological evidence for the disease in the Americas than there is for the disease in Europe at the time of Columbus's expeditions.

Animal Paleopathology

In archaeology, the study of the diseases of animals has not been as wide and extensive as those of humans. Baker and Brothwell's seminal work was published in 1980 and is still considered a classic text, being frequently referred to within the discipline. However, this position of importance has largely come about, not because of its comprehensive coverage, but because there has been no real alternative. Most palaeopathological literature is to be found in periodicals or compiled publications of conference papers. No synthesis of the research in the field as a whole has been attempted for the last twenty-five years.

The study of dinosaur paleopathology has undergone a resurgence in the past two decades. An extensive bibliography of dinosaur paleopathology was released in 2002

Measures of Disease Frequency and Disease Burden

A principal role of epidemiology is to describe and explain differences in the distribution of disease or other health outcomes of interest between populations. Examples of health outcomes measured in epidemiological studies include:

1. Morbidity
2. Mortality
3. Infectious disease incidence
4. Birth defects
5. Disability
6. Injuries
7. Vaccine efficacy
8. Utilisation of hospital services

Measures of disease frequency are used to describe how common an illness (or other health event) is with reference to the size of the population (the population at risk) and a measure of time.

There are two main measures of disease frequency:

Prevalence	Measures existing cases of disease and is expressed as a proportion
Incidence	Measures new cases of disease and is expressed in person-time units

Prevalence

Prevalence measures the proportion of individuals in a defined population that have a disease or other health outcomes of interest at a specified point in time (point prevalence) or during a specified period of time (period prevalence).

$$\text{Point Prevalence} = \frac{\text{Number of cases in a defined population at one point in time}}{\text{Number of persons in a defined population at the same point in time}}$$

Example

Of 10,000 female residents in town A on 1st January 2006, 1,000 have hypertension. The prevalence of hypertension among women in town A on this date is calculated as:

1,000/10,000 = 0.1 or 10%

- Prevalence is a useful measure for quantifying the burden of disease in a population at a given point in time
- Calculating prevalence of various conditions across different geographical areas or amongst different sub-groups of the population and then examining prevalence of other potential risk factors can be of particular use when planning health services
- Prevalence is not a useful measure for establishing the determinants of disease in a population

Incidence

In contrast to prevalence, incidence is a measure of the number of new cases of a disease (or other health outcome of interest) that develops in a population at risk during a specified time period.

Table: *There are two main measures of incidence*

Risk (or cumulative incidence)	Is related to the population at risk at the beginning of the studyperiod
Rate	Is related to a more precise measure of the population at risk during the study period and is measured in person-time units.

Risk

Risk is the proportion of individuals in a population (initially free of disease) who develop the disease within a specified time interval. Incidence risk is expressed as a percentage (or if small as per 1000 persons).

$$\text{Incidence Risk} = \frac{\text{Number of new cases of disease in a specified period of time}}{\text{Number of disease free persons at the beginning of that time period}}$$

Incidence Risk = Number of new cases of disease in a specified period of time

Number of disease free persons at the beginning of that time period

The incidence risk assumes that the entire population at risk at the beginning of the study period has been followed for the specified time period for the development of the outcome under investigation. However, in a cohort study participants may be lost during follow-up.

For example, some participants may:

- Develop the outcome under investigation
- Refuse to continue to participate in the study
- Migrate
- Die
- Enter the study some time after it starts

To account for these variations during follow up, a more precise measure can be calculated, the incidence rate .

Incidence Rate

Incidence rates also measure the frequency of new cases of disease in a population. However, incidence rates take into account the sum of the time that each person remained under observation and at risk of developing the outcome under investigation.

$$\text{Incidence Risk} = \frac{\text{Number of new cases of disease in a geven time period}}{\text{Total person-time at risk during the follow up perid}}$$

Calculation of Person-time at Risk

The denominator in an incidence rate is the sum of each individual's time at risk and is commonly expressed in person years at risk. The incidence rate is the rate of contracting the disease among those still at risk.

When a study subject develops the disease, dies or leaves the study they are no longer at risk and will no longer contribute person-time units at risk. Person-time at risk is a measure of the number of persons at risk during the given time-period.

In the graph below, different numbers of persons are at risk (N-d) during the time-period t. The total person-time at risk is represented by the area below the line (Y). Persons who have developed the disease (d) are no longer considered at risk (as they already have the disease).

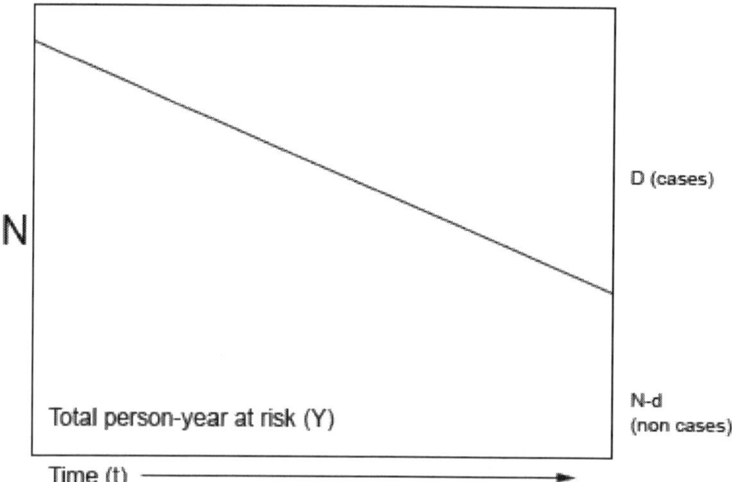

N = population initially at risk, Y = person years at risk, D = number of new cases, incidence rate = d/Y, risk (cumulative incidence) = d/N

For example:

Person-time (years) at risk for 5 individuals in a hypothetical cohort study between 2000-2004.

Year	2000	2001	2002	2003	2004	Years at risk
Persons						
1	----------	----------	----------	----------	-----------	5.0
2	----------	----------	----------	----------	-----x	4.5
3	----------	----------	----------	-----x		3.5
4		----------	-----x			1.5
5	----------	----------	----------	-----L		3.5
Total	4	5	4.5	3	1.5	18

= time at risk, X = disease, L = person lost to follow up

Figure illustrates the calculation of person-time units (years) at risk of a hypothetical population of 5 individuals in a 5 year cohort study. In the above example the incidence rate for disease (X) is calculated as:

$$\text{Incidence Risk} = \frac{\text{Number of new cases of disease in a geven time period}}{\text{Total person-time at risk during the study perid}}$$

3/18 = 0.167 per person year or 16.7 per 100 person years.

Note that for most rare diseases, risks and rates are numerically similar because the number at risk will approximately equal the total population at all times.

Issues in Defining the Population at Risk

- For any measure of disease frequency, precise definition of the denominator is essential for accuracy and clarity
- The population at risk (denominator) should include all persons at risk of developing the outcome under investigation. Therefore, individuals who currently have the disease under study or who are immune (e.g. due to immunization) should be excluded from the denominator. However, this is not always possible in practice
- Note that when individuals not at risk of the disease are included in the denominator (population at risk) the resultant measure of disease frequency will underestimate the true incidence of disease in the population under investigation

The Relationship Between Prevalence and Incidence

The proportion of the population that has a disease at a point in time (prevalence) and the rate of occurrence of new disease during a period of time (incidence) are closely related.

Prevalence depends on:

1. The incidence rate (r)
2. The duration of disease (T)

For example, if the incidence of a disease is low but the duration of disease (i.e. until recovery or death) is long, the prevalence will be high relative to the incidence. For example diseases like leprosy or tuberculosis tend to persist for a longer duration, from months to years, hence the prevalence (old and new cases) would be longer than the incidence.

Conversely, if the incidence of a disease is high and the duration of the disease is short, the prevalence will be low relative to the incidence. For example, acute conditions like diarrhoea have a relatively short duration (a few days).

A change in the duration of a disease, for example the development of a new treatment which prevents death but does not result in a cure will lead to an increase in prevalence. Fatal diseases or diseases from which a rapid recovery is common have a low prevalence, whereas diseases with a low incidence may have a high prevalence if they are incurable but rarely fatal and have a long duration.

The relationship between incidence and prevalence can be expressed as:

$P = ID$

P = Prevalence

I = Incidence Rate

D = Average duration of the disease

A population in which the numbers of people with and without the disease remain stable is known as a steady-state population. In such (theoretical) circumstances, the point prevalence of disease is approximately equal to the product of the incidence rate and the mean duration of disease (i.e. length of time from diagnosis to recovery or death), providing that prevalence is less than about 0.11.

That is Prevalence = Incidence x Duration

As a result, when two of the measures are known, the third can be calculated by substitution.

Measures of Effect

Measures of effect are used in epidemiological studies to assess the strength of an association between a putative risk factor and the subsequent occurrence of disease. This requires that the incidence of disease in a group of persons exposed to a potential risk factor is compared with the incidence in a group of persons not exposed to the potential risk factor. This comparison can be summarized by calculating either the ratio of measures of disease frequency for the two groups or the difference between the two, and reflects the increase in frequency of disease in one population compared with another, treated as baseline.

These Measures are Often Collectively Referred to as Measures of Relative Risk

The relative risk is a measure of the strength of an association between an exposure and disease and can be used to assess whether a valid observed association is likely to be causal. The most commonly used measure of effect is the ratio of incidence rates that is:

Rate (or risk) in exposed group

Rate (or risk) in unexposed group

Interpreting Measures of Relative Risk (RR)

A relative risk of 1.0 - indicates that the incidence of disease in the exposed and unexposed groups is identical and that there is no association observed between the disease and risk factor/exposure. A relative risk > 1.0 occurs when the risk of disease is greater among those exposed and indicates a positive association, or an increased risk among those exposed to the risk factor compared with those unexposed. A relative risk of 1.3 means a 30% rise in risk for those exposed to the risk factor compared to those who were unexposed.

A Relative Risk

Note: Rate ratios and risk ratios tend to be numerically similar for rare diseases.

The choice of a ratio measure or a difference measure should be based on our understanding of the mechanism by which a risk factor increases the incidence of disease

Measuring Health and Disease

Sources of Routine Data

Various sources of routinely collected data are available for use in epidemiological studies.

These include:

- Demographic data from census and population registers
- Death certificates
- Cancer registrations
- Birth registrations
- Congenital malformations registrations
- Infectious disease notifications
- Hospital episode data
- Health surveys
- Royal College of General Practitioners weekly returns

Some of these data are collected routinely on a national or regional basis such as deaths, cancer registrations, births, fertility and infectious disease notifications. However, the availability and quality of routine health statistics that can be utilised for epidemiological investigations may vary considerably.

- Health statistics may be collected on a systematic and ongoing basis, or may only be collected intermittently (such as in health surveys).
- They may be collected for the entire population or for a sample of the population.
- They may be available nationally, regionally or locally.
- They may be cohort or cross-sectional in concept.
- They may be person or episode based.
- Much of the mortality and morbidity data in the UK is collected separately for England, Wales, Scotland and Northern Ireland, making comparisons between countries more problematic, particularly as data collection may not be standardized between countries.
- The ability to compare mortality or morbidity between countries, for example cancer rates or cancer survival, may prove problematic, as coverage, the methods of data collection, and the classification of certain cancers may vary significantly.

In England most health statistics are published by the Office for National Statistics (ONS), of which a large amount is available electronically.

Demographic Data

Basic demographic data are essential for any epidemiological investigation, as they form the baseline count of the total population being studied. Reliable denominators are necessary for the calculation of the various measures of disease frequency in epidemiological studies.

The primary source of denominator data in the UK is derived from the national census which is carried out every 10 years. The last UK census was held in 2001 and the next national census is scheduled for 2011. In addition to population counts by age and sex the national census also collects data for a number of socio-economic characteristics of the population including: ethnicity (since 1991), country of birth, accommodation, education, employment and information on limiting long term illness (since 1991).

As no central agency of statistics exists for all four countries in the UK, separate simultaneous censuses are taken by each of the three government census agencies in England and Wales, Scotland and Northern Ireland.

- England and Wales: In England and Wales the census is conducted by the Office for National Statistics (ONS).
- Scotland; In Scotland the census is conducted by the General Register Office for Scotland (GROS).
- Northern Ireland: Census data in Northern Ireland is conducted by the Northern Ireland Statistics and Research Agency.

Issues in the Use of Census Data

In the UK, the census is conducted every 10 years. As a result, population data can become quickly out of date and may lead to spurious measures of disease frequency and effect. In addition, data may be incomplete for some population sub-groups.

However, annual mid-year population estimates, based on updates from the most recent census and taking into account births, deaths, net migration, and ageing of the population, are produced by the Office for National Statistics. Mid-year population estimates are also available for Scotland and Northern Ireland. In some, particularly urban settings, there may be a significant issue with migration rates, which can lead to potential inaccuracy in some local population projection estimates.

Morbidity Data

Sources of Routine Morbidity Data: Routine data on morbidity is less readily available than data relating to mortality. However, a range of morbidity data that may be utilised in epidemiological studies is available, and includes:

- Cancer registrations.
- Statutory notifications of infectious disease.

- Laboratory reporting of microbiological data.
- General practitioner reporting of clinical data.
- Hospital episode data.
- Data from health surveys.
- Morbidity surveys from general practice.
- Royal College of General Practitioner weekly returns.

Cancer Statistics – England

Cancer registrations are conducted by 9 independent regional registries that collect, on a voluntary basis, data on cancer incidence in residents of their regions. Regional registries supply cancer data to the ONS for the provision of cancer statistics.

These data are published annually by the ONS (3-4 years after the year in which the cancer was diagnosed) in:

- Cancer Statistics: Registration Series MB1.

Available Online: National and regional information on cancer incidence. Statistical tables of numbers and rates of newly diagnosed cases of cancer by site, age-group and sex are presented. Age standardized rates (using the European standard population) for the latest ten year period by cancer site and sex are also included.

- Cancer Registrations Wales: Cancer registrations in Wales are co-coordinated by the Welsh Cancer Intelligence and Surveillance Unit (WCIS).
- Cancer Registrations Scotland: The cancer registration system in Scotland is coordinated by the information and statistics division (ISD) of the NHS in Scotland.

Interpretation of Cancer Registration Data

Care is needed when examining trends over time or between different regions (ONS). For example, cancer registries may differ with respect to methods of data collection, completeness of registrations or recording of data items. In addition, misclassification of cancer cases or changes in coding systems over time may affect the reliability of the data, particularly when examining trends over time.

Hospital Episode Statistics (HES)

The Department of Health Hospital Episodes Statistics (HES) provides a wide range of information for inpatient treatment delivered by NHS hospitals in England. HES have been collected since 1989 and comprise patient-based records of finished consultant episodes (ordinary admissions and day cases) by diagnosis, operation and speciality from NHS hospitals in England. More than 12 million new records are generated each year, containing a range of information about an individual patients admitted, including:

- Clinical information about diagnoses and operations
- Data on age-group, sex and ethnicity
- Geographical information on where the patient was treated and the area in which they live.
- Date of admission, length of stay and time waited.
- Whether the patient was on a waiting list or was admitted as an emergency

Note that prior to the introduction of the HES in 1989, the hospital in-patient enquiry (HIPE) collected data on discharges and deaths, which is not directly comparable to HES data. Detailed information regarding the format and analysis of HES is available online

Statutory Notifiable Diseases

In England and Wales specified infectious diseases are statutorily notifiable. Notification data on infectious disease are analysed and published by the Health Protection Agency Centre for Infections (CfI). In addition to notifications a wide range of microbiological data are also collected. Health Protection Agency

Vital Statistics for England and Wales

Vital statistics for England and Wales are produced by the ONS and include data for the number of conceptions, live births, stillbirths and cause of death for persons in England and Wales by age and sex. Individual studies for specific diseases are also presented. Data are presented by local authorities, health authorities and wards.

Health Surveys

The UK General Household Survey: The General Household Survey (GHS) started in 1971 and is carried out annually by the Social Service Division of the ONS. It comprises a random sample of 13,000 households in the UK. Data are collected for a number of socio-economic factors including health, use of health services, the prevalence of smoking and drinking, alcohol consumption, fertility history, employment, education and income.

The Health Survey for England

The Health Survey for England (HSE) was established in 1991 by the Department of Health and comprises a series of annual surveys of the nation's health. The HSC is designed to be representative of the general population in England and aims to provide a measure of the health status of the population. Annual surveys cover the adult population aged 16 and older living in private households. Children have been included in the survey since 1995. Each year the survey focuses on different demographic groups or on diseases and their risk factors, and looks at health indicators including cardiovascular disease, physical activity and eating habits. In addition to completing a health questionnaire, those surveyed receive a nurse visit, during which various physical measurements including blood pressure, lung function tests, blood and saliva are collected. The Health Survey for England is available online from the Department of Health

Uses of Routine Health Statistics

Routine health statistics may be utilised for a variety of epidemiological investigations, including descriptive studies (cross sectional surveys or comparative mortality or morbidity studies) and disease surveillance. For example, cancer registration data may be used to examine trends in cancer incidence over time or variations in the incidence of specific cancers by age, sex, socio-economic status or geographic area. Cancer registration data may also be used to evaluate the effectiveness of cancer screening programmes or cancer care.

Routine or vital health statistics may also be utilised for use in analytical studies. However, their usefulness will depend on their completeness, accuracy, coverage and comparability between different regions or countries.

Strengths and Weaknesses of Routine Data

Data collected specifically by an investigator for use in epidemiological studies are subject to their control. This is less true for routinely collected data, and therefore they may be more likely to be subject to incompleteness, bias, and measurement error.

Strengths	***Weaknesses***
Readily available	Lack of completeness, with potential bias
Low cost	Often poorly presented and analysed
Useful for establishing baseline characterisitcs	Limited data on risk factors
Identify cases in a case-control study	Data may not be collected in a uniform way across the entire population
Generating aetiological (casual) hypotheses	Techniques of data collection may vary geographically, e.g. Recording data, coding.
Derive expected numbers in a cohort study or as a source for ascertaining outcome in a cohort study	Equivalent data not always available for all countries
Useful for examining trends of disease over time and by place	Delay between collection and publication

Errors in Epidemiological Measurements

Random Error (Chance)

Chance is a random error appearing to cause an association between an exposure and an outcome. A principal assumption in epidemiology is that we can draw an inference about the experience of the entire population based on the evaluation of a sample of the population. However a problem with drawing such an inference is that the play of chance may affect the results of an epidemiological study because of the effects of random variation from sample to sample.

The effect of random error may produce an estimate that is different from the true underlying value. Note that the effect of random error may result in either an underestimation or overestimation of the true value.

Sampling Error

Because of chance, different samples will produce different results and therefore must be taken into account when using a sample to make inferences about a population. This difference is referred to as the sampling error and its variability is measured by the standard error.

Sampling Error may Result in

A Type I error - Rejecting the null hypothesis when it is true

A Type II error - Accepting the null hypothesis when it is false

For example, when comparing the mean weights of primary class students in a government school and private school, it is generally assumed that students in government schools have a poorer nutrition and less weight (hypothesis). To prove the same, the null hypothesis is stated, no difference in the weights of students in either schools. However, because of sampling errors, there is a statistical probability of identifying a difference when truly there is no difference. This is called a type 1 error, and by convention it is fixed at 5% or below (p value = the probability of an event occurring by chance). On the other hand, a type 2 error is when we fail to observe a difference when there is a difference due to say, inadequate sample.

Reducing Sampling Error

Sampling error cannot be eliminated but with an appropriate study design can be reduced to an acceptable level. One of the major determinants to the degree to which chance affects the findings in a study is sample size. In general, sampling error decreases as the sample size increases. Therefore, use of an appropriate sample size will reduce the degree to which chance variability may account for the results observed in a study. The role of chance can be assessed by performing appropriate statistical tests and by calculation of confidence intervals. Note that the value of p will depend on both the magnitude of the association and on the study size. Confidence intervals are more informative than p values because they provide a range of values, which is likely to include the true population effect. They also indicate whether a non-significant result is or is not compatible with a true effect that was not detected because the sample size was too small.

Measurement Error (Reliability and Validity)

All epidemiological investigations involve the measurement of exposures, outcomes and other characteristics of interest (e.g. potential confounding factors).

Types of measures may include:

- Responses to self-administered questionnaires
- Responses to interview questions
- Laboratory results
- Physical measurements
- Information recorded in medical records
- Diagnosis codes from a database

Responses to Self-administered Questionnaires

All these measures may be subject to some degree of measurement error and therefore result in the introduction of bias into the study. The research instruments used to measure exposure, disease status and other variables of interest should be both valid and reliable.

Validity

The degree to which an instrument is capable of accurately measuring what it purports to measure is referred to as its validity. An examples would be how well a questionnaire measures exposure or outcome in a prospective cohort study, or the accuracy of a diagnostic test.

Assessing Validity

Assessing validity requires that an error free reference test or gold standard is available to which the measure can be compared.

Reliability (Repeatability)

Reliability refers to the consistency of the performance of an instrument over time and among different observers.

Assessing Reliability

1. Intra measurement reliability: Repeated measurements by the same observer on the same subject.
2. Inter-observer measurement carried out on the same subject by two or more observers and the results compared.

Misclassification (Information Bias)

Misclassification refers to the classification of an individual, a value or an attribute into a category other than that to which it should be assigned. The misclassification of exposure or disease status can be considered as either differential or non-differential.

Non-differential (random) misclassification occurs when classifications of disease status or exposure occurs equally in all study groups being compared. That is, the probability of exposure being misclassified is independent of disease status and the probability of disease status being misclassified is independent of exposure status.

Non-differential misclassification increases the similarity between the exposed and non-exposed groups, and may result in an underestimate (dilution) of the true strength of an association between exposure and disease.

Differential (non-random) misclassification occurs when the proportions of subjects misclassified differ between the study groups. That is, the probability of exposure being misclassified is dependent on disease status, or the probability of disease status being misclassified is dependent on exposure status. This type of error is considered a more serious problem, as the effect of differential misclassification is that the observed estimate of effect can be biased in the direction of producing either an overestimate or under-estimate of the true association.

Differential misclassification may be introduced in a study as a result of:

- Recall bias
- Observer/interviewer bias

Study Designs - Geographical Studies

Types of Geographical Studies are as Follows

- Descriptive studies
- Correlation studies
- Health surveillance

- Studies of disease clustering
- Health intervention studies

Descriptive Studies

An example of this kind of study would be examining variations in health status between populations.

Correlation Studies

These look at correlations between variables. For example, a study may investigate the body shape of a group of patients. In doing this it might correlate the height and weight of a number of people. One would expect that as people got taller so they would be heavier. Therein lies the correlation.

Health Surveillance

There is more than one definition for health surveillance. Under one definition it is thought to comprise those strategies and methods to detect and systematically record the adverse effects of work on the health of workers. Secondly, it has been used to include systematic assessments of fitness for work, and/or of health status that is not directly related to occupation.

Disease Cluster

This is a geographical region where an above average percentage of the population has, or has had, a particular disease.

Strengths and Weaknesses

It is important to consider the strengths and weaknesses of Geographical studies. These are listed below.

Strengths

- Cheap and simple to conduct.
- Utilise routinely collected health statistics.
- Exposure data often only available at area level.
- Differences in exposure between areas may be bigger than at the individual level.
- Utilise geographical information systems to examine spatial framework of disease and exposure.
- Generate hypotheses to examine at the individual level.

Weaknesses

- Measures of exposure are only a proxy based on the average in the population. Caution needed when applying grouped results to the individual level (ecological fallacy - the ecological fallacy is a widely recognised error in the interpretation of statistical data in an ecological study, whereby inferences about the nature of individuals are based solely upon aggregate statistics collected for the group to which those individuals belong. This fallacy assumes that all members of a group exhibit characteristics of the group at large).

- Potential for systematic differences between areas in recording disease frequency. For example, there may be differences in disease coding and classification, or in diagnosis and completeness of reporting.
- Potential for systematic differences between areas in the measurement of exposures.
- Lack of available data on confounding factors.

Cross-sectional Studies

A cross-sectional study examines the relationship between disease (or other health related state) and other variables of interest as they exist in a defined population at a single point in time or over a short period of time (e.g. calendar year).

Cross-sectional studies can be thought of as providing a snapshot of the frequency of a disease or other health related characteristics (e.g. exposure variables) in a population at a given point in time. Cross-sectional studies are used to assess the burden of disease or health needs of a population and are particularly useful in informing the planning and allocation of health resources.

Types of Cross-sectional Study

Descriptive

A cross-sectional survey may be purely descriptive and used to assess the burden of a particular disease in a defined population. For example a random sample of schools across London may be used to assess the prevalence of asthma among 12-14 year olds.

Analytical

Analytical cross-sectional surveys may also be used to investigate the association between a putative risk factor and a health outcome. However this type of study is limited in its ability to draw valid conclusions as to the association between a risk factor and health outcome. In a cross-sectional survey the risk factors and outcome are measured simultaneously, and therefore it may be difficult to determine whether the exposure proceeded or followed the disease. In practice, cross-sectional studies will include an element of both types of design.

Issues in the Design of Cross-sectional Surveys

Choosing a Representative Sample

A cross-sectional study should be representative of the population if generalizations from the findings are to have any validity. For example, a study of the prevalence of diabetes among women aged 40-60 years in Town A should comprise a random sample of all women aged 40-60 years in that town.

Sample Size

The sample size should be sufficiently large enough to estimate the prevalence of the conditions of interest with adequate precision. Sample size calculations can be carried out using sample size tables or statistical packages such as Epi Info.

Potential bias in cross-sectional studies

Non-response is a particular problem affecting cross-sectional studies and can result in bias of the measures of outcome. This is a particular problem when the characteristics of non-responders differ from responders.

Analysis of Cross-sectional Studies

In a cross-sectional study all factors (exposure, outcome, and confounders) are measured simultaneously. The main outcome measure obtained from a cross-sectional study is prevalence, that is:

$$\text{Prevalence} = \frac{\text{Number of cases in a defined population at one point in time}}{\text{Number of persons in a defined population at the same point in time}}$$

Note that for continuous variables such as blood pressure or weight, prevalence may only be calculated when the variable is divided into those which fall below or above a particular pre-determined level. Alternatively, mean or median levels may be calculated. In analytical cross-sectional studies, the odds ratio can be used to assess the strength of an association between a risk factor and health outcome of interest, provided that the current exposure accurately reflects the past exposure.

Strengths and Weaknesses of Cross-sectional Studies

Strengths

- Relatively quick and easy to conduct (no long periods of follow-up).

- Data on all variables is only collected once.
- Able to measure prevalence for all factors under investigation.
- Multiple outcomes and exposures can be studied.
- The prevalence of disease or other health related characteristics are important in public health for assessing the burden of disease in a specified population and in planning and allocating health resources.
- Good for descriptive analyses and for generating hypotheses.

Weaknesses

- Difficult to determine whether the outcome followed exposure in time or exposure resulted from the outcome.
- Not suitable for studying rare diseases or diseases with a short duration.
- As cross-sectional studies measure prevalent rather than incident cases, the data will always reflect determinants of survival as well as aetiology.
- Unable to measure incidence.
- Associations identified may be difficult to interpret.
- Susceptible to bias due to low response and misclassification due to recall bias.

Case-control Studies

Case-control studies start with the identification of a group of cases (individuals with a particular health outcome) in a given population and a group of controls (individuals without the health outcome) to be included in the study.

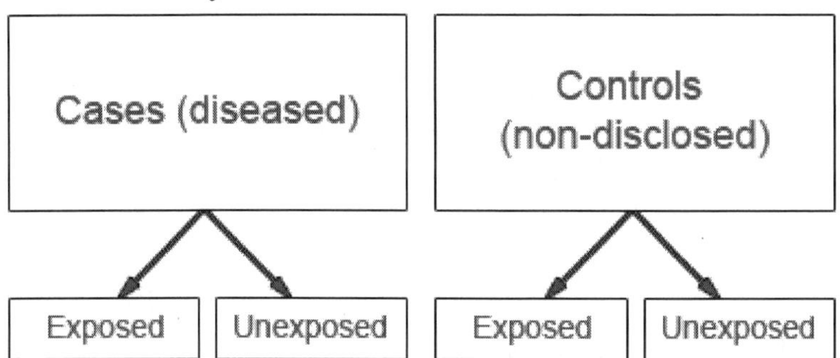

In a case-control study the prevalence of exposure to a potential risk factor(s) is compared between cases and controls. If the prevalence of exposure is more common among cases than controls, it may be a risk factor for the outcome under investigation. A major characteristic of case-control studies is that data on potential risk factors are collected retrospectively and as a result may give rise to bias. This is a particular problem associated with case-control studies and therefore needs to be carefully considered during the design and conduct of the study.

Issues in the Design of Case-control Studies

Formulation of a Clearly Defined Hypothesis

As with all epidemiological investigations the beginning of a case-control study should begin with the formulation of a clearly defined hypothesis. Case definition It is essential that the case definition is clearly defined at the outset of the investigation to ensure that all cases included in the study are based on the same diagnostic criteria. Source of cases The source of cases needs to be clearly defined.

Selection of Cases

Case-control studies may use incident or prevalent cases.

Incident Cases

Comprise cases newly diagnosed during a defined time period. The use of incident cases is considered as preferential, as the recall of past exposure(s) may be more accurate among newly diagnosed cases. In addition, the temporal sequence of exposure and disease is easier to assess among incident cases.

Prevalent Cases

comprise individuals who have had the outcome under investigation for some time. The use of prevalent cases may give rise to recall bias as prevalent cases may be less likely to accurately report past exposures(s). As a result, the interpretation of results based on prevalent cases may prove more problematic, as it may be more difficult to ensure that reported events relate to a time before the development of disease rather than to the consequence of the disease process itself. For example, individuals may modify their exposure following the onset of disease. In addition, unless the effect of exposure on duration of illness is known, it will not be possible to determine the extent to which a particular characteristic is related to the prognosis of the disease once it develops rather than to its cause.

Source of Cases

Cases may be recruited from a number of sources; for example they may be recruited from a hospital, clinic, GP registers or may be population bases. Population based case control studies are generally more expensive and difficult to conduct.

Selection of Controls

A particular problem inherent in case-control studies is the selection of a comparable control group. Controls are used to estimate the prevalence of exposure in the population which gave rise to the cases. Therefore, the ideal control group would comprise a random sample from the general population that gave rise to the cases. However, this is not always possible in practice.

The goal is to select individuals in whom the distribution of exposure status would be the same as that of the cases in the absence of an exposure disease association. That is, if there is no true association between exposure and disease, the cases and controls should have the same distribution of exposure. The source of controls is dependent on the source of cases. In order to minimize bias, controls should be selected to be a representative sample of the population which produced the cases. For example, if cases are selected from a defined population such as a GP register, then controls should comprise a sample from the same GP register.

In case-control studies where cases are hospital based, it is common to recruit controls from the hospital population. However, the choice of controls from a hospital setting should not include individuals with an outcome related to the exposure(s) being studied. For example, in a case-control study of the association between smoking and lung cancer the inclusion of controls being treated for a condition related to smoking (e.g. chronic bronchitis) may result in an underestimate of the strength of the association between exposure (smoking) and outcome. Recruiting more than one control per case may improve the statistical power of the study, though including more than 4 controls per case is generally considered to be no more efficient.

Measuring Exposure Status

Exposure status is measured to assess the presence or level of exposure for each individual for the period of time prior to the onset of the disease or condition under investigation when the exposure would have acted as a causal factor. Note that in case-control studies the measurement of exposure is established after the development of disease and as a result is prone to both recall and observer bias. Various methods can be used to ascertain exposure status. These include:

- Standardized questionnaires
- Biological samples
- Interviews with the subject
- Interviews with spouse or other family members

- Medical records
- Employment records
- Pharmacy records

The procedures used for the collection of exposure data should be the same for cases and controls.

Common Sources of Bias in Case-control Studies

Due to the retrospective nature of case-control studies, they are particularly susceptible to the effects of bias, which may be introduced as a result of a poor study design or during the collection of exposure and outcome data. Because the disease and exposure have already occurred at the outset of a case control study, there may be differential reporting of exposure information between cases and controls based on their disease status. For example, cases and controls may recall past exposure differently (recall bias). Similarly, the recording of exposure information may vary depending on the investigator's knowledge of an individual's disease status (interviewer/observer bias). Therefore, the design and conduct of the study must be carefully considered, as there are limited options for the control of bias during the analysis. Selection bias in case-control studies Selection bias is a particular problem inherent in case-control studies, where it gives rise to non-comparability between cases and controls. Selection bias in case control studies may occur when: 'cases (or controls) are included in (or excluded from) a study because of some characteristic they exhibit which is related to exposure to the risk factor under evaluation'. The aim of a case-control study is to select study controls who are representative of the population which produced the cases. Controls are used to provide an estimate of the exposure rate in the population. Therefore, selection bias may occur when those individuals selected as controls are unrepresentative of the population that produced the cases.

The potential for selection bias in case control studies is a particular problem when cases and controls are recruited exclusively from hospital or clinics. Hospital patients tend to have different characteristics than the population, for example they may have higher levels of alcohol consumption or cigarette smoking. If these characteristics are related to the exposures under investigation, then estimates of the exposure among controls may be different from that in the reference population, which may result in a biased estimate of the association between exposure and disease. Berkesonian bias is a bias introduced in hospital based case-control studies, due to varying rates of hospital admissions. As the potential for selection bias is likely to be less of a problem in population based case-control studies, neighbourhood controls may be a preferable choice when using cases from a hospital or clinic setting. Alternatively, the potential for selection bias may be minimized by selecting controls from more than one source, such as by using both hospital and neighbourhood controls. Selection bias may also be introduced in case-control studies when exposed cases are more likely to be selected than unexposed cases.

Analysis of Case-control Studies

The odds ratio (OR) is used in case-control studies to estimate the strength of the association between exposure and outcome. Note that it is not possible to estimate the incidence of disease from a case control study unless the study is population based and all cases in a defined population are obtained. The results of a case-control study can be presented in a 2x2 table as follow:

	Cases	Controls	Total
Exposed	a	b	a+b
Unexposed	c	d	c+d
Total	a+c	b+d	a+b+c+d

The odds ratio is a measure of the odds of disease in the exposed compared to the odds of disease in the unexposed (controls) and is calculated as:

$$OR = \frac{a/c}{b/d} = \frac{ad}{bc}$$

Example: Calculation of the OR from a hypothetical case-control study of smoking and cancer of the pancreas among 100 cases and 400 controls.

Table: *Hypothetical case-control study of smoking and cancer of the pancreas.*

	Cases	Controls	Total
Smokers	60 (a)	100 (b)	160
Non-smokers	40 (d)	300 (d)	340
Total	100	400	500

OR = 60 x 300 100 x 40 OR = 4.5 The OR calculated from the hypothetical data in above table estimates that smokers are 4.5 times more likely to develop cancer of the pancreas than non-smokers. NB: The odds ratio of smoking and cancer of the pancreas has been performed without adjusting for potential confounders. Further analysis of the data would involve stratifying by levels of potential confounders such as age. The 2x2 table can then be extended to allow for stratum specific rates of the confounding variable(s) to be calculated and, where appropriate, an overall summary measure, adjusted for the effects of confounding, and a statistical test of significance can also be calculated. In addition, confidence intervals for the odds ratio would also be presented.

Strengths and Weaknesses of Case-control Studies

Strengths

- Cost effective relative to other analytical studies such as cohort studies.
- Case-control studies are retrospective, and cases are identified at the beginning of the study; therefore there is no long follow up period (as compared to cohort studies).
- Efficient for the study of diseases with long latency periods.
- Efficient for the study of rare diseases.
- Good for examining multiple exposures.

Weaknesses

- Particularly prone to bias; especially selection, recall and observer bias.
- Case-control studies are limited to examining one outcome.
- Unable to estimate incidence rates of disease (unless study is population based).
- Poor choice for the study of rare exposures.
- The temporal sequence between exposure and disease may be difficult to determine.

Cohort Studies

In a cohort study, a group of individuals exposed to a putative risk factor and a group who are unexposed to the risk factor are followed over time (often years) to determine the occurrence of disease. The incidence of disease in the exposed group is compared with the incidence of disease in the unexposed group. The relative risk (incidence risk or incidence rate) is used to assess whether the exposure and disease are causally linked. Cohort studies may be prospective or retrospective. A prospective cohort study is also called a concurrent cohort study, where the subjects have been followed up for a period and the outcomes of interest are recorded.

In a retrospective cohort study both the exposure and outcome have already occurred at the outset of the study. While this type of cohort study is less time consuming and costly than a prospective cohort study, it is more susceptible to the effects of bias. For example, the exposure may have occurred some years previously and adequate reliable data on exposure may be unavailable or incomplete. In addition, information on confounding variables may be unavailable, inadequate or difficult to collect.

Issues in the Design of Cohort Studies

Selection of Study Groups

The aim of a cohort study is to select study participants who are identical with the exception of their exposure status. All study participants must be free of the outcome under investigation and have the potential to develop the outcome under investigation.

Measuring Exposure

Levels of exposure (e.g. packs of cigarettes smoked per year) are measured for each individual at baseline at the beginning of the study and assessed at intervals during the period of follow-up. When several exposures are being considered simultaneously, the non-exposed group should comprise all those with none of the risk factors under investigation.

A particular problem occurring in cohort studies is whether individuals in the control group are truly unexposed. For example, study participants may start smoking or they may fail to correctly recall past exposure. Similarly, those in the exposed group may change their behaviour in relation to the exposure such as diet, smoking or alcohol consumption.

Exposure data may be obtained from a number of sources including medical or employment records, standardized questionnaires, interviews and by physical examination.

Measuring Outcome

Outcome measures may be obtained from various sources, including routine surveillance of cancer registry data, death certificates, medical records or directly from the participant. Note that the method used to ascertain outcome must be identical for both exposed and unexposed groups.

Methods of follow-up

The follow-up of study participants in a cohort study is a major challenge. A great deal of cost and time is required to ensure follow-up of cohort members and to update measures of exposures and confounders, in addition to monitoring participants' health outcomes. The failure to collect outcome data for all members of the cohort will affect the validity of study results.

Potential Sources of Bias in Cohort Studies

A major source of potential bias in cohort studies is due to losses to follow-up. Cohort members may die, migrate, change jobs or refuse to continue to participate in the study. In addition, losses to follow-up may be related to the exposure, outcome or both. For example, individuals who develop the outcome may be less likely to continue to participate in the study. The degree to which losses to follow-up are correlated with exposure and outcome will lead to serious bias in the measures of effect of exposure and outcome.

A major source of potential bias in cohort studies arises from the degree of accuracy with which subjects have been classified with respect to their exposure or disease status. Differential misclassification can lead to an over or underestimate of the effect between exposure and outcome.

Selection Bias in Cohort Studies

Selection bias is a potential problem in case-control studies. Selection bias may be introduced when the completeness of follow-up or case ascertainment differs between exposure categories. This can be minimized by ensuring that a high level of follow-up is maintained among all study groups.

The Healthy Worker Effect

The healthy worker effect is another potential form of selection bias in cohort studies, particularly affecting occupational studies. In an occupational cohort study where disease rates among individuals from a particular occupational group are compared with an external standard population, bias may be introduced if membership of the exposed cohort is partly dependent upon health (which may be related to the presence or absence of the health outcome under investigation).

Individuals who are employed, for example, are generally healthy by nature of their ability to work. Therefore, mortality or morbidity rates in the occupation group cohort may be initially lower than in the population as a whole, which includes individuals who are too ill to work.

In order to minimize the potential for this form of bias, a comparison group may be selected from a group of workers with different jobs performed at different locations within a single facility. For example, a group of non-exposed office workers. Alternatively, the comparison group may be selected from an external population of employed individuals.

Analysis of Cohort Studies

Analysis of a cohort study uses either the risk or the rate ratio of disease in the exposed cohort compared with the rate or risk in the unexposed cohort. Note that the risk ratio uses as a denominator the entire group recruited at the start of the study, while the rate ratio uses as a denominator the person years, which takes account of losses to follow-up.

Table: *Calculation of the rate ratio from a hypothetical cohort study of smoking and cancer of the pancreas followed for 1 year.*

	Cancer of the pancreas	No disease	Total	Incidence rate
Smokers	42	27,000	27,042	1.5/1000/yr
Non-smokers	7	63,000	63,007	0.1/1000/yr
Total	49	90,000	90,049	

From the data in table, taken from a hypothetical cohort study to investigate the association between smoking and cancer of the pancreas, the relative and attributable risk can be calculated as follows:

Rate Ratio = Incidence rate in exposed group (r1)

Incidence rate in unexposed group (r0)

RR = 1.5/0.1 = 15

The relative risk of 15 indicates that the risk of cancer of the pancreas is 15 times higher among smokers than non-smokers.

Strengths and Weaknesses of Cohort Studies

Strengths

- Multiple outcomes can be measured for any one exposure.
- Can look at multiple exposures.
- Exposure is measured before the onset of disease (in prospective cohort studies).
- Good for measuring rare exposures, for example among different occupations.

- Demonstrate direction of causality.
- Can measure incidence and prevalence.

Weaknesses

- Costly and time consuming.
- Prone to bias due to loss to follow-up.
- Prone to confounding.
- Participants may move between one exposure category.
- Knowledge of exposure status may bias classification of the outcome.
- Being in the study may alter participant's behaviour.
- Poor choice for the study of a rare disease.
- Classification of individuals (exposure or outcome status) can be affected by changes in diagnostic procedures.

Intervention Studies and Randomised Controlled Trials

Intervention studies are considered to provide the most reliable evidence in epidemiological research. Intervention studies can generally be considered as either preventative or therapeutic.

Therapeutic trials are conducted among individuals with a particular disease to assess the effectiveness of an agent or procedure to diminish symptoms, prevent recurrence, or reduce mortality from the disease.

Preventative trials are conducted to evaluate whether an agent or procedure reduces the risk of developing a particular disease among individuals free from that disease at the beginning of the trial, for example, vaccine trials. Preventative trials may be conducted among individuals or among entire communities

Types of experimental interventions may include:

- Therapeutic agents
- Prophylactic agents
- Diagnostic agents
- Surgical procedures
- Health service strategies

Characteristics of an Intervention Study

- A distinguishing characteristic of an intervention study is that the intervention (the preventative or therapeutic measure) being tested is allocated by the investigator to a group of two or more study subjects (individuals, households, communities).

- Subjects are followed prospectively to compare the intervention vs. the control (standard treatment, no treatment or placebo). The main intervention study design is the randomised controlled trial (RCT).

Cross-over Trials

A pre-post clinical trial/cross-over trial is one in which the subjects are first assigned to the treatment group and, after a brief interval for cessation of residual effect of the drug, are shifted into the placebo/ alternative group. Thus, the subjects act as their own control at the end of the study. However, such studies are not feasible if there is mortality, or if the disease is easily cured by one of the interventions.

Randomised Controlled Trials

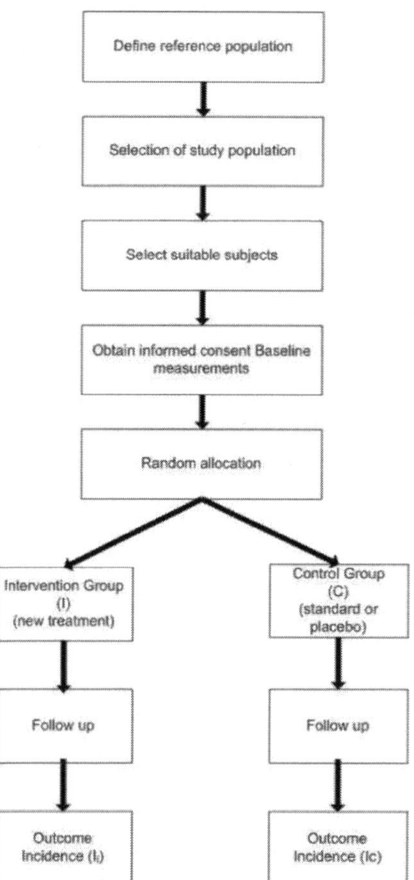

Figure: *General outline of a two armed randomised controlled trial.*

The randomised controlled trial is considered as the most rigorous method of determining whether a cause-effect relationship exists between an intervention and outcome. The strength of the RCT lies in the process of randomisation that is unique to this type of epidemiological study design.

Generally, in a randomised controlled trial, study participants are randomly assigned to one of two groups: the experimental group receiving the intervention that is being tested and a comparison group (controls) which receives a conventional treatment or placebo. These groups are then followed prospectively to assess the effectiveness of the intervention compared with the standard or placebo treatment.

The random allocation of subjects is used to ensure that the intervention and control groups are similar in all respects (distribution of potential confounding factors) with the exception of the therapeutic or preventative measure being tested. The choice of comparison treatments may include an existing standard treatment or a placebo (a treatment which resembles the intervention treatment in all respects except that it contains no active ingredients).

Note that ethical constraints limit the choice of comparison treatments.

Basic Outline of the Design of a Randomised Controlled Trial

1. Development of a comprehensive study protocol. The study protocol will include:
   - Aim and rationale of the trial
   - Proposed methodology/data collection
   - Definition of the hypothesis
   - Ethical considerations
   - Background/review of published literature
   - Quality assurance and safety
   - Treatment schedules, dosage, toxicity data etc.
2. Formulation of hypothesis.
3. Objectives of the trial.
4. Sample size calculations.
5. Define reference population.
6. Choice of a comparison treatment - placebo or current available best treatment.

7. Selection of intervention and control groups, including source, inclusion and exclusion criteria, and methods of recruitment.
8. Informed consent procedures.
9. Collection of baseline measurements, including all variables considered or known to affect the outcome(s) of interest.
10. Random allocation of study participants to treatment groups (standard or placebo vs. new).
11. Follow-up of all treatment groups, with assessment of outcomes continuously or intermittently.
12. Monitor compliance and losses to follow-up.
13. Interim analysis.
14. Analysis - comparison of treatment groups.
15. Interpretation (assess the strength of effect, alternative explanations such as sampling variation, bias).
16. Publication.

Randomisation

The aim of randomisation is to ensure that any observed differences between the treatment groups are due to differences in the treatment alone and not due to the effects of confounding (known or unknown) or bias. That is, that the groups are similar in all respects with the exception of the intervention under investigation. Methods of random allocation are used to ensure that all study participants have the same chance of allocation to the treatment or control group, and that the likelihood of receiving an intervention is equal regardless of when the participant entered the study. Therefore, the probability of any participant receiving the intervention or the standard treatment/placebo is independent of any other participant being assigned that treatment.

The assignment of study subjects to each intervention is determined by formal chance process and cannot be predicted or influenced by the investigator or participant. In a well designed RCT, random allocation is determined in advance.

Methods of Randomisation - allocation of subjects to intervention and control groups

Simple Randomisation: For example, computer generated random number tables. Simple randomisation is rarely used.

Block Randomisation: Block randomisation is a method used to ensure that the numbers of participants assigned to each group is equally distributed and is commonly used in smaller trials.

Stratified Randomisation: Stratified randomisation is used to ensure that important baseline variables (potential confounding factors) are more evenly distributed between groups than chance alone may assure. However, there are a limited number of baseline variables that can be balanced by stratification because of the potential for small numbers of subjects within each stratum.

Minimized Randomisation: This method may be used when the study is sufficiently small and simple randomisation will not result in balanced groups.

Note that deterministic methods of allocation such as by date of birth or alternate assignment to each group are not considered as random.

Advantages of Randomisation

- Eliminates confounding - tends to create groups that are comparable for all factors that influence outcome, known, unknown or difficult to measure. Therefore, the only difference between the groups should be the intervention.
- Eliminates selection bias.
- Gives validity in statistical tests based on probability theory.
- Any baseline differences that exist between study groups are attributable to chance rather than bias. Though this should still be considered as a potential concern.

Disadvantages of Randomisation

Does not guarantee comparable groups as differences in confounding variables may arise by chance.

Blinding in Randomised Controlled Trials

Blinding is a process where the critical information on allocation of treatment is hidden either from the patients, or from observer or the evaluator in the study. The method of blinding in RCT is used to ensure that there are no differences in the way in which each group is assessed or managed, and therefore minimize bias. Bias may be introduced, for example, if the investigator is aware of which treatment a subject is receiving, as this may influence (intentionally or unintentionally) the way in which outcome data is measured or interpreted. Similarly, a subject's knowledge of treatment assignment may influence their response to a specific treatment.

Blinding also involves ensuring that the intervention and standard or placebo treatment appears the same.

Double blinding is when neither the investigator nor the study participant is aware of treatment assignments. However, this design is not always possible.

A single blind RCT is when the investigator but not the study participants know which treatment has been allocated.

Strengths of a Randomised Controlled Trial

- A well designed randomised control trial provides the strongest evidence of any epidemiological study design that a given intervention has a postulated effectiveness and is safe.
- A RCT provides the best type of epidemiological study from which to draw conclusions on causality.
- Randomisation provides a powerful tool for controlling for confounding, even by factors that may be unknown or difficult to measure. Therefore, if well designed and conducted, a RCT minimizes the possibility that any observed association is due to confounding.
- Clear temporal sequence - exposure clearly precedes outcome.
- Provides a strong basis for statistical inference.
- Enables blinding and therefore minimizes bias.
- Can measure disease incidence and multiple outcomes.

Weaknesses of a Randomised Controlled Trial

- Ethical constraints - for example, it is not always possible or ethical to manipulate exposure at random.
- Expensive and time consuming.
- Requires complex design and analysis if unit of allocation is not the individual.
- Inefficient for rare diseases or diseases with a delayed outcome.
- Generalisability - subjects in a RCT may be more willing to comply with the treatment regimen and therefore may not be representative of all individuals who might be given the treatment.

Developing a Questionnaire

Questionnaires are a commonly used tool in epidemiological studies. They may be used as the sole instrument for the collection of study data, such as in a cross-sectional design, or in combination with other instruments of data collection. The degree to which a questionnaire produces data that are relevant and valid to a study's goals and objectives will depend on how well the questionnaire is designed, how well questions are constructed, and how well the questionnaire is administered.

A valid questionnaire measures what it claims to measure. For example, a self-completed questionnaire that seeks to measure people's food intake may be invalid because it measures what they say they have eaten, not what they have actually eaten.

Basic Guidelines for Constructing a Valid Questionnaire

Careful consideration of a study's objectives and aims in the design of a questionnaire are essential if it is to yield responses that are both valid and reliable.

Types of Questions

Questionnaire items may be open or closed ended and be presented in various formats.

Closed questions are questions which limit the response to a specified list of possible answers. The use of closed questions offers a number of advantages to the researcher, including providing a set of standard responses that enable researchers to produce aggregated data quickly. However, the range of possible answers is set by the researchers not respondents, and therefore the richness of potential responses is lower. In addition, if a closed question fails to include all potential responses then important information relating to the overall study objectives may be omitted, leading to biased results. Where appropriate, closed questions should include an opened ended question for 'Other' and an option for 'Don't Know'. In contrast, open questions allow the respondent to answer freely. However, if opened ended questions are used, then the methods for analysing these responses should be considered during the design of the questionnaire.

Piloting

Piloting the questionnaire among a representative sample of the target population in the same way that it will be administered in the main study is essential and will help identify potential problems with the design or layout of the questionnaire. Piloting will:

- Help determine whether questions are ambiguous and allow questions to be rephrased.
- Check that instructions are clear and easy to follow.
- Test whether the questionnaire can be administered in a reasonable amount of time.

- Enable investigators to eliminate questions that do not produce usable data.
- Assess whether each question provides an adequate range of responses.
- Enable investigators to rephrase questions or replace existing scales where appropriate.
- Determine whether responses can be interpreted in terms of the objectives of the study.
- Determine whether the questionnaire is culturally acceptable to study participants.

Maximising Response Rates

- Notify participants in advance with a letter of introduction that outlines the purpose and importance of the study.
- Include clear instructions of how to complete the questionnaire.
- Clear and simple layout.
- Questions should be clear and concise and avoid the use of technical jargon and long, leading or negative questions.
- Inclusion of a stamped, addressed envelope if conducting a postal survey.
- Ensure anonymity where possible.
- Highlight the public health importance.
- Follow-up of non-responders by telephone or letter.
- Use of a researcher who is available to answer questions.
- Collection of questionnaires where feasible by the researcher.

Causation in Epidemiology: Association and Causation

A principal aim of epidemiology is to assess the cause of disease. However, since most epidemiological studies are by nature observational rather than experimental, a number of possible explanations for an observed association need to be considered before we can infer a cause-effect relationship exists. That is, the observed association may in fact be due to the effects of one or more of the following:

- Chance (random error)
- Bias (systematic error)
- Confounding

Therefore, an observed statistical association between a risk factor and a disease does not necessarily lead us to infer a causal relationship.

Conversely, the absence of an association does not necessarily imply the absence of a causal relationship.

The judgement as to whether an observed statistical association represents a cause-effect relationship between exposure and disease requires inferences far beyond the data from a single study and involves consideration of criteria that include the magnitude of the association, the consistency of findings from other studies and biologic credibility.

The Bradford-Hill criteria are widely used in epidemiology as providing a framework against which to assess whether an observed association is likely to be causal.

The Bradford-Hill Criteria (J Roy Soc Med 1965:58:295-300)

Strength of the Association: According to Hill, the stronger the association between a risk factor and outcome, the more likely the relationship is to be causal.

Consistency of Findings: Have the same findings must be observed among different populations, in different study designs and different times?

Specificity of the Association: There must be a one to one relationship between cause and outcome.

Temporal Sequence of Association: Exposure must precede outcome.

Biological Gradient: Change in disease rates should follow from corresponding changes in exposure (dose-response).

Biological Plausibility: Presence of a potential biological mechanism.

Coherence: Does the relationship agree with the current knowledge of the natural history/biology of the disease?

Experiment: Does the removal of the exposure alter the frequency of the outcome?

According to Rothman, while Hill did not propose these criteria as a checklist for evaluating whether a reported association might be interpreted as causal, they have been widely applied in this way. Rothman contends that the Bradford - Hill criteria fail to deliver on the hope of clearly distinguishing causal from non-causal relations.

For example, the first criterion 'strength of association' does not take into account that not every component cause will have a strong association with the disease that it produces and that strength of association depends on the prevalence of other factors.

In terms of the third criterion, 'specificity', which suggests that a relationship is more likely to be causal if the exposure is related to a single outcome, Rothman argues that this criterion is misleading as a cause may have many effects, for example smoking.

The fifth criterion, biological gradient, suggests that a causal association is increased if a biological gradient or dose-response curve can be demonstrated. However, such relationships may result from confounding or other biases. According to Rothman, the only criterion that is truly a causal criterion is 'temporality', that is, that the cause preceded the effect. Note that it may be difficult, however, to ascertain the time sequence for cause and effect.

The process of causal inference is complex, and arriving at a tentative inference of a causal or non-causal nature of an association is a subjective process. For a comprehensive discussion on causality refer to Rothman.

Role of Chance, Bias and Confounding in Epidemiological Studies

While the results of an epidemiological study may reflect the true effect of an exposure(s) on the development of the outcome under investigation, it should always be considered that the findings may in fact be due to an alternative explanation. Such alternative explanations may be due to the effects of chance (random error), bias or confounding, which may produce spurious results, leading us to conclude the existence of a valid statistical association when one does not exist, or alternatively the absence of an association when one is truly present.

Observational studies are particularly susceptible to the effects of chance, bias and confounding, and these need to be considered at both the design and analysis stage of an epidemiological study so that their effects can be minimized.

Confounding, Interaction and Effect Modification

Confounding involves the possibility that an observed association is due, totally or in part, to the effects of differences between the study groups (other than the exposure under investigation) that could affect their risk of developing the outcome being studied.

Confounding occurs when the effects of two associated exposures have not been separated, resulting in the interpretation that the effect is due to one variable rather than the other. The consequence of confounding is that the estimated association is not the same as the true effect.

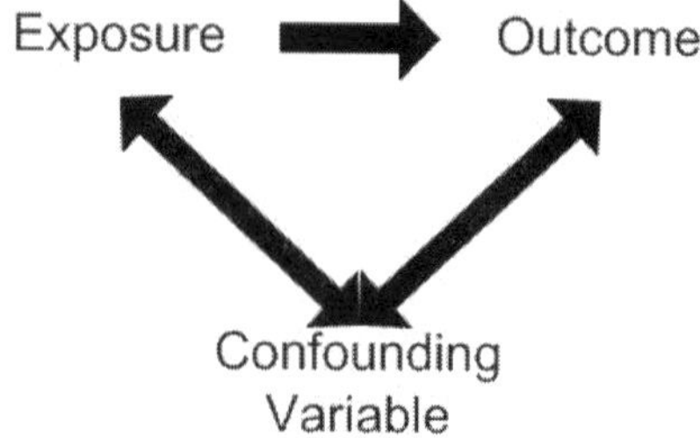

In Order for a Variable to be Considered as a Confounder

1. The variable must be independently associated with the outcome (i.e. be a risk factor).
2. The variable must be associated with the exposure under study in the source population.
3. It should not lie on the causal pathway between exposure and disease.

Examples of confounding

A study found alcohol consumption to be associated with the risk of Coronary Heart Disease. However, smoking may have confounded the association between alcohol and CHD. For example smoking is independently associated with CHD (is a risk factor) and is also associated with alcohol consumption (smokers tend to drink more than non-smokers).

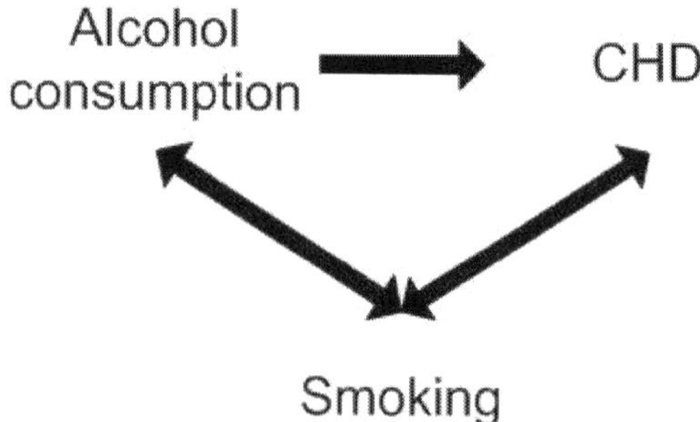

Figure: *Controlling for the potential confounding effect of smoking may in fact show no association between alcohol consumption and CHD.*

Effects of Confounding

Confounding factors, if not controlled for, cause bias in the estimate of the impact of the exposure being studied.

The effects of confounding can result in:

- An observed difference between study populations when no real difference exists.
- No observed difference between study populations when a true association does exist.

- An underestimate of an effect.
- An overestimate of an effect.

Residual Confounding

Residual confounding occurs when a confounder has not been adequately adjusted for in the analysis, for example by using too large age groups.

Bias

Bias may be defined as any systematic error in an epidemiological study that results in an incorrect estimate of the association between exposure and risk of disease.

- Bias results from systematic errors in the research methodology.
- Limited scope exists for the adjustment of most forms of bias at the analysis stage. As a result careful consideration and control of the ways in which bias may be introduced during the design and conduct of the study is essential in order to limit the effects on the validity of the study results.

Common Types of Bias in Epidemiological Studies

Information Bias: Information bias results from systematic differences in the way data on exposure or outcome are obtained from the various study groups. Types of information bias include:

Observer Bias

Observer bias occurs when there are systematic differences in the way information is collected for the groups being studied. Observer bias may occur as a result of the investigator's prior knowledge of the hypothesis under investigation or knowledge of an individual's exposure or disease status. Such information may result in differences in the way information is collected, measured or interpretation by the investigator for each of the study groups.

Minimizing Observer Bias

- Where possible, observers should be blinded to the exposure and disease status of the individual.
- Blind observers to the hypothesis under investigation.
- In a randomised controlled trial, blind investigators and participants to treatment and control group (double blind randomised controlled trial).
- Development of a protocol for the collection, measurement and interpretation of information.

- Use of standardized questionnaires.
- Training of interviewers.

Losses to Follow-up

Loss to follow-up is a particular problem associated with cohort studies. Bias may be introduced if the individuals lost to follow-up differ with respect to the exposure and outcome from those persons who remain in the study.

Recall Bias

In a case-control study, data on exposure are collected retrospectively. The quality of the data, therefore, is determined to a large extent by the patient's ability to accurately recall past exposure(s). Recall bias may occur when the information provided on exposure is different between the cases and controls. For example, an individual with the outcome under investigation (case) may report their exposure experience differently than an individual without the outcome (control) under investigation. That is, cases may tend to have a better recall on past exposures than controls. Recall bias may result in either an underestimate or overestimate of the association between exposure and outcome. Methods to minimize recall bias include: the collection of exposure data from work or medical records or to blind the study participants as to the hypothesis under investigation.

Selection Bias

Selection bias occurs when the two groups being compared differ systematically. That is, there are differences in the characteristics between those who are selected for a study and those who are not selected, and where those characteristics are related to either the exposure or outcome under investigation. While the results of an epidemiological study may reflect the true effect of an exposure(s) on the development of the outcome under investigation, it should always be considered that the findings may in fact be due to an alternative explanation. Such alternative explanations may be due to the effects of chance (random error), bias or confounding, which may produce spurious results, leading us to conclude the existence of a valid statistical association when one does not exist, or alternatively the absence of an association when one is truly present.

Observational studies are particularly susceptible to the effects of chance, bias and confounding, and these need to be considered at both the design and analysis stage of an epidemiological study so that their effects can be minimized.

Chapter 5

Social Epidemiology

Social epidemiology is defined as "The branch of epidemiology that studies the social distribution and social determinants of health," that is, "both specific features of, and pathways by which, societal conditions affect health." Social epidemiology may focus on individual-level measures, or on emergent social properties that have no correlation at the individual level; simultaneous analysis at both levels may be warranted. Use of such multilevel models (also known as hierarchical and mixed effects models) has grown in recent years, but as for all observational epidemiology, this approach suffers from theoretical and practical concerns.

Social epidemiology overlaps with fields in the social sciences, most notably medical anthropology, medical sociology, and medical geography. However, these latter fields often use health and disease in order to explain specifically social phenomenon (such as the growth of lay health advocacy movements), while social epidemiologists generally use social concepts in order to explain patterns of health in the population.

Genetic Epidemiology

Genetic epidemiology is the study of the role of genetic factors in determining health and disease in families and in populations, and the interplay of such genetic factors with environmental factors. In slightly more formal language, genetic epidemiology was defined by Morton as "a science which deals with the etiology, distribution, and control of disease in groups of relatives and with inherited causes of disease in populations". It is closely allied to both molecular epidemiology and statistical genetics, but these overlapping fields each have distinct emphases, societies and journals. Traditionally, the study of the role of genetics in disease progresses through the following study designs, each answering a slightly different question:

- Familial aggregation studies: Is there a genetic component to the disease, and what are the relative contributions of genes and environment?
- Segregation studies: What is the pattern of inheritance of the disease (e.g. dominant or recessive)?
- Linkage studies: On which part of which chromosome is the disease gene located?
- Association studies: Which allele of which gene is associated with the disease?

This traditional approach has proved highly successful in identifying monogenic disorders and locating the genes responsible.

More recently, the scope of genetic epidemiology has expanded to include common diseases for which many genes each make a smaller contribution (polygenic, multifactorial or multigenic disorders). This has developed rapidly in the first decade of the 21st century following completion of the Human Genome Project, as advances in genotyping technology and associated reductions in cost has made it feasible to conduct large-scale genome-wide association studies that genotype many thousands of single nucleotide polymorphisms in thousands of individuals. These have led to the discovery of many genetic polymorphisms that influence the risk of developing many common diseases.

Environmental Epidemiology

Environmental epidemiology is the branch of epidemiology concerned with the discovery of the environmental exposures that contribute to or protect against injuries, illnesses, developmental conditions, disabilities, and deaths; and identification of public health and health care actions to manage the risks associated with harmful exposures. Environmental epidemiology studies external factors that affect the incidence, prevalence, and geographic range of health conditions. These factors may be naturally occurring or may be introduced into environments where people live, work, and play. Environmental exposures are involuntary and thus generally exclude occupational exposures and voluntary exposures such as active smoking, medications, and diet.

Environmental exposures can be broadly categorized into those that are proximate (e.g., directly leading to a health condition), including chemicals, physical agents, and microbiological pathogens, and those that are more distal, such as social conditions, climate change, and other broad-scale environmental changes. Proximate exposures occur through air, food, water, and skin contact. Distal exposures cause adverse health conditions directly by altering proximate exposures, and indirectly through changes in ecosystems and other support systems for human health.

Environmental epidemiology research can inform risk assessments; development of standards and other risk management activities; and estimates of the co-benefits and co-harms of policies designed to reduce global environment change, including policies implemented in other sectors (e.g. food and water) that can affect human health.

Vulnerability is the summation of all risk and protective factors that ultimately determine whether an individual or subpopulation experiences adverse health outcomes when an exposure to an environmental agent occurs. Sensitivity is an individual's or subpopulation's increased responsiveness, primarily for biological reasons, to that exposure. Biological sensitivity may be related to developmental stage, pre-existing medical conditions, acquired factors, and genetic factors. Socioeconomic factors also play a critical role in altering vulnerability and sensitivity to environmentally mediated factors by increasing the likelihood of exposure to harmful agents, interacting with biological factors that mediate risk, and/or leading to differences in the ability to prepare for or cope with exposures or early phases of illness. Populations living in certain regions may be at increased risk due to location and the environmental characteristics of a region.

Epidemic Model

An epidemic model is a simplified means of describing the transmission of communicable disease through individuals. The outbreak and spread of disease has been questioned and studied for many years. The ability to make predictions about diseases could enable scientists to evaluate inoculation or isolation plans and may have a significant effect on the mortality rate of a particular epidemic. The modelling of infectious diseases is a tool which has been used to study the mechanisms by which diseases spread, to predict the future course of an outbreak and to evaluate strategies to control an epidemic (Daley & Gani, 2005).

The first scientist who systematically tried to quantify causes of death was John Graunt in his book *Natural and Political Observations made upon the Bills of Mortality*, in 1662. The bills he studied were listings of numbers and causes of deaths published weekly. Graunt's analysis of causes of death is considered the beginning of the "theory of competing risks" which according to Daley and Gani (Daley & Gani, 2005, p. 2) is "a theory that is now well established among modern epidemiologists".

The earliest account of mathematical modelling of spread of disease was carried out in 1766 by Daniel Bernoulli. Trained as a physician, Bernoulli created a mathematical model to defend the practice of inoculating against smallpox (Hethcote, 2000). The calculations from this model showed that universal inoculation against smallpox would increase the life expectancy from 26 years 7 months to 29 years 9 months (Bernoulli & Blower, 2004).

Daniel Bernoulli's work, of course, preceded our modern understanding of germ theory, and it was not until the research of Ronald Ross into the spread of malaria, that modern theoretical epidemiology began. This was soon followed by the acclaimed work of A. G. McKendrick and W. O. Kermack, whose paper *A Contribution to the Mathematical Theory of Epidemics* was published in 1927. A simple deterministic (compartmental) model was formulated in this paper. The model was successful in predicting the behaviour of outbreaks very similar to that observed in many recorded epidemics (Brauer & Castillo-Chavez, 2001).

Types of Epidemic Models

Stochastic

"Stochastic" means being or having a random variable. A stochastic model is a tool for estimating probability distributions of potential outcomes by allowing for random variation in one or more inputs over time. Stochastic models depend on the chance variations in risk of exposure, disease and other illness dynamics. They are used when these fluctuations are important, as in small populations (Trottier & Philippe, 2001).

Deterministic

When dealing with large populations, as in the case of tuberculosis, deterministic or compartmental mathematical models are used. In the deterministic model, individuals in the population are assigned to different subgroups or compartments, each representing a specific stage of the epidemic. Letters such as M, S, E, I, and R are often used to represent different stages. The transition rates from one class to another are mathematically expressed as derivatives, hence the model is formulated using differential equations. While building such models, it must be assumed that the population size in a compartment is differentiable with respect to time and that the epidemic process is deterministic. In other words, the changes in population of a compartment can be calculated using only the history used to develop the model (Brauer & Castillo-Chavez, 2001).

Another approach is through discrete analysis on a lattice (such as a two-dimensional square grid), where the updating is done through asynchronous single-site updates (Kinetic Monte Carlo) or synchronous updating (Cellular Automata). The lattice approach enables inhomogeneities and clustering to be taken into account. Lattice systems are usually studied through computer simulation, and are discussed in the Wikipedia page Epidemic models on lattices.

Terminology

The following is a summary of the notation used in this and the next sections.

- M : Passively immune infants
- S : Susceptibles
- E : Exposed individuals in the latent period
- I : Infectives
- R : Removed with immunity
- β : Contact rate
- μ : Average death rate
- B : Average birth rate
- $1/\varepsilon$: Average latent period
- $1/\gamma$: Average infectious period
- R_0 : Basic reproduction number
- N : Total population
- f : Average loss of immunity rate of recovered individuals
- δ : Average temporary immunity period

Deterministic Compartmental Models

The SIR Model

In 1927, W. O. Kermack and A. G. McKendrick created a model in which they considered a fixed population with only three compartments: susceptible, $S(t)$; infected, $I(t)$; and removed, $R(t)$. The compartments used for this model consist of three classes:

- $S(t)$ is used to represent the number of individuals not yet infected with the disease at time t, or those susceptible to the disease.
- $I(t)$ denotes the number of individuals who have been infected with the disease and are capable of spreading the disease to those in the susceptible category.
- $R(t)$ is the compartment used for those individuals who have been infected and then removed from the disease, either due to immunization or due to death. Those in this category are not able to be infected again or to transmit the infection to others.

The flow of this model may be considered as follows:

$$\mathcal{S} \to \mathcal{I} \to \mathcal{R}$$

Using a fixed population, $N = S(t) + I(t) + R(t)$, Kermack and McKendrick derived the following equations:

$$\frac{dS}{dt} = -\frac{\beta SI}{N}$$

$$\frac{dI}{dt} = \frac{\beta SI}{N} - \gamma$$

$$\frac{dR}{dt} = \gamma I$$

Several assumptions were made in the formulation of these equations: First, an individual in the population must be considered as having an equal probability as every other individual of contracting the disease with a rate of β, which is considered the contact or infection rate of the disease. Therefore, an infected individual makes contact and is able to transmit the disease with βN others per unit time and the fraction of contacts by an infected with a susceptible is S / N. The number of new infections in unit time per infective then is $\beta N(S / N)$, giving the rate of new infections (or those leaving the susceptible category) as $\beta N(S / N)I = \beta SI$ (Brauer & Castillo-Chavez, 2001). For the second and third equations, consider the population leaving the susceptible class as equal to the number entering the infected class. However, a number equal to the fraction (γ which represents the mean recovery/death rate, or $1 / \gamma$ the mean infective period) of infectives are leaving this class per unit time to enter the removed class. These processes which occur simultaneously are referred to as the Law of Mass Action, a widely accepted idea that the rate of contact between two groups in a population is proportional to the size of each of the groups concerned (Daley & Gani, 2005). Finally, it is assumed that the rate of infection and recovery is much faster than the time scale of births and deaths and therefore, these factors are ignored in this model.

The SIR Model with Births and Deaths

Using the case of measles, for example, there is an arrival of new susceptible individuals into the population. For this type of situation births and deaths must be included in the model. The following differential equations represent this model, assuming a death rate μ and birth rate equal to the death rate:

$$\frac{dS}{dt} = -\frac{\beta SI}{N} + \mu(N - S)$$

$$\frac{dI}{dt} = \frac{\beta SI}{N} - \gamma I - \mu I$$

$$\frac{dR}{dt} = \gamma I - \mu R$$

The SIS Model with Births and Deaths

The SIS model can be easily derived from the SIR model by simply considering that the individuals recover with no immunity to the disease, that is, individuals are immediately susceptible once they have recovered.

$$\mathcal{S} \rightarrow \mathcal{I} \rightarrow \mathcal{S}$$

Removing the equation representing the recovered population from the SIR model and adding those removed from the infected population into the susceptible population gives the following differential equations:

$$\frac{dS}{dt} = -\frac{\beta SI}{N} + \mu(N - S) + \gamma I$$

$$\frac{dI}{dt} = \frac{\beta SI}{N} - \gamma I - \mu I$$

The SIRS Model

This model is simply an extension of the SIR model as we will see from its construction.

$$\mathcal{S} \rightarrow \mathcal{I} \rightarrow \mathcal{R} \rightarrow \mathcal{S}$$

The only difference is that it allows members of the recovered class to be free of infection and rejoin the susceptible class.

$$\frac{dS}{dt} = -\frac{\beta SI}{N} + \mu(N - S) + fR$$

$$\frac{dI}{dt} = \frac{\beta SI}{N} - \gamma I - \mu I$$

$$\frac{dR}{dt} = \gamma I - \mu R - fR$$

Models with More Compartments

The SEIS Model

The SEIS model takes into consideration the exposed or latent period of the disease, giving an additional compartment, E(t).

$$\mathcal{S} \rightarrow \mathcal{E} \rightarrow \mathcal{I} \rightarrow \mathcal{S}$$

In this model an infection does not leave any immunity thus individuals that have recovered return to being susceptible again, moving back into the $S(t)$ compartment. The following differential equations describe this model:

$$\tfrac{dS}{dT} = B - \beta SI - \mu S + \gamma I$$

$$\tfrac{dE}{dT} = \beta SI - (\epsilon + \mu)E$$

$$\tfrac{dI}{dT} = \varepsilon E - (\gamma + \mu)I$$

The SEIR Model

The SIR model discussed above takes into account only those diseases which cause an individual to be able to infect others immediately upon their infection. Many diseases have what is termed a latent or exposed phase, during which the individual is said to be infected but not infectious.

$$\mathcal{S} \rightarrow \mathcal{E} \rightarrow \mathcal{I} \rightarrow \mathcal{R}$$

In this model the host population (N) is broken into four compartments: susceptible, exposed, infectious, and recovered, with the numbers of individuals in a compartment, or their densities denoted respectively by $S(t)$, $E(t)$, $I(t)$, $R(t)$, that is $N = S(t) + E(t) + I(t) + R(t)$

$$\tfrac{dS}{dT} = B - \beta SI - \mu S$$

$$\tfrac{dE}{dT} = \beta SI - (\varepsilon + \mu)E$$

$$\tfrac{dI}{dT} = \varepsilon E - (\gamma + \mu)I$$

$$\tfrac{dR}{dT} = \gamma I - \mu R$$

The MSIR Model

There are several diseases where an individual is born with a passive immunity from its mother.

$$\mathcal{M} \rightarrow \mathcal{S} \rightarrow \mathcal{I} \rightarrow \mathcal{R}$$

To indicate this mathematically, an additional compartment is added, M(t), which results in the following differential equations:

$$\frac{dM}{dT} = B - \delta M - \mu M$$

$$\frac{dS}{dT} = \delta M - \beta SI - \mu S$$

$$\frac{dI}{dT} = \beta SI - \gamma I - \mu I$$

$$\frac{dR}{dT} = \gamma I - \mu R$$

The MSEIR Model

For the case of a disease, with the factors of passive immunity, and a latency period there is the MSEIR model.

$$\mathcal{M} \rightarrow \mathcal{S} \rightarrow \mathcal{E} \rightarrow \mathcal{I} \rightarrow \mathcal{R}$$

$$\frac{dM}{dT} = B - \delta M - \mu M$$

$$\frac{dS}{dT} = \delta M - \beta SI - \mu S$$

$$\frac{dE}{dT} = \beta SI - (\varepsilon + \mu)E$$

$$\frac{dI}{dT} = \varepsilon E - (\gamma + \mu)I$$

$$\frac{dR}{dT} = \gamma I - \mu R$$

The MSEIRS Model

An MSEIRS model is similar to the MSEIR, but the immunity in the R class would be temporary, so that individuals would regain their susceptibility when the temporary immunity ended.

$$\mathcal{M} \rightarrow \mathcal{S} \rightarrow \mathcal{E} \rightarrow \mathcal{I} \rightarrow \mathcal{R} \rightarrow \mathcal{S}$$

Reproduction Number

There is a threshold quantity which determines whether an epidemic occurs or the disease simply dies out. This quantity is called the basic reproduction number, denoted by R_0, which can be defined as the number of secondary infections caused by a single infective introduced into a population made up entirely of susceptible individuals ($S(0) \approx N$) over the course of the infection of this single infective. This infective individual makes βN contacts per unit time producing new infections with a mean infectious period of $1/\gamma$.

Therefore, the basic reproduction number is

$$R_0 = (\beta N)/\gamma.$$

This value quantifies the transmission potential of a disease. If the basic reproduction number falls below one ($R_0 < 1$), i.e. the infective may not pass the infection on during the infectious period, the infection dies out. If $R_0 > 1$ there is an epidemic in the population. In cases where $R_0 = 1$, the disease becomes endemic, meaning the disease remains in the population at a consistent rate, as one infected individual transmits the disease to one susceptible (Trottier & Philippe, 2001).

In cases of diseases with varying latent periods, the basic reproduction number can be calculated as the sum of the reproduction number for each transition time into the disease. An example of this is tuberculosis. Blower et al. (1995) calculated from a simple model of TB the following reproduction number:

$$R_0 = R_0^{FAST} + R_0^{SLOW}$$

In their model, it is assumed that the infected individuals can develop active TB by either direct progression (the disease develops immediately after infection) considered above as FAST tuberculosis or endogenous reactivation (the disease develops years after the infection) considered above as SLOW tuberculosis.

Other Considerations Within Compartmental Epidemic Models

Vertical Transmission

In the case of some diseases such as AIDS and Hepatitis B, it is possible for the offspring of infected parents to be born infected. This transmission of the disease down from the mother is called Vertical Transmission. The influx of additional members into the infected category can be considered within the model by including a fraction of the newborn members in the infected compartment (Brauer & Castillo-Chavez, 2001).

Vector transmission

Diseases transmitted from human to human indirectly, i.e. malaria spread by way of mosquitoes, are transmitted through a vector. In these cases, the infection transfers from human to insect and an epidemic model must include both species, generally requiring many more compartments than a model for direct transmission.

Others

Other occurrences (taken from *Mathematical Models in Population Biology and Epidemiology* by Fred Brauer and Carlos Castillo-Chavez

) which may need to be considered when modelling an epidemic include things such as the following:

- Nonhomogeneous mixing
- Age-structured populations
- Variable infectivity
- Distributions that are spatially non-uniform
- Diseases caused by macroparasites
- Acquired immunity through vaccinations

Mathematical Modelling of Infectious Disease

Mathematical models can project how infectious diseases progress to show the likely outcome of an epidemic and help inform public health interventions. Models use some basic assumptions and mathematics to find parameters for various infectious diseases and use those parameters to calculate the effects of possible interventions, like mass vaccination programmes.

History

Early pioneers in infectious disease modelling were William Hamer and Ronald Ross, who in the early twentieth century applied the law of mass action to explain epidemic behaviour. Lowell Reed and Wade Hampton Frost developed the Reed–Frost epidemic model to describe the relationship between susceptible, infected and immune individuals in a population.

Concepts

R_0, the basic reproduction number

The average number of other individuals each infected individual will infect in a population that has no immunity to the disease.

S: The proportion of the population who are susceptible to the disease (neither immune nor infected).

A: The average age at which the disease is contracted in a given population.

L: The average life expectancy in a given population.

Assumptions

Models are only as good as the assumptions on which they are based. If a model makes predictions which are out of line with observed results and the mathematics is correct, the initial assumptions must change to make the model useful.

- Rectangular and stationary age distribution, i.e., everybody in the population lives to age L and then dies, and for each age (up to L) there is the same number of people in the population. This is often well-justified for developed countries where there is a low infant mortality and much of the population lives to the life expectancy.
- Homogeneous mixing of the population, i.e., individuals of the population under scrutiny assort and make contact at random and do not mix mostly in a smaller subgroup. This assumption is rarely justified because social structure is widespread, for example, most people in London, only make contact with other Londoners, and within London then there will be smaller subgroups such as the Turkish community or teenagers (just to give two examples) who will mix with each other more than people outside their group. However, homogeneous mixing is a standard assumption to make the mathematics tractable.

Endemic Steady State

An infectious disease is said to be endemic when it can be sustained in a population without the need for external inputs. This means that, on average, each infected person is infecting *exactly* one other person (any more and the number of people infected will grow exponentially and there will be an epidemic, any less and the disease will die out). In mathematical terms, that is:

$$R_0 = 1.$$

The basic reproduction number (R_0) of the disease, assuming everyone is susceptible, multiplied by the proportion of the population that is actually susceptible (S) must be one (since those who are not susceptible do not feature in our calculations as they cannot contract the disease). Notice that this relation means that for a disease to be in the endemic steady state, the higher the basic reproduction number, the lower the proportion of the population susceptible must be, and vice versa.

Assume the rectangular stationary age distribution and let also the ages of infection have the same distribution for each birth year. Let the average age of infection be A, for instance when individuals younger than A are susceptible and those older than A are immune (or infectious). Then it can be shown by an easy argument that the proportion of the population that is susceptible is given by:

$$S = \frac{A}{L}.$$

But the mathematical definition of the endemic steady state can be rearranged to give:

$$S = \frac{1}{R_0}.$$

Therefore, since things equal to the same thing are equal to each other:

$$\frac{1}{R_0} = \frac{A}{L} \Rightarrow R_0 = \frac{L}{A}.$$

This provides a simple way to estimate the parameter R_0 using easily available data. For a population with an exponential age distribution,

$$R_0 = 1 + \frac{L}{A}.$$

This allows for the basic reproduction number of a disease given A and L in either type of population distribution.

Infectious Disease Dynamics

Mathematical models need to integrate the increasing volume of data being generated on host-pathogen interactions. Many theoretical studies of the population dynamics, structure and evolution of infectious diseases of plants and animals, including humans, are concerned with this problem.

Research topics include:

- transmission, spread and control of infection
- epidemiological networks
- spatial epidemiology
- persistence of pathogens within hosts
- intra-host dynamics
- immuno-epidemiology
- virulence
- Strain (biology) structure and interactions
- antigenic shift
- phylodynamics
- pathogen population genetics
- evolution and spread of resistance
- role of host genetic factors

- statistical and mathematical tools and innovations
- role and identification of infection reservoirs

Mathematics of Mass Vaccination

If the proportion of the population that is immune exceeds the herd immunity level for the disease, then the disease can no longer persist in the population. Thus, if this level can be exceeded by vaccination, the disease can be eliminated. An example of this being successfully achieved worldwide is the global smallpox eradication, with the last wild case in 1977. The WHO is carrying out a similar vaccination campaign to eradicate polio.

The herd immunity level will be denoted q. Recall that, for a stable state:

$$R_0 \cdot S = 1.$$

S will be $(1 - q)$, since q is the proportion of the population that is immune and $q + S$ must equal one (since in this simplified model, everyone is either susceptible or immune). Then:

$$R_0 \cdot (1-q) = 1,$$

$$1 - q = \frac{1}{R_0},$$

$$q = 1 - \frac{1}{R_0}.$$

Remember that this is the threshold level. If the proportion of immune individuals *exceeds* this level due to a mass vaccination programme, the disease will die out.

We have just calculated the critical immunisation threshold (denoted q_c). It is the minimum proportion of the population that must be immunised at birth (or close to birth) in order for the infection to die out in the population.

$$q_c = 1 - \frac{1}{R_0}$$

When Mass Vaccination Cannot Exceed the Herd Immunity

If the vaccine used is insufficiently effective or the required coverage cannot be reached (for example due to popular resistance), the programme may fail to exceed q_c. Such a programme can, however, disturb the balance of the infection without eliminating it, often causing unforeseen problems.

Suppose that a proportion of the population q (where $q < q_c$) is immunised at birth against an infection with $R_0 > 1$. The vaccination programme changes R_0 to R_q where

$$R_q = R_0(1-q)$$

This change occurs simply because there are now fewer susceptibles in the population who can be infected. R_q is simply R_0 minus those that would normally be infected but that cannot be now since they are immune. As a consequence of this lower basic reproduction number, the average age of infection A will also change to some new value A_q in those who have been left unvaccinated.

Recall the relation that linked R_0, A and L. Assuming that life expectancy has not changed, now:

$$R_q = \frac{L}{A_q},$$

$$A_q = \frac{L}{R_q} = \frac{L}{R_0(1-q)}.$$

But $R_0 = L/A$ so:

$$A_q = \frac{L}{(L/A)(1-q)} = \frac{AL}{L(1-q)} = \frac{A}{1-q}.$$

Thus the vaccination programme will raise the average age of infection, another mathematical justification for a result that might have been intuitively obvious. Unvaccinated individuals now experience a reduced force of infection due to the presence of the vaccinated group.

However, it is important to consider this effect when vaccinating against diseases that are more severe in older people. A vaccination programme against such a disease that does not exceed q_c may cause more deaths and complications than there were before the programme was brought into force as individuals will be catching the disease later in life. These unforeseen outcomes of a vaccination programme are called perverse effects.

When Mass Vaccination Exceeds the Herd Immunity

If a vaccination programme causes the proportion of immune individuals in a population to exceed the critical threshold for a significant length of time, transmission of the infectious disease in that population will stop. This is known as elimination of the infection and is different from eradication.

Elimination: Interruption of endemic transmission of an infectious disease, which occurs if each infected individual infects less than one other, is achieved by maintaining vaccination coverage to keep the proportion of immune individuals above the critical immunisation threshold.

Eradication: Reduction of infective organisms in the wild worldwide to zero. So far, this has only been achieved for smallpox and rinderpest. To get to eradication, elimination in all world regions must be achieved.

Compartmental Models in Epidemiology

The establishment and spread of infectious diseases is a complex phenomenon with many interacting factors, e.g., the environment with which the pathogen and hosts are situated in, the population(s) it is exposed to, and the intra- and inter-dynamics of the population it is exposed to. The role of mathematical epidemiology is to model the establishment and spread of pathogens. A predominant method of doing so, is to use the notion of abstracting the population into *compartments* under certain assumptions, which represent their health status with respect to the pathogen in the system. One of the cornerstone works to achieve success in this method was done by Kermack and McKendrick in the early 1900s.

These models are known as compartmental models in epidemiology, and serve as a base mathematical framework for understanding the complex dynamics of these systems, which hope to model the main characteristics of the system. These compartments, in the simplest case, can stratify the population into two health states: susceptible to the infection of the pathogen (often denoted by S); and infected by the pathogen (given the symbol I). The way that these compartments interact is often based upon phenomenological assumptions, and the model is built up from there. These models are usually investigated through ordinary differential equations (which are deterministic), but can also be viewed in more realistic stochastic framework (for example, the Gillespie model). To push these basic models to further realism, other compartments are often included, most notably the recovered/removed/immune compartment (denoted R).

Once one is able to model an infectious pathogen with compartmental models, one can predict the various properties of the pathogen spread, for example the prevalence (total number of infected from the epidemic) and the duration of the epidemic. Also, one can understand how different situations may affect the outcome of the epidemic, e.g., what is the best technique for issuing a limited number of vaccines in a given population?

The SIR Model

The SIR model labels these three compartments S = number susceptible, I =number infectious, and R =number recovered (immune). This is a good and simple model for many infectious diseases including measles, mumps and rubella.

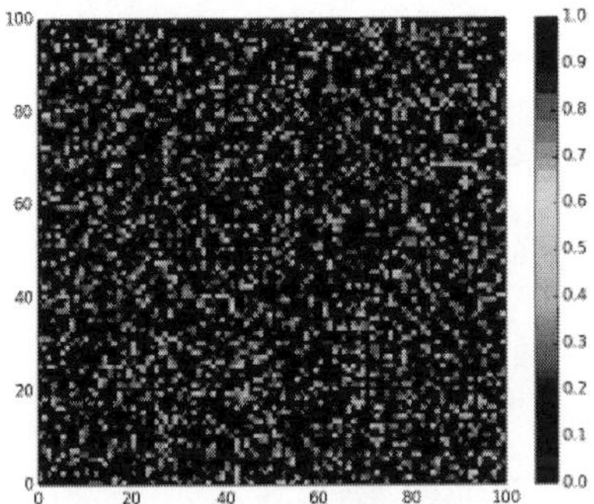

Figure: *SIR model simulated using python. N=1 Recovered, N<1 Susceptible, N>0.5 Infected*

The letters also represent the number of people in each compartment at a particular time. To indicate that the numbers might vary over time (even if the total population size remains constant), we make the precise numbers a function of *t* (time): S(*t*), I(*t*) and R(*t*). For a specific disease in a specific population, these functions may be worked out in order to predict possible outbreaks and bring them under control.

The SIR Model is Dynamic in Three Senses

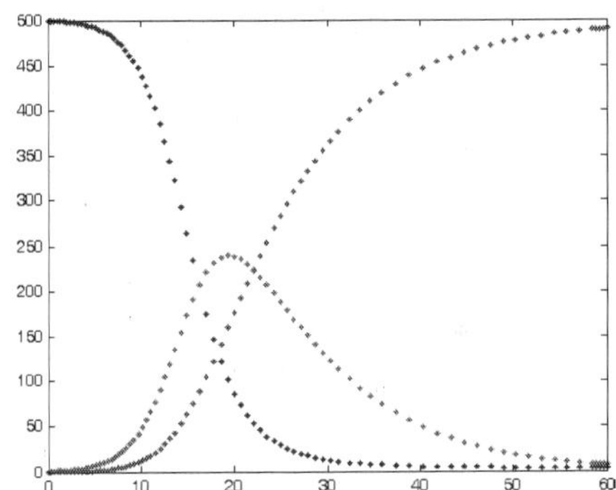

Figure: *Blue=Susceptible, Green=Infected, and Red=Recovered*

As implied by the variable function of *t*, the model is dynamic in that the numbers in each compartment may fluctuate over time. The importance of this dynamic aspect is most obvious in an endemic disease with a short infectious period, such as measles in the UK prior to the introduction of a vaccine in 1968. Such diseases tend to occur in cycles of outbreaks due to the variation in number of susceptibles (S(*t*)) over time. During an epidemic, the number of susceptible individuals falls rapidly as more of them are infected and thus enter the infectious and removed compartments. The disease cannot break out again until the number of susceptibles has built back up as a result of offspring being born into the susceptible compartment.

Each member of the population typically progresses from susceptible to infectious to removed. This can be shown as a flow diagram in which the boxes represent the different compartments and the arrows the transition between compartments.

Transition Rates

For the full specification of the model, the arrows should be labelled with the transition rates between compartments. Between S and I, the transition rate is β I, where β is the contact rate, which takes into account the probability of getting the disease in a contact between a susceptible and an infectious subject.

Between I and R, the transition rate is ν (simply the rate of recovery or death). If the duration of the infection is denoted D, then $\nu = 1/D$, since an individual experiences one recovery in D units of time.

It is assumed that the permanence of each single subject in the epidemic states is a random variable with exponential distribution. More complex and realistic distributions (such as Erlang distribution) can be equally used with few modifications.

Bio-mathematical Deterministic Treatment of the SIR Model

The SIR Model Without Vital Dynamics

The dynamics of an epidemic, for example the flu, are often much faster than the dynamics of birth and death, therefore, birth and death are often omitted in simple compartmental models. The SIR system without so-called vital dynamics (birth and death, sometimes called demography) described above can be expressed by the following set of ordinary differential equations:

$$\frac{dS}{dt} = -\frac{\beta IS}{N},$$

$$\frac{dI}{dt} = \frac{\beta IS}{N} - \gamma I,$$

$$\frac{dR}{dt} = \gamma I .$$

This model was for the first time proposed by O. Kermack and Anderson Gray McKendrick as a special case of what we now call Kermack-McKendrick theory, and followed work McKendrick had done with the Ronald Ross. This system is non-linear, and does not admit a generic analytic solution. Nevertheless, significant results can be derived analytically. Firstly note that from:

$$\frac{dS}{dt} + \frac{dI}{dt} + \frac{dR}{dt} = 0 ,$$

it follows that:

$$S(t) + I(t) + R(t) = \text{Constant} = N ,$$

expressing in mathematical terms the constancy of population N. Note that the above relationship implies that one need only study the equation for two of the three variables.

Secondly, we note that the dynamics of the infectious class depends on the following ratio:

$$R_0 = N\frac{\beta}{\gamma} ,$$

the so-called basic reproduction number (also called basic reproduction ratio). This ratio is derived as the expected number of new infections (these new infections are sometimes called secondary infections) from a single infection in a population where all subjects are susceptible. This idea can probably be more readily seen if we say that the typical time between contacts is $T_c = \beta^{-1}$, and the typical time until recovery is $T_r = \gamma^{-1}$. From here it follows that, on average, the number of contacts by an infected individual with others *before* the infected has recovered is: T_r / T_c.

By dividing the first differential equation by the third, separating the variables and integrating we get

$$S(t) = S(0)e^{-R_0 (R(t)-R(0))} ,$$

(where S(0) and R(0) are the initial numbers of, respectively, susceptible and removed subjects). Thus, in the limit $t \to +\infty$, the proportion of recovered individuals obeys the transcendental equation

$$R_\infty = 1 - S(0)e^{-R_0 (R_\infty - R(0))} .$$

This equation shows that at the end of an epidemic, unless S(0)=0, not all individuals of the population have recovered, so some must remain susceptible. This means that the end of an epidemic is caused by the decline in the number of infected individuals rather than an absolute lack of susceptible subjects. The role of the basic reproduction number is extremely important.

In fact, upon rewriting the equation for infectious individuals as follows:

$$\frac{dI}{dt} = (R_0 S / N - 1)\gamma I ,$$

it yields that if:

$$R_0 > \frac{N}{S(0)},$$

then:

$$\frac{dI}{dt}(0) > 0,$$

i.e., there will be a proper epidemic outbreak with an increase of the number of the infectious (which can reach a considerable fraction of the population). On the contrary, if

$$R_0 < \frac{N}{S(0)},$$

then

$$\frac{dI}{dt}(0) < 0,$$

i.e., independently from the initial size of the susceptible population the disease can never cause a proper epidemic outbreak. As a consequence, it is clear that the basic reproduction number is extremely important.

The Force of Infection

Note that in the above model the function:

$$F = \beta I,$$

models the transition rate from the compartment of susceptible individuals to the compartment of infectious individuals, so that it is called the force of infection. However, for large classes of communicable diseases it is more realistic to consider a force of infection that does not depend on the absolute number of infectious subjects, but on their fraction (with respect to the total constant population N):

$$F = \beta \frac{I}{N}.$$

Capasso and, afterwards, other authors have proposed nonlinear forces of infection to model more realistically the contagion process.

The SIR Model with Vital Dynamics and Constant Population

Considering a population characterized by a death rate μ and birth rate equal to the death rate, and where a communicable disease is spreading. The model is:

$$\frac{dS}{dt} = \mu N - \mu S - \beta \frac{I}{N} S$$

$$\frac{dI}{dt} = \beta \frac{I}{N} S - (\gamma + \mu) I$$

$$\frac{dR}{dt} = \gamma I - \mu R$$

for which it holds:

$$S + I + R = N.$$

Also in this case we may define a basic reproduction number :

$$R_0 = \frac{\beta}{\mu + \gamma},$$

which has threshold properties. In fact, independently from biologically meaningful initial values:

$$\left(S(0), I(0), R(0)\right) \in \left\{(S, I, R) \in [0, N]^3 : S + I + R = N\right\}$$

one can show that:

$$R_0 \leq 1 \Rightarrow \lim_{t \to +\infty} \left(S(t), I(t), R(t)\right) = \text{DFE} = \left(N, 0, 0\right)$$

$$R_0 > 1, I(0) > 0 \Rightarrow \lim_{t \to +\infty} \left(S(t), I(t), R(t)\right) = \text{EE} = \left(\frac{N}{R_0}, \frac{\mu}{\beta}(R_0 - 1) N, \frac{\gamma}{\beta}(R_0 - 1) N\right).$$

The point DFE is called the disease free equilibrium, whereas the point EE is called the Endemic Equilibrium. Since, with heuristic arguments, one may show that R_0 may be read as the average number of infections caused by a single infectious subject in a wholly susceptible population, the above relationship biologically means that if this number is less or equal than one the disease get extinct, whereas if this number is greater than one the disease will remain permanently endemic in the population.

Variable Contact Rates and Pluriannual or Chaotic Epidemics

It is well known that the probability of getting a disease is not constant in the time. Some diseases are seasonal, such as the common cold viruses, which are more prevalent during winter. With childhood diseases, such as measles, mumps, and rubella, there is a strong correlation with the school calendar, so that during the school holidays the probability of getting such a disease dramatically decreases.

As a consequence, for many classes of diseases one should consider a force of infection with periodically ('seasonal') varying contact rate

$$F = \beta(t)\frac{I}{N}, \beta(t+T) = \beta(t)$$

with period T equal to one year.

Thus, our model becomes

$$\frac{dS}{dt} = \mu N - \mu S - \beta(t)\frac{I}{N}S$$

$$\frac{dI}{dt} = \beta(t)\frac{I}{N}S - (\gamma + \mu)I$$

(the dynamics of recovered easily follows from $R = N - S - I$), i.e. a nonlinear set of differential equations with periodically varying parameters. It is well known that this class of dynamical systems may undergo very interesting and complex phenomena of nonlinear parametric resonance. It is easy to see that if:

$$\frac{1}{T}\int_0^T \frac{\beta(t)}{\mu + \gamma}dt < 1 \Rightarrow \lim_{t \to +\infty}\left(S(t), I(t)\right) = DFE = \left(N, 0\right),$$

whereas if the integral is greater than one the disease will not die out and there may be such resonances. For example, considering the periodically varying contact rate as the 'input' of the system one has that the output is a periodic function whose period is a multiple of the period of the input. This allowed to give a contribution to explain the poly-annual (typically biennial) epidemic outbreaks of some infectious diseases as interplay between the period of the contact rate oscillations and the pseudo-period of the damped oscillations near the endemic equilibrium. Remarkably, in some cases the behaviour may also be quasi-periodic or even chaotic.

The SIS Model

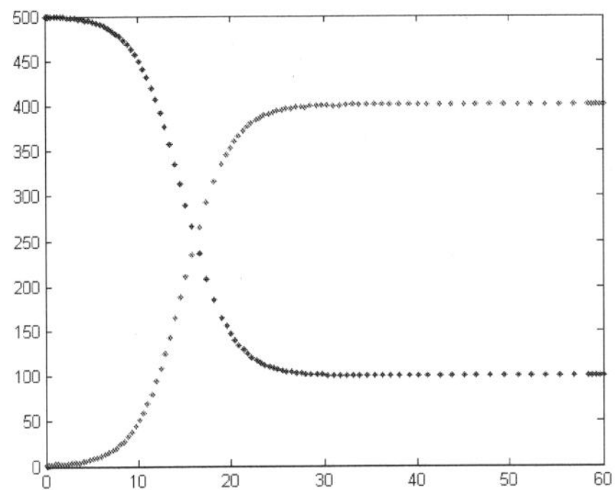

***Figure:** Susceptibles and infected get equilibrated.*

Some infections, for example those from the common cold and influenza, do not confer any long lasting immunity. Such infections do not give immunization upon recovery from infection, and individuals become susceptible again.

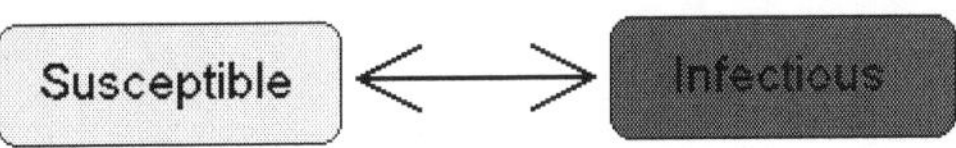

We have the model:

$$\frac{dS}{dt} = -\frac{\beta SI}{N} + \gamma I$$

$$\frac{dI}{dt} = \frac{\beta SI}{N} - \gamma I$$

Note that denoting with N the total population it holds that: $\frac{dS}{dt} + \frac{dI}{dt} = 0 \Rightarrow S(t) + I(t) = N$ it follows that:

$$\frac{dI}{dt} = (\beta N - \gamma)I - \beta I^2$$

i.e. the dynamics of infectious is ruled by a logistic equation, so that $\forall I(0) > 0$:

$$\frac{\beta N}{\gamma} \leq 1 \Rightarrow \lim_{t \to +\infty} I(t) = 0$$

$$\frac{\beta N}{\gamma} > 1 \Rightarrow \lim_{t \to +\infty} I(t) = \frac{\beta N - \gamma}{\beta}$$

Fortunately, it is possible to find an analytical solution to this model (by making a transformation of variables: $I = y^{-1}$ and substituting this into the mean-field equations), such that the basic reproduction rate is greater than unity. The solution is given as

$$I(t) = \frac{I_\infty}{1 + Ve^{-\chi(t-t_0)}}$$

where $I_\infty = \chi N / \beta$ is the endemic infected population, $\chi = \beta - \gamma$, and $V = I_\infty / I_0 - 1$. As the system is assumed to be closed, the susceptible population is then $S(t) = N - I(t)$.

Elaborations on the Basic SIR Model

The MSIR Model

For many infections, including measles, babies are not born into the susceptible compartment but are immune to the disease for the first few months of life due to protection from maternal antibodies (passed across the placenta and additionally through colostrum). This added detail can be shown by including an M class (for maternally derived immunity) at the beginning of the model.

Carrier State

Some people who have had an infectious disease such as tuberculosis never completely recover and continue to carry the infection, whilst not suffering the disease themselves. They may then move back into the infectious compartment and suffer symptoms (as in tuberculosis) or they may continue to infect others in their carrier state, while not suffering symptoms.

The most famous example of this is probably Mary Mallon, who infected 22 people with typhoid fever. The carrier compartment is labelled C.

The SEIR Model

For many important infections there is a significant incubation period during which the individual has been infected but is not yet infectious themselves. During this period the individual is in compartment E (for exposed).

Assuming that the incubation period is a random variable with exponential distribution with parameter a (i.e. the average incubation period is a^{-1}), and also assuming the presence of vital dynamics with birth rate equal to death rate, we have the model:

$$\frac{dS}{dt} = \mu N - \mu S - \beta \frac{I}{N} S$$

$$\frac{dE}{dt} = \beta \frac{I}{N} S - (\mu + a)E$$

$$\frac{dI}{dt} = aE - (\gamma + \mu)I$$

$$\frac{dR}{dt} = \gamma I - \mu R.$$

Of course, we have that $S + E + I + R = N$.

For this model, the basic reproduction number is:

$$R_0 = \frac{a}{\mu + a} \frac{\beta}{\mu + \gamma}.$$

Similarly to the SIR model, also in this case we have a Disease-Free-Equilibrium (N,0,0,0) and an Endemic Equilibrium EE, and one can show that, independently form biologically meaningful initial conditions

$$(S(0), E(0), I(0), R(0)) \in \left\{(S, E, I, R) \in [0, N]^4 : S \geq 0, E \geq 0, I \geq 0, R \geq 0, S + E + I + R = N\right\}$$

it holds that:

$$R_0 \leq 1 \Rightarrow \lim_{t \to +\infty} \left(S(t), E(t), I(t), R(t)\right) = DFE = \left(N, 0, 0, 0\right)$$

$$R_0 > 1, I(0) > 0 \Rightarrow \lim_{t \to +\infty} \left(S(t), E(t), I(t), R(t)\right) = EE.$$

In case of periodically varying contact rate $\beta(t)$ the condition for the global attractiveness of DFE is that the following linear system with periodic coefficients:

$$\frac{dE_1}{dt} = \beta(t) I_1 - (\gamma + a)E_1$$

$$\frac{dI_1}{dt} = aE_1 - (\gamma + \mu)I_1$$

is stable (i.e. it has its Floquet's eigenvalues inside the unit circle in the complex plane).

Modelling Mass Vaccination Programmes

Vaccinating the Newborns

In presence of a communicable diseases, one of main tasks is that of eradicating it via prevention measures and, if possible, via the establishment of a mass vaccination programme.

Let us consider a disease for which the newborn are vaccinated (with a vaccine giving lifelong immunity) at a rate $P \in (0,1)$:

$$\frac{dS}{dt} = \mu N(1-P) - \mu S - \beta \frac{I}{N} S$$

$$\frac{dI}{dt} = \beta \frac{I}{N} S - (\mu + \gamma) I$$

$$\frac{dV}{dt} = \mu NP - \mu V$$

where V is the class of vaccinated subjects. It is immediate to show that:

$$\lim_{t \to +\infty} V(t) = NP,$$

thus we shall deal with the long term behaviour of S and I, for which it holds that:

$$R_0(1-P) \le 1 \Rightarrow \lim_{t \to +\infty} \left(S(t), I(t)\right) = DFE = \left(N\left(1-P\right), 0\right)$$

$$R_0(1-P) > 1, I(0) > 0 \Rightarrow \lim_{t \to +\infty} \left(S(t), I(t)\right) = EE = \left(\frac{N}{R_0(1-P)}, N\left(R_0(1-P)-1\right)\right).$$

In other words if

$$P \ge P^* = 1 - \frac{1}{R_0}$$

the vaccination programme is successful in eradicating the disease, on the contrary it will remain endemic, although at lower levels than the case of absence of vaccinations. This means that the mathematical model suggests that for a disease whose basic reproduction number may be as high as 18 one should have to vaccinate 94.4% of newborns in order to eradicate the disease.

Vaccination and Information

Modern societies are facing the challenge of "rational" exemption, i.e. the family's decision to not vaccinate children as a consequence of a "rational" comparison between the perceived risk from infection and that from getting damages from the vaccine. In order to assess whether this behaviour is really rational, i.e. if it can equally lead to the eradication of the disease, one may simply assume that the vaccination rate is an increasing function of the number of infectious subjects:

$$P = P(I), P'(I) > 0.$$

In such a case the eradication condition becomes:

$$P(0) \geq P^*,$$

i.e. the baseline vaccination rate should be greater than the "mandatory vaccination" threshold, which, in case of exemption, cannot hold.

Thus, "rational" exemption might be myopic since it is based only on the current low incidence due to high vaccine coverage, instead taking into account future resurgence of infection due to coverage decline.

Vaccination of Non Newborns

In case there also are vaccinations of non newborn at a rate ρ the equation for the susceptible and vaccinated subject has to be modified as follows:

$$\frac{dS}{dt} = \mu N(1-P) - \mu S - \rho S - \beta \frac{I}{N} S$$

$$\frac{dV}{dt} = \mu NP + \rho S - \mu V$$

leading to the following eradication condition:

$$P \geq 1 - \left(1 + \frac{\rho}{\mu}\right)\frac{1}{R_0}$$

Pulse Vaccination Strategy

This strategy repeatedly vaccinates a defined age-cohort (such as young children or the elderly) in a susceptible population over time. Using this strategy, the block of susceptible individuals is then immediately removed, making it possible to eliminate an infectious disease, (such as measles), from the entire population.

Every T time units a constant fraction p of susceptible subjects is vaccinated in a relatively short (with respect to the dynamics of the disease) time. This leads to the following impulsive differential equations for the susceptible and vaccinated subjects:

$$\frac{dS}{dt} = \mu N - \mu S - \beta \frac{I}{N} S, S(nT^+) = (1-p)S(nT^-) n = 0,1,2,\ldots$$

$$\frac{dV}{dt} = -\mu V, V(nT^+) = V(nT^-) + pS(nT^-) n = 0,1,2,\ldots$$

It is easy to see that by setting $I = 0$ one obtains that the dynamics of the susceptible subjects is given by:

$$S^*(t) = 1 - \frac{p}{1-(1-p)E^{-\mu T}} E^{-\mu MOD(t,T)}$$

and that the eradication condition is:

$$R_0 \int_0^T S^*(t)dt < 1$$

The Influence of Age: Age-structured Models

Age has a deep influence on the disease spread rate in a population, especially the contact rate. This rate summarizes the effectiveness of contacts between susceptible and infectious subjects. Taking into account the ages of the epidemic classes $s(t,a), i(t,a), r(t,a)$ (to limit ourselves to the susceptible-infectious-removed scheme) such that:

$$S(t) = \int_0^{a_M} s(t,a)da$$

$$I(t) = \int_0^{a_M} i(t,a)da$$

$$R(t) = \int_0^{a_M} r(t,a)da$$

(where $a_M \leq +\infty$ is the maximum admissible age) and their dynamics is not described, as one might think, by "simple" partial differential equations, but by integro-differential equations:

$$\partial_t s(t,a) + \partial_a s(t,a) = -\mu(a)s(a,t) - s(a,t)\int_0^{a_M} k(a,a_1;t)i(a_1,t)da_1$$

$$\partial_t i(t,a) + \partial_a i(t,a) = s(a,t)\int_0^{a_M} k(a,a_1;t)i(a_1,t)da_1 - \mu(a)i(a,t) - \gamma(a)i(a,t)$$

$$\partial_t r(t,a) + \partial_a r(t,a) = -\mu(a)r(a,t) + \gamma(a)i(a,t)$$

where:

$$F(a,t,i(\cdot,\cdot)) = \int_0^{a_M} k(a,a_1;t)i(a_1,t)da_1$$

is the force of infection, which, of course, will depend, though the contact kernel $k(a,a_1;t)$ on the interactions between the ages.

Complexity is added by the initial conditions for newborns (i.e. for a=0), that are straightforward for infectious and removed:

$$i(t,0) = r(t,0) = 0$$

but that are nonlocal for the density of susceptible newborns:

$$s(t,0) = \int_0^{a_M} \left(\varphi_s(a)s(a,t) + \varphi_i(a)i(a,t) + \varphi_r(a)r(a,t)\right)da$$

where $\varphi_j(a), j = s,i,r$ are the fertilities of the adults. Moreover, defining now the density of the total population $n(t,a) = s(t,a) + i(t,a) + r(t,a)$ one obtains:

$$\partial_t n(t,a) + \partial_a n(t,a) = -\mu(a)n(a,t)$$

In the simplest case of equal fertilities in the three epidemic classes, we have that in order to have demographic equilibrium the following necessary and sufficient condition linking the fertility $\varphi(.)$ with the mortality $\mu(a)$ must hold:

$$1 = \int_0^{a_M} \varphi(a)\exp\left(-\int_0^a \mu(q)dq\right)da$$

and the demographic equilibrium is

$$n^*(a) = C\exp\left(-\int_0^a \mu(q)dq\right),$$

automatically ensuring the existence of the disease-free solution:

$$DFS(a) = \left(n^*(a),0,0\right).$$

A basic reproduction number can be calculated as the spectral radius of an appropriate functional operator.

Deterministic Versus Stochastic Epidemic Models

It is important to stress that the deterministic models presented here are valid only in case of sufficiently large populations, and as such should be used cautiously.

To be more precise, these models are only valid in the thermodynamic limit, where the population is effectively infinite. In stochastic models, the long-time endemic equilibrium derived above, does not hold, as there is a finite probability that the number of infected individuals drops below one in a system. In a true system then, the pathogen may not propagate, as no host will be infected. But, in deterministic mean-field models, the number of infecteds can take on real, namely, non-integer values of infected hosts, and the pathogen may still persist in the system with a finite number of infected hosts, less than one but greater than zero.

Transmission Risks and Rates

Transmission of an infection requires three conditions:

- an infectious individual
- a susceptible individual
- an effective contact between them

An effective contact is defined as any kind of contact between two individuals such that, if one individual is infectious and the other susceptible, then the first individual infects the second. Whether or not a particular kind of contact will be effective depends on the infectious agent and its route of transmission.

The effective contact rate (denoted β) in a given population for a given infectious disease is measured in effective contacts per unit time. This may be expressed as the total contact rate (the total number of contacts, effective or not, per unit time, denoted γ), multiplied by the risk of infection, given contact between an infectious and a susceptible individual. This risk is called the transmission risk and is denoted p. Thus:

$$\beta = \gamma \times p$$

The total contact rate, γ, will generally be greater than the effective contact rate, β, since not all contacts result in infection. That is to say, p is almost always less than 1 and it can never be greater than 1, since it is effectively the probability of transmission occurring.

This relation formalises the fact that the effective contact rate depends not only on the social patterns of contact in a particular society (γ) but also on the specific types of contact and the pathology of the infectious organism (p).

For example, it has been shown that a concurrent sexually transmitted infection can substantially increase the probability (p) of infecting a susceptible with HIV. Therefore, one way to reduce the value of p (and hence lower HIV transmission rates) might be to treat other sexually transmitted infections.

There are a number of difficulties in using this relation. The first is that it is very difficult to measure contact rates because they vary widely between individuals and groups, and within the same group at different times. For sexually transmitted infections, large scale studies of sexual behaviour have been set up to estimate the contact rate.

In developed countries for serious diseases such as AIDS or tuberculosis, contact tracing is often carried out when a patient is diagnosed (the patient and medical authorities try to inform every possible contact the patient may have made since infection). This, however, is not so much a research tool and more to alert the contacts to the possibility that they may be infected and so can seek medical treatment and avoiding passing on the disease if they have contracted it.

A second consideration is that it is generally thought unethical to carry out direct experiments to establish per-contact infection risks as this would require the deliberate exposure of individuals to infectious agents. The Common Cold Unit that researched cold transmission in the UK between 1946 and 1989 was a notable exception. It is also possible to estimate the transmission risk in certain circumstances where exposures to infection have been documented, for example the rate of infection among nurses who have accidentally pricked their fingers with a needle that had previously been used with contaminated blood.

A more direct assessment of transmission risks can be provided by a contact study, which is often carried out because of an outbreak (such a study was carried out during the SARS outbreak of 2002–3). The first (or primary) case within a defined group (such as a school or family) is identified and people infected by this individual (called secondary cases) are documented. If the number of susceptibles in the group is n and the number of secondary cases is x, then an estimation of the transmission risk is

$$p=xn.$$

Here, p is the same parameter as before but it has been calculated in a different way. To reflect this, it is called the secondary attack rate (it is really a risk, of course, and not a rate, but the term is still commonly used). Even if the whole group in question is susceptible, x is generally smaller than the basic reproduction number for the disease. That is defined as the number of individuals each infected individual will go on to infect themselves, in a population with no resistance to the disease. The basic reproduction number includes all secondary cases infected by a primary case, while x is only the number of secondary cases within the group in question.

Secondary attack rates are useful for comparisons between vaccinated and unvaccinated groups and hence assessing the efficacy of vaccinations against the disease under inspection. However, there are inevitably complications with such contact studies. It is not always obvious which members of the group are susceptible and distinguishing between secondary and subsequent cases (for example, those infected by the secondary cases are tertiary cases and so on) can be difficult. Also, the possibility of infection from an outsider must be ignored.

Despite these problems, the parameters p and β are powerful tools in the mathematical modelling of epidemics. But it should always be remembered that a model is only as good as the assumptions on which it is based and the data from which its parameters are calculated.

GIS and Public Health

Geographic information systems (GISs) and geographic information science (GIScience) combine computer-mapping capabilities with additional database management and data analysis tools. Commercial GIS systems are very powerful and have touched many applications and industries, including environmental science, urban planning, agricultural applications, and others.

Public health is another focus area that has made increasing use of GIS techniques. A strict definition of public health is difficult to pin down, as it is used in different ways by different groups. In general, public health differs from personal health in that it is (1) focused on the health of populations rather than of individuals, (2) focused more on prevention than on treatment, and (3) operates in a mainly governmental (rather than private) context. These efforts fall naturally within the domain of problems requiring use of spatial analysis as part of the solution, and GIS and other spatial analysis tools are therefore recognised as providing potentially transformational capabilities for public health efforts.

This article presents some history of use of geographic information and geographic information systems in public health application areas, provides some examples showing the utilisation of GIS techniques in solving specific public health problems, and finally addresses several potential issues arising from increased use of these GIS techniques in the public health arena.

History

Public health efforts have been based on analysis and use of spatial data for many years. Dr. John Snow (physician), often credited as the father of epidemiology, is arguably the most famous of those examples. Dr. Snow used a hand-drawn map to analyse the geographic locations of deaths related to cholera in London in the mid-1850s. His map, which superimposed the locations of cholera deaths with those of public water supplies, pinpointed the Broad Street pump as the most likely source of the cholera outbreak. Removal of the pump handle led to a rapid decline in the incidence of cholera, helping the medical community to eventually conclude that cholera was a water-borne disease.

Dr. Snow's work provides an indication of how a GIS could benefit public health investigations and other research. He continued to analyse his data, eventually showing that the incidence rate of cholera was also related to local elevation as well as soil type and alkalinity. Low-lying areas, particularly those with poorly draining soil, were found to have higher incidence rates for cholera, which Dr. Snow attributed to the pools of water that tended to collect there, again showing evidence that cholera was in fact a water-borne disease (rather than one borne by 'miasma' as was commonly believed at the time.

This is an early example of what has come to be known as disease diffusion mapping, an area of study based on the idea that a disease starts from some source or central point and then spreads throughout the local area according to patterns and conditions there. This is another area of research where the capabilities of a GIS have been shown to be of help to practitioners.

GIS for Public Health

Today's public health problems are much larger in scope than those Dr. Snow faced, and researchers today depend on modern GIS and other computer mapping applications to assist in their analyses.

Public health informatics (PHI) is an emerging speciality which focuses on the application of information science and technology to public health practice and research. As part of that effort, a GIS – or more generally a spatial decision support system (SDSS) – offers improved geographic visualization techniques, leading to faster, better, and more robust understanding and decision-making capabilities in the public health arena.

For example, GIS displays have been used to show a clear relationship between clusters of emergent Hepatitis C cases and those of known intravenous drug users in Connecticut. Causality is difficult to prove conclusively – collocation does not establish causation – but confirmation of previously established causal relationships (like intravenous drug use and Hepatitis C) can strengthen acceptance of those relationships, as well as help to demonstrate the utility and reliability of GIS-related solution techniques. Conversely, showing the coincidence of potential causal factors with the ultimate effect can help suggest a potential causal relationship, thereby driving further investigation and analysis (source needed?).

Alternately, GIS techniques have been used to show a lack of correlation between causes and effects or between different effects. For example, the distributions of both birth defects and infant mortality in Iowa were studied, and the researchers found no relationship in those data. This led to the conclusion that birth defects and infant mortality are likely unrelated, and are likely due to different causes and risk factors. GIS can support public health in different ways as well. First and foremost, GIS displays can help inform proper understanding and drive better decisions.

For example, elimination of health disparities is one of two primary goals of Healthy People 2010, one of the preeminent public health programmes in existence today in the US. GIS can play a significant role in that effort, helping public health practitioners identify areas of disparities or inequities, and ideally helping them identify and develop solutions to address those shortcomings. GIS can also help researchers integrate disparate data from a wide variety of sources, and can even be used to enforce quality control measures on those data.

Much public health data is still manually generated, and is therefore subject to human-generated mistakes and miscoding. For example, geographic analysis of health care data from North Carolina showed that just over 40% of the records contained errors of some sort in the geographic information (city, county, or zip code), errors that would have gone undetected without the visual displays provided by GIS. Correction of these errors led not only to more correct GIS displays, but also improved ALL analyses using those data.

Issues with GIS for Public Health

There are also concerns or issues with use of GIS tools for public health efforts. Chief among those is a concern for privacy and confidentiality of individuals. Public health is concerned about the health of the population as a whole, but must use data on the health of individuals to make many of those assessments, and protecting the privacy and confidentiality of those individuals is of paramount importance. Use of GIS displays and related databases raises the potential of compromising those privacy standards, so some precautions are necessary to avoid pinpointing individuals based on spatial data. For example, data may need to be aggregated to cover larger areas such as a zip code or county, helping to mask individual identities. Maps can also be constructed at smaller scales so that less detail is revealed. Alternately, key identifying features (such as the road and street network) can be left off the maps to mask exact location, or it may even be advisable to intentionally offset the location markers by some random amount if deemed necessary.

It is well established in the literature that statistical inference based on aggregated data can lead researchers to erroneous conclusions, suggesting relationships that in fact do not exist or obscuring relationships that do in fact exist. This issue is known as the modifiable areal unit problem. For example, New York public health officials worried that cancer clusters and causes would be misidentified after they were forced to post maps showing cancer cases by ZIP code on the internet. Their assertion was that ZIP codes were designed for a purpose unrelated to public health issues, and so use of these arbitrary boundaries might lead to inappropriate groupings and then to incorrect conclusions.

Summary

Use of GIS in public health is an application area still in its infancy. Like most new applications, there is a lot of promise, but also a lot of pitfalls that must be avoided along the way. Many researchers and practitioners are concentrating of this effort, hoping that the benefits outweigh the risks and the costs associated with this emerging application area for modern GIS techniques.

Chapter 6

Environment and Health

Framing the Issue

There is a growing body of evidence that the environment can affect human health and that human health care can affect the environment. Thus, the traditional divide between clinical medicine and environmental protection is disappearing. This change has created a need for bioethical reflection on all levels of interaction between human health and the environment.

The questions that span medical and environmental ethics are complex, diverse, frequently global in scope, and not able to be answered without collaboration among environmental scientists, physicians, public health professionals, ethicists, lawyers, and policymakers. Where should a county place a solid waste facility? Should emergency health care workers be vaccinated against smallpox? Should new housing developments have sidewalks and bike paths to help prevent obesity? Should any use of DDT be permitted to control malaria? Should the United States increase foreign aid to help impoverished nations improve their water supplies? Are transgenic plants an acceptable alternative to pesticides and chemical fertilizers? How much of their limited resources for environmental health should the nations of the world allocate to preventing and adapting to global climate change? Finding satisfactory answers to questions like these will become increasingly important as the environmental impacts of human activities continue to mount.

The Science: Environmental Health and Hazards

All organisms depend on their environments for energy and the materials needed to sustain life: clean air, potable water, nutritious food, and safe places to live. For most of human history, increases in longevity were due to improved access to these necessities. Advances in agriculture, sanitation, water treatment, and hygiene have had a far greater impact on human health than medical technology.

Although the environment sustains human life, it can also cause disease. Lack of basic necessities is a significant cause of human mortality. In 2004, lack of access to safe drinking water was responsible for 1.8 million deaths (mostly small children) from diarrhea. That same year, lack of adequate sanitation caused 160 million people to become infected with schistosomiasis, which can cause malnutrition and organ damage. Approximately 1.1 billion people currently lack access to safe drinking water, and 2.6 billion do not have proper sanitation. Environmental hazards increase the risk of cancer, heart disease, asthma, and many other illnesses. These hazards can be physical, such as pollution and food contaminants, or they can be social, including dangerous work conditions and poverty.

By contrast, activities that promote health and extend human life can have adverse environmental effects. For example, food production causes environmental damage from pesticides and fertilizers, soil salinization, waste produced by livestock, carbon emissions from food manufacturing and transportation, and overfishing. Health care facilities also have adverse environmental impacts. Hospitals use large quantities of electricity and fossil fuels and produce medical wastes. To prevent some diseases, it may be necessary to damage the environment. For example, malaria was eradicated in the United States and other developed nations in the 1940s and 1950s as a result of draining wetlands and spraying DDT to kill mosquitoes. A reduction in mortality from starvation or disease can lead to overpopulation, which stresses the environment in many different ways—increasing use of fossil fuels, clearing land, generating pollution and waste, and so on.

Bioethical, Social, and Legal Considerations

Relationships between human health and the environment raise many ethical, social, and legal dilemmas by forcing people to choose among competing values. These considerations can be grouped into the following categories.

Managing Benefits and Risks

Many of the issues at the intersection of health and the environment have to do with managing benefits and risks. For example, pesticides play an important role in increasing crop yields, but they can also pose hazards to human health and the environment.

Alternatives to pesticide use create trade-offs in health. The extreme action of stopping all pesticide use could significantly reduce agricultural productivity, leading to food shortages and increased food prices that would, in turn, increase starvation in some parts of the world. Public health authorities have opted to regulate the use of pesticides to enhance food production while minimizing damage to the environment and human health.

No issue demands greater care in balancing benefits and risks than global warming. A significant percentage of global climate change is due to the human production of greenhouse gases. Climate change is likely to cause tremendous harm to the environment and human health, but taking steps to drastically reduce greenhouse gases could have adverse consequences for global, national, and local economies, which would result in a general decline in human health and health care. For example, greatly increasing gasoline taxes would encourage greater fuel efficiency and lower carbon dioxide emissions, but it would also increase the price of transportation, leading to widespread inflation and reduced consumer spending power.

For many years some politicians and scholars have argued that we should wait for more evidence of global warming, since the steps needed to prevent or minimize it could have disastrous economic consequences. Others have argued that society cannot afford to wait for complete evidence because the consequences of global climate change could be catastrophic and irreversible. This difference of opinion raises a fundamental question about the ethics of benefit/risk management: What is the role of scientific evidence in decision-making?

Most regulatory agencies in the United States make benefit/risk decisions based on information from scientific studies, such as chemical analyses, cell studies, animal experiments, and controlled clinical trials. Agencies often refrain from making regulatory decisions until they have adequate scientific evidence. Many commentators and organisations endorse an alternative approach, the precautionary principle. The idea is that society should take reasonable steps to prevent or minimize significant, irreversible harm, even when scientific evidence is incomplete. Although the precautionary principle has many adherents, especially in Europe and California, it remains controversial.

Social Justice

Managing benefits and risks raises social justice concerns. In general, people with lower socioeconomic status have greater exposure to detrimental environmental conditions in their homes or at work, such as lead, mercury, or smoke produced by factories. Communities and nations should minimize such injustices when making decisions, such as choosing a site for a factory, a power plant, or waste dump, or regulating safety in the workplace. The decision-making process should be fair, open, and democratic, so that people who will be affected by environmental risks have a voice in these deliberations and can make their concerns known. When drafting and implementing environmental health regulations, it is important to consider vulnerable subpopulations. A vulnerable subpopulation is a group with an increased susceptibility to the adverse effects of an environmental risk factor due to age, genetics, health status, or some other condition. For example, children are more susceptible to the effects of lead, mercury, and some pesticides than adults. Some people have a genetic mutation that increases their susceptibility to cancer caused by passive smoking.

If an environmental regulation is designed to protect average members of the population, it may fail to adequately protect vulnerable populations. Justice demands that we take care of people who are vulnerable. But almost everyone in the population has an above-average susceptibility to at least one environmental risk factor. Since providing extra protections to everyone would be costly and impractical, protections must be meted out carefully, and the populations who are vulnerable to a particular environmental risk factor must be defined clearly. For example, about 0.4% of the U.S. population is severely allergic to peanuts. Banning the sale of peanuts would be a costly and impractical way to protect these people, but requiring that products containing peanuts be labelled as such would be reasonable.

Social justice must be a factor in allocating resources for health care. Governments spend billions of dollars trying to improve the health of citizens and to prevent disease. These funds go to biomedical research, overseeing the safety of foods and drugs, enforcing environmental or occupational health regulations, and running programmes for disaster preparedness, public health, health education, sanitation, water treatment, and so on. In the United States, the lion's share of health resources goes to providing medical diagnosis and treatment, but one might argue that it would be wiser to shift some resources to disease prevention programmes, such as environmental protection, public health, and health education, since prevention is generally more cost-effective than treatment.

Human Rights

Various public health strategies pit the rights of individuals against the good of society. These include mandatory treatment, vaccination, or diagnostic testing; isolation and quarantine; and disease surveillance. The main argument for these public health strategies is that individual human rights may have to be limited to prevent the transmission of infectious diseases, such as tuberculosis, SARS, HIV/AIDS, and pneumonia. But restrictions on rights should be carefully considered and safeguards put in place to prevent public health authorities from overstepping their bounds. Protecting the public's health should not come at the expense of human rights.

Some health and environmental protections also limit property rights. The owner of a coal-burning power plant must deal with many laws concerning the operation of the plant, workplace safety, and carbon emissions. A developer who plans to build 150 new homes with land he has purchased may also have to deal with laws concerning storm drainage, water and sewage lines, gas lines, sidewalks, and so on. Restrictions on property rights are justified to protect human health and the environment. But opponents of these restrictions argue that they are often excessive or not adequately supported by scientific evidence.

Human rights issues also come up in research on environmental health that involves human subjects. For such research to be ethical, human subjects must give consent, and great care must be taken to ensure that they understand that they can opt out of the research project. Since the late 1990s, some pesticide companies have tested pesticides on human subjects to gather data to submit to the government for regulatory purposes. Some commentators charge that these experiments are unethical because they place people at unacceptably high risk without clear benefit to society. Others have argued that the experiments, if properly designed and implemented, could produce important benefits to society by providing useful knowledge about the effects of pesticides, which could lead to stronger regulations.

Emerging Issues Likely to Affect Policy

There are many new developments in science, technology, and industry that are bound to pose benefits and risks to the environment and human health. They include nanotechnology, genetic modification of plants and animals, antibiotic resistance, threats to food safety, and the growing market for biofuels. Longstanding challenges persist, including the preservation of ecosystems and endangered species and questions about animal experimentation. Many more will emerge. To deal with them in a responsible way, we must continue to research the relationship between human health and the environment and to hold fair and democratic public deliberations—community forums, academic conferences, and legislative debates—involving participants with diverse cultural, socioeconomic, philosophical, and scientific perspectives.

Environmental Disease

In epidemiology, environmental diseases are diseases that can be directly attributed to environmental factors (as distinct from genetic factors or infection). Apart from the true monogenic genetic disorders, environmental diseases may determine the development of disease in those genetically predisposed to a particular condition. Stress, physical and mental abuse, diet, exposure to toxins, pathogens, radiation, and chemicals found in almost all personal care products and household cleaners are possible causes of a large segment of non-hereditary disease. If a disease process is concluded to be the result of a combination of genetic and *environmental factor* influences, its etiological origin can be referred to as having a multifactorial pattern.

There are many different types of environmental disease including:

- Lifestyle disease such as cardiovascular disease, diseases caused by substance abuse such as alcoholism, and smoking-related disease
- Disease caused by physical factors in the environment, such as skin cancer caused by excessive exposure to ultraviolet radiation in sunlight
- Disease caused by exposure to chemicals in the environment such as toxic metals

Categories of Environmental Disease

- First, there are those caused by the ancient metals : lead and mercury.
- Then there are those caused by the other metals: arsenic, phosphorus, and zinc.
- The newer metals can also cause environmental disease: beryllium, cadmium, chromium, manganese, nickel, cobalt, osmium, platinum, selenium, tellurium, thallium, uranium, and vanadium.

There are many other diseases likely to have been caused by common anions found in natural drinking water. Fluoride is one of the most common found in drier climates where the geology favours release of fluoride ions to soil as the rocks decompose. In Sri Lanka, 90% of the country is underlain by crystalline metamorphic rocks of which most carry mica as a major mineral. Mica carries fluoride in their structure and releases to soil when decomposes. In the dry and arid climates, fluoride concentrates on top soil and slowly dissolves in shallow groundwater. This has been the cause of high fluoride levels in drinking water where the majority of the rural Sri Lankans obtain their drinking water from backyard wells.

High fluoride in drinking water has caused very high incidence of fluorosis among dry zone population in Sri Lanka. However, in the wet zone, high rainfall effectively removes fluoride from soils where no fluorosis is evident.

The iodine deficiency has also been noted in some parts of Sri Lanka which has been identified as a result of iodine fixation by hydrated iron oxide found in lateritic soils in wet coastal lowlands.

- Additionally, there are environmental diseases caused by the aromatic carbon compounds including : benzene, hexachlorocyclohexane, toluene diisocyanate, phenol, pentachlorophenol, quinone and hydroquinone.

  Also included are the aromatic nitro-, amino-, and pyridilium-deratives: nitrobenzene, dinitrobenzene, trinitrotoluene, paramethylaminophenol sulfate (Metol), dinitro-ortho-cresol, aniline, trinitrophenylmethylnitramine (tetryl), hexanitrodiphenylamine (aurantia), phenylenediamine, and paraquat.

  The aliphatic carbon compounds can also cause environmental disease. Included in these are methanol, nitroglycerine, nitrocellulose, dimethylnitrosamine, and the halogenated hydrocarbons: methyl chloride, methyl bromide, trichloroethylene, carbon tetrachloride, and the chlorinated naphthalenes. Also included are glycols: ethylene chlorhydrin and diethylene dioxide as well as carbon disulfide, acrylonitrile, acrylamide, and vinyl chloride.

- Other important chemical causes of environmental diseases are the noxious gases which can be categorized as : Simple asphyxiants, chemical asphyxiants, and irritant gases. The simple asphyxiants are nitrogen, methane, and carbon dioxide.

The chemical asphyxiants are carbon monoxide, sulphuretted hydrogen and hydrogen cyanide.

The irritant gases are sulfur dioxide, ammonia, nitrogen dioxide, chlorine, phosgene, and fluorine and its compounds, which include luroine and hydrofluoric acid, fluorspar, fluorapatite, cryolite, and organic fluorine compounds.

The U.S. Coast Guard has developed a Coast Guard-wide comprehensive system for surveillance of workplace diseases.

The American Medical Association's fifth edition of the Current Medical Information and Terminology (CMIT) was used as a reference to expand the basic list of 50 Sentinel Health Events (Occupational) [SHE(O)] published by the National Institute of Occupational Health and Safety (NIOSH), September, 1983.

The expanded list of 107 sentinel events serves as a framework for the development of a computerized system of occupational health surveillance in the U.S. Coast Guard. This application of SHE(O) surveillance can have application in the early detection and prevention of environmental diseases.

Human Disease

Human disease, an impairment of the normal state of a human being that interrupts or modifies its vital functions.

Health Versus Disease

Before human disease can be discussed, the meanings of the terms health, physical fitness, illness, and disease must be considered. Health could be defined theoretically in terms of certain measured values; for example, a person having normal body temperature, pulse and breathing rates, blood pressure, height, weight, acuity of vision, sensitivity of hearing, and other normal measurable characteristics might be termed healthy. But what does normal mean, and how is it established? It is well known that if the temperatures are taken of a large number of active, presumably healthy, individuals the temperatures will all come close to 98.6 °F (37 °C). The great preponderance of these values will fall between 98.4 °F (36.9 °C) and 98.8 °F (37.1 °C). Thus, health could in part be defined as having a temperature within this narrow range. Similarly, a normal range can be established for pulse, blood pressure, and height. In some healthy individuals, however, the body temperature may range below 98.4 °F or above 98.8 °F. These low and high temperatures fall outside the limits defined above as normal and are instances of biological variability.

Biological criteria of normality are based on statistical concepts. Body height may be used as an example. If the heights of every individual in a large sample were plotted on a graph, the many points would fall on a bell-shaped curve. At one end of the curve would be the very short people, and at the other extreme the few very tall people. The majority of the points of the sample population would fall on the dome of the bell-shaped curve. At the peak of the dome would be those individuals whose height approaches the average of all the heights. Scientists use curves in determining what they call normal criteria. By accepted statistical criteria, 95 percent of the population measured would be included in the normal range—that is, 47.5 percent above and 47.5 percent below the mean at the very centre of the bell. Looked at in another way, in any given normal biological distribution 5 percent will be considered outside the normal range. Thus the 7-foot (213-cm) basketball player would be considered abnormally tall, but that which is abnormal must be distinguished from that which represents disease. The basketball player might be abnormally tall but still have excellent health. Thus, in any statistical analysis of health, the possibility of biological variation must be recognised.

A better example than height of how problems can arise with biological variability is heart size. If the heart is subjected to a greater than normal burden over a long period, it can respond by growing larger (the process is known as hypertrophy). This occurs in certain forms of heart disease, especially in those involving long-standing high blood pressure or structural defects of the heart valves. A large heart, therefore, may be a sign of disease. On the other hand, it is not uncommon for athletes to have large hearts. Continuous strenuous exercise requires a greater output of blood to the tissues, and the heart adapts to this demand by becoming larger. In some cases the decision as to whether an abnormally large heart represents evidence of disease or is simply a biological variant may tax the diagnostic abilities of the physician.

The effects of age introduce yet another difficulty in the attempt to define health in theoretical measured norms. It is well known that muscular strength diminishes in the advanced years of life, the bones become more delicate and more easily fractured, vision and hearing become less sharp, and a variety of other retrogressive changes occur. There is some basis for considering this general deterioration as a disease, but, in view of the fact that it affects virtually everyone, it can be accepted as normal. Theoretical criteria for health, then, would have to be set for virtually every year of life. Thus, one would have to say that it is normal for a man of 80 to be breathless after climbing two flights of stairs, while such breathlessness would be distinctly abnormal in an agile child of 10 years of age. Moreover, an individual's general level of physical activity significantly alters his ability to respond to the ordinary demands of daily life. The amount of muscular strength possessed by an 80-year-old man who has remained physically active would be considerably more than that of his fragile friend who has led a confined life because of his dislike of activity. There are, therefore, many difficulties in establishing criteria for health in terms of absolute values.

Health might be defined better as the ability to function effectively in complete harmony with one's environment. Implied in such a definition is the capability of meeting—physically, emotionally, and mentally—the ordinary stresses of life. In this definition health is interpreted in terms of the individual's environment. Health to the construction worker would have a dimension different from health to the bookkeeper. The healthy construction worker expects to be able to do manual labour all day, while the bookkeeper, although perfectly capable of performing sedentary work, would be totally incapable of such heavy labour and indeed might collapse from the physical strain; yet both individuals might be termed completely healthy in terms of their own way of life.

The term physical fitness, although frequently used, is also exceedingly difficult to define. In general it refers to the state of optimal maintenance of muscular strength, proper function of the internal organs, and youthful vigour. The champion athlete prepared to cope not only with the commonplace stresses of life but also with the unusual illustrates the concept of physical fitness. To be in good physical condition is to have the ability to swim a mile to save one's life or to slog home through snowdrifts when a car breaks down in a storm. Some experts in fitness insist that the state of health requires that the individual be in prime physical condition. They prefer to divide the spectrum of health and disease into (1) health, (2) absence of disease, and (3) disease. In their view, those who are not in prime condition and are not physically fit cannot be considered as healthy merely because they have no disease.

Health involves more than physical fitness, since it also implies mental and emotional well-being. Should the angry, frustrated, emotionally unstable person in excellent physical condition be called healthy? Certainly this individual could not be characterized as effectively functioning in complete harmony with the environment. Indeed, such an individual is incapable of good judgement and rational response. Health, then, is not merely the absence of illness or disease but involves the ability to function in harmony with one's environment and to meet the usual and sometimes unusual demands of daily life.

The definitions of illness and disease are equally difficult problems. Despite the fact that these terms are often used interchangeably, illness is not to be equated with disease. A person may have a disease for many years without even being aware of its presence. Although diseased, this person is not ill. Similarly, a person with diabetes who has received adequate insulin treatment is not ill. An individual who has cancer is often totally unaware of having the disorder and is not ill until after many years of growth of the tumour, during which time it has caused no symptoms. The term illness implies discomfort or inability to function optimally. Hence it is a subjective state of lack of well-being produced by disease. Regrettably, many diseases escape detection and possible cure because they remain symptomless for long years before they produce discomfort or impair function.

Disease, which can be defined at the simplest level as any deviation from normal form and function, may either be associated with illness or be latent. In the latter circumstance, the disease will either become apparent at some later time or will render the individual more susceptible to illness. The person who fractures an ankle has an injury—a disease—producing immediate illness. Both form and function have been impaired. The illness occurred at the instant of the development of the injury or disease. The child who is infected with measles, on the other hand, does not become ill until approximately 10 days after exposure (the incubation period). During this incubation period the child is not ill but has a viral infectious disease that is incubating and will soon produce discomfort and illness. Some diseases render a person more susceptible to illness only when the person is under stress. Some diseases may consist of only extremely subtle defects in cells that render the cells more susceptible to injury in certain situations.

The blood disease known as sickle cell anemia, for example, results from a hereditary abnormality in the production of the red oxygen-carrying pigment (hemoglobin) of the red cells of the blood. The child of a mother and father who both have sickle cell anemia will probably inherit an overt form of sickle cell anemia and will have the same disease as the parents. If only one parent has sickle cell anemia, however, the child may inherit only a tendency to sickle cell anemia. This tendency is referred to by physicians as the sickle cell trait. Individuals having such a trait are not anemic but have a greater likelihood of developing such a disease. When they climb a mountain and are exposed to lower levels of oxygen in the air, red blood cells are destroyed and anemia develops. This can serve as an example of a disease or a disease trait that renders the affected person more susceptible to illness.

Disease, defined as any deviation from normal form and function, may be trivial if the deviation is minimal. A minor skin infection might be considered trivial, for example. On the eyelid, however, such an infection could produce considerable discomfort or illness. Any departure from the state of health, then, is a disease, whether health be measured in the theoretical terms of normal measured values or in the more pragmatic terms of ability to function effectively in harmony with one's environment.

Maintenance of Health

Health is not a static condition but represents a fluid range of physical and emotional well-being continually subjected to internal and external challenges such as worry, overwork, varying external temperatures, mechanical stresses, and infectious agents. These constantly changing conditions require the adjustment of the function of the various systems within the body. Mechanisms are continually at work to maintain a constant internal environment called by the French scientist Claude Bernard the *milieu intérieur*. The maintenance of this relatively constant internal environment is known as homeostasis. On a hot summer day, for example, the body is challenged to maintain its normal temperature of 98.6 °F (37 °C). Sweating represents a mechanism by which the skin is kept moist. By the evaporation of the moisture, heat is lost more rapidly. The hot day, therefore, represents a challenge to homeostasis. On a cold day gooseflesh may develop, an example of a homeostatic response that is a throwback to mechanisms in lower animals. In fur-bearing ancestors of humans, cold external environments caused the individual hair shafts to rise and, in effect, produce a heavier, thicker insulation of the body against the external chill. Humans still develop this primitive gooseflesh response but, regrettably, lack the luxuriant pelt to protect themselves.

Bacteria, viruses, and other microbiological agents are obvious challenges to health. The body is able, to a considerable extent, to protect itself and adjust to challenges, and, to the extent that it is successful, the state of health is maintained. While health is often thought of as fragile and subject to many onslaughts, it is, in fact, a ruggedly guarded state protected by a host of highly efficient internal mechanisms.

Some of the mechanisms vital to the maintenance of health include (1) the maintenance of the internal environment, or homeostasis, (2) adaptation to stress situations, (3) defence against microbiological agents, such as bacteria and viruses, (4) repair and regeneration of damaged tissue or cells, and (5) clotting of the blood to prevent excessive bleeding. Each of these areas will be discussed briefly. Despite these separate considerations, the commonality of purpose—the preservation and maintenance of health—must not be lost sight of. Insofar as each of these mechanisms works to maintain a constant internal environment, it can be considered as a homeostatic mechanism. Later, when disease is discussed, it will be apparent that to a considerable extent disease represents a failure of homeostasis and the other defencive responses listed above.

Homeostasis

As noted earlier, the term homeostasis refers to the maintenance of the internal environment of the body within narrow and rigidly controlled limits. The major functions important in the maintenance of homeostasis are fluid and electrolyte balance, acid-base regulation, thermoregulation, and metabolic control.

Fluid and Electrolyte Balance

This term refers to the controlled partition of water and major chemical constituents among the cells and the extracellular fluids of the body. The human body is basically a collection of cells grouped together into organ systems and bathed in fluids, most notably the blood. The intracellular fluid is the fluid contained within cells. The extracellular fluid—the fluid outside the cells—is divided into that found within the blood and that found outside the blood; the latter fluid is known as the interstitial fluid. These fluids are not simply water but contain varying amounts of solutes (electrolytes and other bioactive molecules). An electrolyte (sodium chloride, for example) is defined as any molecule that in solution separates into its ionic components and is capable of conducting an electric current. Cations are electrolytes that migrate towards the negative pole of an electric field; anions migrate towards the positive pole.

extracellular fluid*		***intracellular fluid*****	
Cations (+ electrical charge)			
sodium (Na^+)	142 mEq/l***	sodium (Na^+)	10 mEq/l
potassium (K^+)	4 mEq/l	potassium (K^+)	160 mEq/l
calcium (Ca^{2+})	5 mEq/l		
magnesium (Mg^{2+})	3 mEq/l	magnesium (Mg^{2+})	35 mEq/l
total	154 mEq/l	total	205 mEq/l
Anions (? electrical charge)			
chloride ($Cl^{?}$)	103 mEq/l	chloride ($Cl^{?}$)	2 mEq/l
bicarbonate ($HCO_3^{?}$)	27 mEq/l	bicarbonate ($HC0_3^{?}$)	8 mEq/l
phosphate ($PO_4^{3?}$)	2 mEq/l	($PO_4^{3?}$)	140 mEq/l
sulfate ($SO_4^{2?}$)	1 mEq/l		
protein	16 mEq/l	protein	55 mEq/l
organic acid	5 mEq/l		
total	154 mEq/l	total	205 mEq/l
*Approximate values in the blood plasma. **Approximate values for the muscle cells. ***mEq/l = milliequivalents per litre.			

It is apparent from this table that the ionic compositions of the intracellular and extracellular fluids are significantly different. The major cation of extracellular fluid is sodium. The major anion of the extracellular fluid is chloride, while bicarbonate is the second most important. In contrast, the major cation of the intracellular fluid is potassium, and the major anions are proteins and organic phosphates. The marked differences in sodium and potassium concentrations between the intracellular and extracellular fluid of cells are not fortuitous but are due to active transport by energy-dependent ion pumps located in cell membranes. The pumps continuously move sodium ions out of the cell and potassium ions into the cell. The intracellular and extracellular compartments are thus closely integrated and interdependent: changes in one have immediate effects on the other. In clinical medicine most measurements of electrolyte concentration are performed on the extracellular fluid compartment, notably the blood serum. The concentrations remain fairly constant on a day-to-day basis, in spite of various dietary intakes of food and water.

It is the primary task of the kidneys to regulate the various ionic concentrations of the body. Any abnormality in these concentrations can produce serious disease; for instance, the normal sodium concentration in the serum (the blood minus its cells and clotting factors) ranges from 136 to 142 milliequivalents per litre, while the normal potassium level in the serum is kept within the narrow range of 3.5 to 5 milliequivalents per litre. A rise in the serum potassium to perhaps 6.2 milliequivalents per litre, as can occur when large numbers of cells are severely injured or die and potassium ions are released, could cause serious abnormalities in the performance of the heart by disturbing the regularity of the nervous impulses that maintain the heart's rhythm.

The total amount of body water is also maintained at fairly constant levels from day to day by the combined action of the central nervous system and the kidneys. If one were to refrain from drinking any water for a few days, the thirst centre, located in the hypothalamus deep within the brain, would send out messages that would be translated into the feeling of thirst. At the same time a hormone from the posterior pituitary gland known as antidiuretic hormone (ADH; vasopressin) would be secreted. This hormone, released into the bloodstream, would reach the kidneys, where it would signal the kidneys to retain water and not excrete it. Should too much water be ingested, ADH secretion would be turned off, and the kidneys would promptly excrete the excess amount.

Acid-base Equilibrium

The acidity of the body fluids is maintained within narrow limits. This acidity is expressed in terms of the pH of a solution, values exceeding 7 representing alkalinity and less than 7 acidity. The pH of a solution is an expression of the amount of hydrogen ion present. Increases in hydrogen ion concentration cause a lowering of the pH, and, conversely, decreases in the hydrogen ion concentration raise the pH. Any abnormal process raising the hydrogen ion concentration in the body fluids produces a state of disease referred to as acidosis; one that causes the concentration to be lowered results in alkalosis.

In health the blood is slightly alkaline, being kept at a pH of 7.35 to 7.45, a narrow range which must be maintained for the optimum operation of the many chemical reactions that go on constantly in the body. Alterations in the blood pH occur in many diseases, particularly of the lungs and kidneys, organs whose functions include regulation of the body pH.

Thermoregulation

As has been said above, the temperature of the body is kept nearly constant at 98.6 °F (37 °C). Fluctuations within a few tenths of a degree are perfectly compatible with health. Wider swings in temperature are usually indicative of disease, and thus body temperature is an important factor in assessing health. Body temperature is regulated by a thermostatic control centre in the hypothalamus. A rise in body temperature initiates a chain of events leading to an increase in the rate of breathing and in sweating, two processes that serve to lower the body temperature. Similarly, a decrease in body temperature, perhaps occasioned by a chilly winter walk, leads to increased heat-producing activity such as the muscular contractions of shivering—again mediated by the thermostatic control centre in the hypothalamus.

Metabolic Control

In essence, metabolism involves all the physical and chemical processes by which cells are produced and maintained. Included under this broad umbrella are the regulation of fluid and electrolytes, the maintenance of plasma protein levels adequate for the building and repair of cells, and control of the amounts of sugar (glucose) and fats (lipids) in the blood so as to provide sufficient amounts for all the energy-producing activities of the cells. (The main treatment of this subject is contained in the article metabolism.)

The control of blood glucose levels is a good example of homeostasis. Most of the glucose utilised by the body is derived from the dietary intake of various forms of sugars and starches. These are digested within the intestinal tract into the simplest forms of carbohydrate (monosaccharides). Glucose, galactose, and fructose are the principal monosaccharides. These are absorbed from the intestines into the blood and enter the liver. Here all are eventually converted to glucose. The glucose may be utilised by the liver cells in part as a source of readily available energy, or it may be polymerized and stored as glycogen, but most of it enters the general circulation of the body and contributes to the blood glucose level. Blood glucose may also be derived in times of need by the conversion of the stored glycogen into glucose.

When food is eaten, there is a temporary rise in the blood glucose level known as alimentary hyperglycemia (high blood glucose level). Mechanisms are activated that stimulate the pancreas to secrete the hormone insulin. This hormone makes it possible for cells to utilise the glucose by facilitating its transport (carriage) across the membranes of cells into their interior, where it can enter the complex chemical reactions that provide the cell with energy. By virtue of insulin secretion, the cells receive adequate amounts of glucose, and the blood glucose levels are returned to the normal range, somewhere between 70 and 110 milligrams per 100 millilitres of blood.

Metabolic controls are exerted similarly for fats and proteins. As will be noted later on, derangements of these controls can lead to serious disease. The state of health implies proper, smooth-running metabolic machinery.

Adaptation

Adaptation refers to the ability of cells to adjust to severe stresses and achieve altered states of equilibrium while preserving a healthy state. In the human body the large bulging muscles of an individual engaged in heavy labour are a good example of cellular adaptation. Because of the heavy demand for work from these muscles, each of the individual muscle cells within the labourer's arms and legs becomes larger (hypertrophic). This enlargement is caused by the formation of increased numbers of tiny fibres (myofilaments) that provide the contractile power of muscles. Thus, while the normal muscle cell might have 2,000 myofilaments, the hypertrophied cell might have 4,000 myofilaments. The workload can now be divided evenly among twice as many myofilaments, and the muscle cell is capable of more work. The cells are completely normal and, in fact, are more robust than their fragile cousins. The individual can do heavy work all day without excessive fatigue, and no cell injury results from the heavy workload. A new level of equilibrium has been achieved by the process of cellular hypertrophy. A person with this type of muscular development can be considered to be in excellent physical condition, capable of meeting emergency situations such as running from a fire or catching a train without the dangers that might be encountered by a person who has not undergone such a development.

Inhabitants of high altitudes adapt to the lowered amounts of oxygen within the air by developing an increased number of red blood cells (a condition called secondary polycythemia). The greater number of red cells in the blood are capable of absorbing more oxygen from the air breathed into the lungs, and thus the person who lives in high altitudes makes better use of the slender oxygen content of the air.

Other examples of adaptation can be given; for example, liver cells, when exposed to drugs (or other chemicals), increase their level of drug-metabolizing enzymes.

Thus, adaptation is a mechanism by which the body preserves and maintains its health by adjusting to alterations in the conditions under which it functions.

Defence Against Biotic Invasion

Human beings are surrounded by a microscopic menagerie of organisms, most of which pose no threat and some of which are beneficial. Organisms capable of producing disease are pathogens. The maintenance of health requires defence against biotic invasion. There are four levels of defence in the body: (1) the intact skin and linings of the various orifices of the body (such as the mouth, nose, throat), (2) a widely dispersed system of cells capable of destroying invaders, (3) the capability of mounting an inflammatory reaction that destroys offenders, and (4) the capability of developing an immune response that helps to bring about further neutralization and destroy any attackers.

Maintenance of the Integrity of Skin and Mucosal Linings

With rare exception, pathogenic organisms cannot penetrate the intact covering and linings of the body. Indeed, if one were to take samples of the bacteria found on the skin, one would find large numbers of potentially harmful organisms that represent no threat unless the skin is punctured or the linings of the body are in some way injured. There are exceptions to this generalization, and a few biotic agents probably can penetrate intact mucosal surfaces. The bacterium *Salmonella typhi* that causes typhoid fever is thought to penetrate the normal lining of the gastrointestinal tract. Nevertheless, the intact skin and mucosal linings are primary protective barriers in the maintenance of health. The skin serves as a barrier to the external world, and the mucus-secreting and ciliated membranes of the upper respiratory tract trap inhaled foreign material and bacteria, transporting them to the pharynx where they are either swallowed or expelled by coughing. Potentially harmful bacteria can be introduced into a cut, which thus provides a portal of entry for organisms that may then cause an infection. By adequate washing, at least sufficient numbers of bacteria are flushed out to prevent the infection. Irritation of the skin from any cause or irritation of the throat by habitual smoking of tobacco impairs the integrity of these barriers and predisposes the area to invasion by potentially harmful organisms. The body has ingeniously contrived to place further roadblocks in the way of invaders. The saliva and the secretions in the stomach, for example, contain enzymes and acids that also destroy most organisms. Thus, humans have an effective enclosing barrier that provides protection against biotic attack.

Phagocytic Cells of the Body

Phagocytosis is the process by which certain cells ingest particulate material. When a phagocytic cell comes in contact with some particle such as a bacterium or even inert material such as dust, the cytoplasm of the cell (the cell substance outside its nucleus) flows around the object and forms a phagocytic vesicle. The phagocytic vesicle containing the particle then fuses with a lysosome (a membrane-enclosed sac that contains digestive enzymes). If the chemical composition of the foreign substance permits its degradation by the enzymes, it is destroyed. If the ingested material is resistant to digestion, it is retained within the phagocyte and is thus effectively removed from further interaction with the host. Phagocytic cells abound in the body; they serve as a second line of defence against most biotic invasion.

There are two groups of phagocytic cells, white blood cells—polymorphonuclear leukocytes—and tissue cells. The white blood cells are able to migrate through blood-vessel walls in areas of inflammation or infection, where they may phagocytize foreign material such as bacteria. Moreover, in inflammatory and infectious states, the total number of white cells in the body increases (leukocytosis). Thus the population of phagocytic cells is expanded when the cells are needed in the body's defence.

The second group of phagocytes consists of cells that are usually firmly fixed within tissues and are known as the reticuloendothelial system. The cells in this system are designated by a variety of names depending on their location (e.g., Kupffer cells in the liver, macrophages or histiocytes in loose connective tissue). They are particularly abundant in the spleen, liver, lymph nodes, and bone marrow but are also scattered throughout the blood vessels and virtually all the other tissues of the body. If, for example, bacteria do find a portal of entry but the bacterial invasion is not too massive and the organisms are not too virulent, these phagocytic cells are capable of engulfing and destroying them before they can cause injury.

The Inflammatory Response

Whenever cells are damaged or destroyed, a series of vascular and cellular events known as the inflammatory response is set in motion. This response is protective of health in that it destroys or walls off injurious influences and paves the way for the restoration of normality. The sequence of events is as follows: in an area of injury (as in a bacterial infection), cells release substances that cause the small blood vessels in the affected area to become dilated (vasodilation) and thus increase the blood flow to the injured area; at the same time, clear fluid leaks out of the vessels into the area; this fluid tends to dilute any harmful substances in the area of injury; next, white cells from the blood flow out of the blood vessels into the damaged area and phagocytize the bacteria and dead cells; the resulting mixture of dead cellular debris and white blood cells is known as pus.

The major signs of inflammation are redness and increased heat (caused by blood-vessel dilation), swelling (resulting from the accumulation of fluid), and pain. The last of these is one of the cardinal signs of all inflammatory responses. Pain in inflammation is caused by substances released by damaged tissues that render local nerve endings more sensitive to stimulation. Inflammation can be classified as either acute or chronic. Acute inflammation, such as may be seen around a skin cut, lasts for only a few days and is characterized microscopically by the presence of polymorphonuclear leukocytes. Chronic inflammation is of longer duration and is characterized microscopically by the presence of lymphocytes, monocytes, and plasma cells and, in general, is associated with little fluid exudation.

Because of the pain and swelling, the inflammatory response is often viewed as an unwelcome event following injury. Yet it is important to recognise that it is the first step in the healing process and represents an important protective response in the maintenance of health.

The Immune Response

The immune reaction is one of the most important defence mechanisms against biotic invasion and is therefore vital to the preservation of health. The devastating effects of acquired immune deficiency syndrome (AIDS) and other conditions that suppress or destroy the immune system are cases in point.

The immune response is a relatively recent evolutionary development found only in vertebrates. This complex system has multiple components, which include antigens, antibodies, complement, and various types of white blood cells such as B and T lymphocytes. The interaction of these components collectively results in a reaction that serves to protect the host from the potentially adverse effects of infectious organisms. Antigens are proteins, polysaccharides (complex carbohydrates), or foreign substances that trigger an immune response; they include molecules that are important constituents of bacteria, viruses, and fungi and substances that mark the surfaces of foreign materials such as pollen or transplanted tissue.

Antibodies, or immunoglobulins, are proteins raised against specific antigens; they are formed in the lymph nodes and bone marrow by mature B lymphocytes called plasma cells and are released into circulation to bind and neutralize antigens located throughout the body. This type of response, called humoral immunity, is active mainly against toxins and free pathogens (those not ingested by phagocytes) in body fluids. A second type of response, called cell-mediated immunity, does not yield antibodies but instead generates T lymphocytes that are reactive against specific antigens. This defence is exhibited against bacteria and viruses that have been taken up by the host's cell as well as against fungi, transplanted tissue, and cancer cells. In each case the immune response prevents the invaders from causing further damage to the host. The complement system is a group of proteins found in the blood that facilitates the immune response by both attracting phagocytes to the area of invasion and forming a complex that results in lysis of the foreign cell.

Two remarkable qualities of the immune system are specificity and memory. When an antigen enters the body, it elicits production of either a specific antibody or specific immunologically competent cells; that is, the antibody or the cells will neutralize only the antigen that evokes them. Furthermore, the system exhibits what appears to be memory: once challenged by an antigen, such as the measles virus, the body "remembers" it for years and perhaps for life. The child who has an attack of measles becomes immune for life. If the child is exposed to this specific antigen at a later date, the immune system recognises it and responds and thereby prevents a reinfection. Indeed, these two characteristics of the immune system, specificity and memory, serve as the basis for preventive immunization. Inoculation of infants or children with inactivated or attenuated biotic agents will cause the immune system to be made alert to such an antigen should it appear at a later date. Poliomyelitis, for example, once dreaded as a cause of paralysis and death, has been effectively controlled if not abolished with the polio vaccine.

What has been said will aid in understanding why certain illnesses (such as measles) seem to affect only children. While these viral diseases can affect persons of any age, most adults have had previous exposure to the antigens (viruses) and are thus immune. Children with no previous exposure have no specific immunity to these invaders and consequently develop the diseases. Thus, the immune system is a vital part of the defence against biotic invasion. However, if it malfunctions, the immune system may also cause disease.

Repair and Regeneration

By replacing damaged or destroyed cells with healthy new cells, the processes of repair and regeneration work to restore an individual's health after injury. Unlike the salamander, which is capable of regenerating a limb if it is lost, human beings cannot regenerate whole organs or limbs. If one kidney is destroyed by disease, it is permanently lost. However, the remaining contralateral kidney, if normal, is capable of limited regeneration to compensate for the decrease in kidney mass. The many cell types of the body have varying capacities for regeneration.

Regeneration is the production of new cells exactly like those destroyed. Of the three categories of human cells—(1) the labile cells, which multiply throughout life, (2) the stable cells, which do not multiply continuously but can do so when necessary, and (3) the permanent cells, incapable of multiplication in the adult—only the permanent cells are incapable of regeneration. These are the brain cells and the cells of the skeletal and heart muscles.

Labile cells are those of the bone marrow, the lymphoid tissues, the skin, and the linings of most ducts and hollow organs of the body.

Stable cells are found in the liver, in many of the glands of the body, such as the pancreas and salivary glands, in the lining of the kidney tubules, and in the connective tissues. Normally these cells do not divide unless some are destroyed by disease or injury and must be replaced. If only a small area of the liver (made up of stable cells) is damaged or destroyed, unaffected cells around the area of injury can replace those that were lost. When large areas of the liver are destroyed, however, cellular regeneration cannot occur, and the area of cell loss is replaced by new healthy connective-tissue cells, which produce scars. If a heart attack occurs, a certain number of heart muscle cells (permanent cells) are killed because of loss of blood supply. Because heart muscle cells cannot regenerate, the area of injury is replaced by a scar (if the patient survives). Such repair is by no means perfect, but it nonetheless permits restoration of reasonable heart function with perhaps only a slightly reduced level of health, depending on the number of heart muscle cells that have been lost.

Cellular regeneration in humans is limited by many other factors, such as the availability of blood supply and a supporting connective tissue. When the blood vessels and supporting cells (connective tissue) are destroyed in the liver along with the liver cells, perfect reconstitution of the liver is not possible. There may be some regrowth of liver cells, but they do not form the normal liver architecture, and the newly regenerated cells cannot function because they do not have an appropriate orientation to the blood vessels and bile ducts.

A review of the events that occur after a simple cut in the skin provides a good example of the processes of regeneration. At first, the area becomes red, swollen, and painful because of the inflammatory reaction. A scab forms. Beneath the scab, while the inflammatory process is going on, the cells from the adjacent healthy skin begin to regenerate by dividing and growing over the damaged area. If the damage is minor, perfect reconstruction of the skin and its appendages is likely to result. If the damage has extended below the skin surface, deeper connective-tissue cells, notably the fibroblasts, proliferate and fill the area. These cells lay down collagen (connective-tissue protein) composed of tough, durable fibrils (minute fibres), and, eventually, scar formation ensues. Once scarring has occurred, it cannot be reversed, although considerable shrinking of the scar may occur. If scar formation is limited, total function will return. On the other hand, if scar tissue formation is excessive, it often leads to a loss of function of the part.

Hemostasis

Another mechanism of defence is hemostasis, the prevention of loss of blood from damaged blood vessels by formation of a clot. (This process is covered more at length in the article blood: Bleeding and blood clotting.) Simply stated, a break in a blood vessel leads to activation of a complex sequence of events that results in the formation of a solid plug of platelets, red blood cells, and fibrin (a fibrous protein formed from fibrinogen). This plug, or clot, seals the damaged vessel and prevents further loss of blood (hemorrhage). The numerous components of the blood called clotting factors contribute in sequential fashion to the formation of the clot. (The clotting factors are commonly referred to by a roman numeral rather than by name. Fibrinogen, for example, is clotting factor I.) A defect in one of these factors can undermine hemostasis; for example, the absence of clotting factor VIII leads to hemophilia A, a disorder of uncontrolled bleeding.

Interrelationship of Defencive Mechanisms

The homeostatic and defencive mechanisms involved in maintaining a constant internal environment are complex and yet wonderfully coordinated. Thus, the normal state of health is not a static condition but exists rather within a narrow range maintained by the coordinated responses of many systems and mechanisms. Health requires the proper function of all these controls. Disease may begin in a single organ or system, but the interdependence and close coordination of the many bodily functions, which cooperate so beautifully in health, may be upset by a chain reaction when one breaks down. A disease of the kidney leading to abnormal retention of sodium, for example, can cause hypertension (high blood pressure). Prolonged hypertension in turn can induce heart failure, and this can result in the abnormal collection of fluid in the lungs. The impairment of respiratory function may then result in a sudden rise in the level of carbon dioxide in the blood, which brings with it further complications. Similarly, if the normal inflammatory response malfunctions, a trivial skin infection (popularly known as a pimple) can enlarge into a boil (a furuncle). The responsible bacterial agents may proliferate in the local site and penetrate small blood vessels to seed the bloodstream, thus causing a generalized infection (septicemia or bacteremia). Such a widespread infection is extremely serious and may cause secondary infections of the heart (endocarditis) or of the coverings of the brain (meningitis) and end in death of the host.

Thus, health implies the proper functioning of the homeostatic mechanisms that have just been described, including those systems involved in the defence of health. The state of disease basically represents a failure of these mechanisms. Although one tends to think of disease in terms of offending agents, these agents are able to produce disease only by their ability to disrupt normal homeostasis, and it is precisely those disruptions that are the manifestations of disease.

Disease: Signs and Symptoms

Disease may be acute, chronic, malignant, or benign. Of these terms, chronic and acute have to do with the duration of a disease, malignant and benign with its potentiality for causing death. An acute disease process usually begins abruptly and is over soon. Acute appendicitis, for example, is characterized by the sudden onset of nausea, vomiting, and pain usually localized in the lower right side of the abdomen. It usually requires immediate surgical treatment. The term chronic refers to a process that often begins very gradually and then persists over a long period. For example, ulcerative colitis—an inflammatory condition of unknown cause that is limited to the colon—is a chronic disease. Its peak incidence is early in the second decade of life. The disease is characterized by relapsing attacks of bloody diarrhea that persist for weeks to months. These attacks alternate with asymptomatic periods that can last from weeks to years.

The terms benign and malignant, most often used to describe tumours, can be used in a more general sense. Benign diseases are generally without complications, and a good prognosis (outcome) is usual. A wart on the skin is a benign tumour caused by a virus; it produces no illness and usually disappears spontaneously if given enough time (often many years). Malignancy implies a process that, if left alone, will result in fatal illness. Cancer is the general term for all malignant tumours.

Diseases usually are indicated by signs and symptoms. A sign is defined as an objective manifestation of disease that can be determined by a physician; a symptom is subjective evidence of disease reported by the patient. Each disease entity has a constellation of signs and symptoms more or less uniquely its own; individual signs such as fever, however, may be found in a great number of diseases. Some of the common manifestations of disease—as they relate to an imbalance of normal homeostasis—are taken up in this section. They are covered more at length in the article diagnosis.

Fever is an abnormal rise in body temperature. It is most often a sign of infection but can be present whenever there is tissue destruction, as, for example, from a severe burn or when large amounts of tissue have died because of lack of blood supply. Body temperature is controlled by the thermostatic centre in the hypothalamus. Certain protein and polysaccharide substances called pyrogens, released either from bacteria or viruses or from destroyed cells of the body, are capable of raising the thermostat and causing a rise in body temperature. Fever is a highly significant indicator of disease.

An increase in the number of circulating phagocytic white blood cells (leukocytosis), mentioned above, is one of the more common manifestations of disease. The stimulus for such an event may be any inflammatory process in the body, such as is caused by bacteria, viruses, or any process that leads to the destruction of cells. Such leukocytosis is reflected in the white blood cell count, which may be substantially elevated above the normal upper value of 10,000 cells per cubic millimetre of blood.

The pulse rate is another easily obtainable and important piece of information. The heart rate varies with the level of physical activity: the heart beats faster during exercise and more slowly during rest. An inappropriate heart rate (or pulse) may be indicative of disease. The heart rate increases in the feverish patient. A weak, rapid pulse rate may be a sign of severe blood loss or of disease within the heart itself. Irregularity of the pulse (arrhythmia) is an important indicator of heart malfunction.

The respiratory rate (rate of breathing) is modified by disease. Persons with fever have an increased respiratory rate (hyperventilation), which serves to lower body temperature (this rapid breathing is analogous to the panting of a dog). Hyperventilation is a common response to painful stress. Any condition leading to acidosis (lowering of body pH) similarly drives the respiratory rate upward. Diseases of the lungs—with the accompanying inability to oxygenate the blood adequately—have a similar effect.

Temperature, pulse, and respiratory rate—called the vital signs—may be important manifestations of disease. A fourth vital sign, blood pressure, is equally significant. Among other things, it indicates the amount of blood in circulation. A decrease in circulating blood volume, as is seen with severe bleeding, lowers the blood pressure and deprives the tissues of adequate blood flow. Reflexes are initiated that compensate for the reduced blood volume and blood pressure. The heart rate increases and compensates to some extent for the sudden reduction in blood volume and pressure; at the same time, peripheral blood vessels in such areas as the abdomen constrict, tending to divert the reduced blood volume to the more vital areas such as the brain and head. Unusual elevation of pressure (hypertension) is a disease by itself.

Fluid and electrolyte imbalances may be further consequences of homeostatic failure and additional significant manifestations of disease. The causes of these abnormalities are complex. Edema, or swelling, results from shifts in fluid distribution within body tissues. Edema may be localized, as when the leg veins are narrowed or obstructed by some disease process. The pressure of the blood in the distended veins rises, and fluid is driven out of the vessels into the tissues, causing swelling of the extremity. Generalized edema is seen in renal (kidney) disease that causes abnormal retention of sodium and water. Heart failure is an additional cause of generalized edema, usually most manifest as swollen feet and ankles. Alterations such as dehydration, hyperventilation, and tissue destruction can all lead to varying fluid and electrolyte derangements. The levels of the serum electrolytes (sodium, potassium, bicarbonate, chloride), determined relatively easily in the laboratory, provide the physician with valuable clues to deranged homeostasis induced by disease.

Finally, the determination of body pH and a number of blood tests designed to evaluate adequate (or inadequate) metabolic regulation provide diagnostic clues of homeostatic failure. These tests include determination of the levels of the blood glucose, blood urea nitrogen, and serum protein.

The disease diabetes mellitus provides an excellent example of failure of the homeostatic mechanisms. Diabetes is a common disease of metabolic-endocrine (ductless gland) origin involving a relative or absolute deficiency of insulin, a hormone that plays a major role in carbohydrate metabolism. Any or all of the homeostatic derangements can be found in this disease. Patients with a severe form of diabetes may at one time be dehydrated because of obligatory excretion of water (osmotic diuresis), be acidotic because of formation of increased amounts of keto acids derived from the oxidation of free fatty acids, be hyperventilating as a result of the acidosis, be comatose because of high levels of blood glucose, have a weak pulse because of severe dehydration, have electrolyte abnormalities, and so on. The signs and symptoms are numerous, all illustrating the interdependence of the homeostatic mechanisms, which, when not functioning properly, provide the manifestations of disease.

At the most elemental level, disease develops when any disruptive or adverse influence overcomes the homeostatic and defencive controls of the body. As will be seen, there are numerous influences that can tip the scales of health towards disease. Viruses and bacteria are obvious threats to health. There are a great many others, some so subtle as to be poorly understood. The following section focuses on the causes of disease rather than on a detailed description of each entity. It represents one method of classification. There is considerable overlap in categories; certain diseases grouped as metabolic-endocrine in origin could also be classified as diseases of genetic origin. Indeed, the interdependence of the organ systems, the metabolic pathways, and the defence systems renders finite classification in medicine difficult. The human body acts as a unit—an individual—both in health and in disease.

The Causes of Disease

The search for the causes (etiologies) of human diseases goes back to antiquity. Hippocrates, a Greek physician of the 4th and 5th centuries bce, is credited with being the first to adopt the concept that disease is not a visitation of the gods but rather is caused by earthly influences. Scientists have since continually searched for the causes of disease and, indeed, have discovered the causes of many. In the development of a disease (pathogenesis) more is involved than merely exposure to a causative agent. A room full of people may be exposed to a sufferer from a common cold, but only one or two may later develop a cold. Many host factors determine whether the agent will induce disease or not. Thus, in the pathogenesis of disease, the resistance, immunity, age, and nutritional state of the person exposed, as well as virulence or toxicity of the agent and the level of exposure, all play a role in determining whether disease develops.

In the following sections the many types of human disease will be divided into categories, and in each only a few examples will be given to establish the nature of the process. These categories are divided on the basis of the presumed etiology of the disease. Many diseases are still of unknown (idiopathic) origin. With others the cause may be suspected but not yet definitively proved. In a few instances the discovery of the etiology of a disease represents the individual achievement of a solitary investigator who may have worked many years on the problem; the story of Louis Pasteur and the discovery of the cause of anthrax is a classic example. More often the individual investigator who makes the final breakthrough stands on the shoulders of hundreds of earlier workers who provided bits and pieces of knowledge vital to the final understanding.

Diseases of Genetic Origin

Certain human diseases result from mutations in the genetic complement (genome) contained in the deoxyribonucleic acid (DNA) of chromosomes. A gene is a discrete linear sequence of nucleotide bases (molecular units) of the DNA that codes for, or directs, the synthesis of a protein; there are an estimated 20,000 to 25,000 genes in the human genome. Proteins, many of which are enzymes, carry out all cellular functions. Any alteration of the DNA may result in the defective synthesis and subsequent malfunctioning of one or more proteins. If the mutated protein is a key enzyme in normal metabolism, the error may have serious or fatal consequences. More than 5,000 distinct diseases have been ascribed to mutations that result in deficiencies of critical enzymes.

Mutations are classified on the basis of the extent of the alteration. Large mutations, which include alterations to chromosome structure and number, are relatively rare because most cause such major disruptions to development that the fetus is naturally aborted. However, certain alterations are not so immediately lethal, and the fetus can survive with a characteristic disorder. Down syndrome is one such case. It involves an error in the division of chromosome 21 that results in trisomy (three copies of a chromosome instead of two are inherited), bringing the total number of chromosomes to 47 instead of 46. Many characteristics such as distinctive facial features and mental retardation result from the presence of this extra chromosome. Smaller mutations are more common and include point mutations, in which substitution of a single nucleotide base occurs, and deletion or insertion mutations, which involve several bases. Point, deletion, and insertion mutations may cause an abnormal protein to be synthesized or may prevent the protein from being made at all.

Mutations that occur in the DNA of somatic (body) cells cannot be inherited, but they can cause congenital malformations and cancers; however, mutations that occur in germ cells—i.e., the gametes, ova and sperm—are transmitted to offspring and are responsible for inherited diseases. Each gamete contributes one set of chromosomes and therefore one copy (allele) of each gene to the resultant offspring. If a gene bearing a mutation is passed on, it may cause a genetic disorder.

Genetic diseases caused by a mutation in one gene are inherited in either dominant or recessive fashion. In dominantly inherited conditions, only one mutant allele, which codes for a defective protein or does not produce a protein at all, is necessary for the disorder to occur. In recessively inherited disorders, two copies of a mutant gene are necessary for the disorder to manifest; if only one copy is inherited, the offspring is not affected, but the trait may continue to be passed on to future offspring. In addition to dominant or recessive transmission, genetic disorders may be inherited in an autosomal or X-linked manner. Autosomal genes are those not located on the sex chromosomes, X and Y; X-linked genes are those located on the X chromosomes that have no complementary genes on the Y chromosome. Females have two copies of the X chromosome, but males have an X and a Y chromosome. Because males have only one copy of the X chromosome, any mutation occurring in a gene on this chromosome will be expressed in male offspring regardless of whether its behaviour is recessive or dominant in females. Autosomal dominant disorders include Huntington's chorea, a degenerative disease of the nervous system that usually does not develop until the carrier is between 30 and 40 years of age. The delayed onset of Huntington's chorea allows this lethal gene to be passed on to offspring. Autosomal recessive diseases are more common and include cystic fibrosis, Tay-Sachs disease, and sickle cell anemia. X-linked dominant disorders are rare, but X-linked recessive diseases are relatively common and include Duchenne's muscular dystrophy and hemophilia A.

Most genetic disorders can be detected at birth because the child is born with characteristic defects. Thus these abnormalities are congenital (existing at birth) genetic disorders. A few genetic defects, such as Huntington's chorea mentioned above, do not become manifest until later in life. Hence it may be said that most but not all genetic diseases are congenital.

Conversely, some congenital diseases are not genetic in origin; instead they may arise from some direct injury to the developing fetus. If a woman contracts the viral disease German measles (rubella) during pregnancy, the virus may infect the fetus and alter its normal development, leading to some malformations, principally of the heart. These malformations constitute a congenital disease that is not genetic.

Further confusion often arises over the terms genetic and familial. A familial disease is hereditary, passed on from one generation to the next. It resides in a genetic mutation that is transmitted by mother or father (or both) through the gametes to their offspring. Not all genetic disorders are familial, however, because the mutation may arise for the first time during the formation of the gametes or during the early development of the fetus. Such an infant will have some genetic abnormality, though the parents themselves do not. Down syndrome is an example of a genetic disease that is not familial.

Factors Relating to Genetic Injury

The causes of mutations are still poorly understood. Certain factors, however, are thought to be important. Maternal age plays an important role in predisposing towards genetic injury. The frequency of Down syndrome and of congenital malformations increases with the age of the mother. This may be so for a variety of reasons. Unlike men, who produce new sperm continually, women are born with all the eggs (ova) they will ever have. Thus the eggs are exposed to the same internal and external agents that the woman comes in contact with. The longer the exposure to such factors (i.e., the older the mother), the greater the chance of genetic injury to the ova. A paternal contribution to the disease also has been discovered—roughly 25 percent of cases may be caused by extra chromosomal material from the father. At present, the nature of the factors responsible for impaired division of chromosomes remains unknown.

Radiation is a well-recognised cause of chromosomal damage. The survivors of the atomic bomb blasts in Japan in 1945 have shown definite chromosomal abnormalities in certain types of their circulating white blood cells. Indeed, a higher incidence of leukemia (a form of cancer of white cells), as well as other cancers, has been reported in this population, suggesting that the chromosomal changes may have played some role in the induction of the disease.

Viruses have been shown to cause mutations in human cells when the cells are grown in tissue culture, but there is no clear evidence that viral infections can cause genetic injury in humans. Instead, current evidence suggests that the oncogenic viruses implicated in some human cancers facilitate genetic mutations rather than cause them directly.

The induction of DNA mutations in cells by drugs and chemicals is complex. It involves metabolism of the drug by detoxification enzymes into reactive intermediates that damage DNA. The mutations that remain are those not removed by DNA repair enzymes. In contrast to viruses, drugs and chemicals have been shown to cause mutations not only in human cells in culture but also in a living host.

Heredity and Environment

Diseases can be spread across a wide spectrum, with predominantly genetic diseases at one extreme of the spectrum and diseases of largely environmental origin at the other. In the genetic part of the spectrum are diseases such as Turner's syndrome; in the environmental part are infectious diseases and chemical poisoning. Between these two extremes lie most human diseases—those with both genetic and environmental causative influences that are significant. Indeed, even at the very extreme ends of the spectrum both factors play some role. The genetic constitution dictates in part the host's response to environmental challenges. Similarly, environmental factors play significant roles in the manifestation of genetically induced disease. Sickle cell anemia, for example, an inherited disease characterized by abnormal red blood cells and hemoglobin, is seriously exacerbated by low levels of oxygen in the air.

Furthermore, there are many disorders in which there is a familial tendency to develop the disease but no formal pattern of inheritance has been delineated. Many forms of cancer, high blood pressure, arthritis, and obesity, for example, seem to have a familial tendency.

Although the exact roles of environmental and genetic factors are unknown in all these diseases, it is strongly felt that both factors contribute to the disease process.

Chemical and Physical Injury

Chemical Injury: Poisoning

A poison is any substance that can cause illness or death when ingested in small quantities. This definition excludes the multitude of substances that cause damage if ingested in large quantities. For example, even oxygen and glucose, so crucial to life, are toxic to cells when administered at high concentrations.

There are several considerations to keep in mind when one discusses poisoning. The first of these, as already suggested, is the degree of toxicity. A substance with a very high toxicity (such as cyanide) need be taken only in minute amounts to cause serious harm or death.

A second consideration is the mechanism by which a poison operates. Each poison acts at particular sites in the cell that are critical for the maintenance of homeostasis. These sites include the genome, whose expression dictates cell structure and function, and the cell membrane, which regulates ion transport, energy metabolism, and synthesis of vital proteins. Each poison also has a characteristic ability to cause damage at particular sites within the body, such as the liver, kidneys, or central nervous system.

A third factor is the body's ability to eliminate the substance. Some chemicals, rapidly excreted in the urine, must act quickly while they remain transiently in the body. Others are poorly eliminated, and, because of this, a chronic ingestion of nontoxic amounts leads to a buildup in the body that can reach toxic levels. Lead poisoning is a good example of this phenomenon.

The route of entry is also important. Many substances are harmless when eaten but become deadly if injected into a vein. There are chemicals and drugs that are highly reactive and interact directly with an important cellular component to cause cell injury or death. Other chemicals or drugs that are not toxic per se become so following their metabolic conversion to toxic intermediates by the host. Similarly, the chemical form of a substance affects its action on the body. Metallic mercury, as found in thermometers, is harmlessly excreted, whereas the chloride salt of the same substance is deadly.

Finally, the condition of the host, the recipient of the poison, is an important consideration. A dose of aspirin (acetylsalicylic acid) that is harmless to an adult may be poisonous to an infant. Similarly, an elderly person's tolerance of a substance may be much lower than that of a healthy young adult.

A wide variety of poisons exist, among which a few stand out as being the most commonly encountered in medical practice. Some are of relatively low toxicity but are important because of their widespread use. Many physicians consider aspirin the most dangerous poison because of its commonplace use and abuse and because it is the leading cause of poisoning in children. In the following paragraphs three groups of agents will be presented: (1) organic chemicals, (2) inorganic chemicals, and (3) drugs.

Organic Chemicals

Among the organic chemicals commonly encountered in instances of poisoning are two forms of alcohol, ethyl alcohol (ethanol) and methyl alcohol (methanol). Ethyl alcohol is the form found in most alcoholic beverages. Methyl alcohol, or wood alcohol, is used for a variety of household purposes.

Acute ethyl alcohol poisoning is encountered after ingestion of large quantities over a relatively short time. The alcohol is quickly absorbed from the gastrointestinal tract, and high blood levels can be achieved in a remarkably short time. Ethyl alcohol acts principally as a central-nervous-system depressant and, fortunately, stupor usually results before fatal doses can be reached. The difference in blood levels between intoxication and fatal stupor is very slight, however, and death may result with the ingestion of large quantities of alcohol from depression of the respiratory centre in the brain.

Methyl alcohol is usually ingested either by accident or with suicidal intent. Once inside the body it is metabolized to formic acid, an extremely toxic substance that selects the nerves in the eye as its target. Without treatment, blindness results. Methyl alcohol also can affect the brain tissue itself.

Carbon monoxide is a nonirritating, inert gas without colour, taste, or odour. A poison responsible for a large number of accidental and suicidal deaths, it is one of the chemical products of any combustion of organic material. Inhalation of a 1 percent concentration can be fatal within 10 to 20 minutes. Carbon monoxide acts as an internal asphyxiant causing oxygen starvation of tissues. It should be noted that exposure to even low concentrations can result in the slow accumulation of this poison over hours, days, or weeks, leading very gradually to toxic or fatal levels.

Inorganic Chemicals

The inorganic chemicals most commonly responsible for poisonings in the United States are cyanide, mercury, arsenic, and lead. While the last three often appear in chemical forms that are quite harmless, it is the soluble salts of the substances that are poisons.

Cyanide is a dangerous substance in any form. It may occur in the form of hydrocyanic gas or as solid compounds such as potassium cyanide. It is one of the most lethal poisons known; an amount of 0.2 gram (0.007 ounce) administered to a 70-kilogram (154-pound) human causes death within minutes. Like carbon monoxide, it acts as a cellular asphyxiant.

Mercury in the pure metallic form is rather harmless, but the salt of the same substance, notably mercuric chloride, is a deadly poison. As little as 0.1 gram is enough to cause damage to body tissues, and 2 grams can cause death in a 70-kilogram person. This agent causes extensive tissue damage wherever high concentrations of the poison are encountered. When the substance is swallowed, the stomach represents the portal of entry.

The mercuric chloride is partially absorbed into the blood, and this portion is excreted through the urine. The remainder affects organs in the digestive tract, principally the stomach and the colon, and the kidneys. Mercuric salts cause death of cells by precipitating the proteins within the cells, a form of cell injury called coagulative necrosis. With careful treatment, affected persons survive with full recovery. Chronic ingestion of smaller amounts of mercuric salts, as is seen in some industrial settings, can result in disease involving the mouth, skin, and nervous system.

Arsenic is contained in many items used around the house. Both odourless and tasteless compounds of arsenic are found in some rat poisons, plant sprays, paints, and other household preparations. Many of these household staples are ingested accidentally by children. Principally affected by arsenic are the blood vessels and the central nervous system; vascular collapse and depression of the central nervous system can be followed by coma and death within hours after ingestion.

The soluble salts of inorganic lead are also strong systemic poisons. They may accumulate within the body over a long period until toxic levels are reached and cell damage ensues. These salts were at one time commonly found in paints, and lead poisoning was frequently seen in children who chewed on their painted cribs or woodwork. Legislation in many countries has outlawed the use of lead-base paints for infants' furniture. Other forms of poisoning are incurred through industrial exposure and ingestion of water from lead pipes. Lead poisoning damages red blood cells and leads to hemolysis (rupturing of red blood cells) with resulting anemia. In the brain, lead accumulation causes the degeneration of nerve cells. This produces such manifestations as mental depression, psychoses, convulsions, and even coma and death. If an early fatality does not occur, the lead is slowly excreted and complete recovery may be anticipated.

Drugs

Drugs are another important cause of poisoning. It is a pharmacological principle that, for any therapeutic gain derived from a drug, a price is paid. There are few drugs used today that have no side effects (i.e., effects unintended when the drug is administered). Although these side effects may be harmless and inconsequential, certain drugs have side effects that are potent. Similarly, a drug may be useful in a certain dose range but harmful when larger doses are taken. Morphine, for example, is an excellent drug for the control of severe pain, but it can depress respiration, and too much of it can cause death. All drugs are, therefore, potentially harmful.

Barbiturates and salicylates are the major drugs commonly found to cause serious illness from overingestion. Barbiturates affect the central nervous system almost exclusively. With toxic levels, the vital centres located within the midbrain are depressed; this leads to profound coma, depression of respiration, oxygen starvation of the tissues, and even shock. The identification of barbiturate poisoning relies almost exclusively on finding the substance in the blood or urine, because there is little anatomic change in tissues. Treatment is directed towards getting the drug out of the system as quickly as possible, either by inducing copious urinary excretion of the drug or by the use of the artificial kidney—a process called hemodialysis.

Aspirin, or acetylsalicylic acid, is a drug that deserves special mention because it is such a common household item and often within the reach of small children. Approximately 10 to 30 grams of aspirin can be fatal in adults, and much smaller amounts can be fatal in children. (A single aspirin tablet of standard size contains approximately one-third gram.) There are many signs and symptoms associated with salicylate poisoning, including headaches, drowsiness, dyspepsia, nausea, vomiting, sweating, and thirst. Salicylate poisoning is an acute medical emergency. Rigorous medical treatment is demanded, and use of the artificial kidney is often required.

Physical Injury

Physical injuries include those caused by mechanical trauma, heat and cold, electrical discharges, changes in pressure, and radiation. Mechanical trauma is an injury to any portion of the body from a blow, crush, cut, or penetrating wound. The complications of mechanical trauma are usually related to fracture, hemorrhage, and infection. They do not necessarily have to appear immediately after occurrence of the injury. Slow internal bleeding may remain masked for days and lead to an eventual emergency. Similarly, wound infection and even systemic infection are rarely detectable until many days after the damage. All significant mechanical injuries must therefore be kept under observation for days or even weeks.

Injuries From cold or Heat

Among physical injuries are injuries caused by cold or heat. Prolonged exposure of tissue to freezing temperatures causes tissue damage known as frostbite. Several factors predispose to frostbite, such as malnutrition leading to a loss of the fatty layer under the skin, lack of adequate clothing, and any type of insufficiency of the peripheral blood vessels, all of which increase the loss of body heat.

When the entire body is exposed to low temperatures over a long period, the result can be alarming. At first blood is diverted from the skin to deeper areas of the body, resulting in anoxia (lack of oxygen) and damage to the skin and the tissues under the skin, including the walls of the small vessels. This damage to the small blood vessels leads to swelling of the tissues beneath the skin as fluid seeps out of the vessels. When the exposure is prolonged, it leads eventually to cooling of the blood itself. Once this has occurred, the results are catastrophic. All the vital organs become affected, and death usually ensues.

Burns may be divided into three categories depending on severity. A first-degree burn is the least destructive and affects the most superficial layer of skin, the epidermis. Sunburn is an example of a first-degree burn. The symptoms are pain and some swelling. A second-degree burn is a deeper and hence more severe injury. It is characterized by blistering and often considerable edema (swelling). A third-degree burn is extremely serious; the entire thickness of the skin is destroyed, along with deeper structures such as muscles. Because the nerve endings are destroyed in such burns, the wound is surprisingly painless in the areas of worst involvement.

The outlook in burn injuries is dependent on the age of the victim and the percent of total body area affected. Loss of fluid and electrolytes and infection associated with loss of skin provide the major causes of burn mortality.

Electrical Injuries

The injurious effects of an electrical current passing through the body are determined by its voltage, its amperage, and the resistance of the tissues in the pathway of the current. It must be emphasized that exposure to electricity can be harmful only if there is a contact point of entry and a discharge point through which the current leaves the body. If the body is well insulated against such passage, at the point of either entry or discharge, no current flows and no injury results. The voltage of current refers to its electromotive force, the amperage to its intensity. With high-voltage discharges, such as are encountered when an individual is struck by lightning, the major effect is to disrupt nervous impulses; death is usually caused by interruption of the regulatory impulses of the heart. In low-voltage currents, such as are more likely to be encountered in accidental exposure to house or industrial currents, death is more often due to the stimulation of nerve pathways that cause sustained contractions of muscles and may in this way block respiration. If the electrical shock does not produce immediate death, serious illness may result from the damage incurred by organs in the pathway of the electrical current passing through the body.

Pressure-change Injuries

Physical injuries from pressure change are of two general types: (1) blast injury and (2) the effects of too-rapid changes in the atmospheric pressure in the environment. Blast injuries may be transmitted through air or water; their effect depends on the area of the body exposed to the blast. If it is an air blast, the entire body is subject to the strong wave of compression, which is followed immediately by a wave of lowered pressure. In effect the body is first violently squeezed and then suddenly overexpanded as the pressure waves move beyond the body. The chest or abdomen may suffer injuries from the compression, but it is the negative pressure following the wave that induces most of the damage, since overexpansion leads to rupture of the lungs and of other internal organs, particularly the intestines. If the blast injury is transmitted through water, the victim is usually floating, and only that part of the body underwater is exposed. An individual floating on the surface of the water may simply be popped out of the water like a cork and totally escape injury.

Decompression sickness is a disease caused by a too-rapid reduction in atmospheric pressure. Underwater divers, pilots of unpressurized aircraft, and persons who work underwater or below the surface of the Earth are subject to this disorder. As the atmospheric pressure lessens, dissolved gases in the tissues come out of solution. If this occurs slowly, the gases diffuse into the bloodstream and are eventually expelled from the body; if this occurs too quickly, bubbles will form in the tissues and blood. The oxygen in these bubbles is rapidly dissolved, but the nitrogen, which is a significant component of air, is less soluble and persists as bubbles of gas that block small blood vessels. Affected individuals suffer excruciating pain, principally in the muscles, which causes them to bend over in agony—hence the term "bends" used to describe this disorder.

Radiation Injury

Radiation can result in both beneficial and dangerous biological effects. There are basically two forms of radiation: particulate, composed of very fast-moving particles (alpha and beta particles, neutrons, and deuterons), and electromagnetic radiation such as gamma rays and X-rays. From a biological point of view, the most important attribute of radiant energy is its ability to cause ionization—to form positively or negatively charged particles in the body tissues that it encounters, thereby altering and, in some cases, damaging the chemical composition of the cells. DNA is highly susceptible to ionizing radiation. Cells and tissues may therefore die because of damage to enzymes, because of the inability of the cell to survive with a defective complement of DNA, or because cells are unable to divide. The cell is most susceptible to irradiation during the process of division. The severity of radiation injury is dependent on the penetrability of the radiation, the area of the body exposed to radiation, and the duration of exposure, variables that determine the total amount of radiant energy absorbed.

When the radiation exposure is confined to a part of the body and is delivered in divided doses, a frequent practice in the treatment of cancer, its effect depends on the vulnerability of the cell types in the body to this form of energy. Some cells, such as those that divide actively, are particularly sensitive to radiation. In this category are the cells of the bone marrow, spleen, lymph nodes, sex glands, and lining of the stomach and intestines. In contrast, permanently nondividing cells of the body such as nerve and muscle cells are resistant to radiation. The goal of radiation therapy of tumours is to deliver a dosage to the tumours that is sufficient to destroy the cancer cells without too severely injuring the normal cells in the pathway of the radiation. Obviously, when an internal cancer is treated, the skin, underlying fat, muscles, and nearby organs are unavoidably exposed to the radiation. The possibility of delivering effective doses of radiation to the unwanted cancer depends on the ability of the normal cells to withstand the radiation. However, as is the case in drug therapy, radiation treatment is a two-edged sword with both positive and negative aspects.

Finally, there are probable deleterious effects of radiation in producing congenital malformations, certain leukemias, and possibly some genetic disorders.

Diseases of Immune Origin

The immune system protects against infectious disease, but it may also at times cause disease. Disorders of the immune system fall into two broad categories: (1) those that arise when some aspect of the host's immune mechanism fails to prevent infection (immune deficiencies) and (2) those that occur when the immune response is directed at an inappropriate antigen, such as a noninfectious agent in an allergic reaction, the body's own antigens in an autoimmune response, or the cells of a transplanted organ in graft rejection.

Immune Deficiencies

The immune system may fail to function for many reasons. Many immunodeficiency disorders are caused by a genetic defect in some component of the system and thus usually manifest early in life. Some deficiencies, however, are acquired through the action of infectious agents such as viruses, through the action of immunosuppressive agents used to treat various medical conditions, and through the effects of certain disease processes such as cancer. Both inherited and acquired immune deficiencies suppress one or many aspects of the immune response, rendering the affected individual unable to resist infection unless treated by administration of immunoglobulins or by bone marrow transplant.

Inherited immune disorders undermine the immune response in a variety of ways: B lymphocytes may be unable to produce antibodies, phagocytes may be unable to digest microbes, or specific complement components may not be produced. Severe combined immunodeficiency (SCID), a condition that arises from several different genetic defects, disrupts the functioning of both the humoral and cell-mediated immune responses.

Acquired immune deficiency syndrome (AIDS) is caused by infection with the human immunodeficiency virus (HIV), which destroys a certain type of T lymphocyte, the helper T cell. An infected individual is susceptible to a variety of infectious organisms, including those called opportunistic pathogens, which may live benignly in the human body and cause disease only when the immune system is suppressed. Certain diseases such as Kaposi's sarcoma and *Pneumocystis carinii* pneumonia, which until recently were rarely encountered by clinicians, have become prevalent in the AIDS population and are often the cause of mortality.

Immune Responses in the Absence of Infection

Allergies

The immune system may react to any foreign substance, and consequently it can respond to innocuous materials in the same way that it responds to infectious agents. If the foreign material poses no threat to the individual, an immune response is unnecessary, but it nevertheless may ensue. This misplaced response is called an allergy, or hypersensitivity, and the foreign material is referred to as an allergen. Common allergens include pollen, dust, bee venom, and various foods such as shellfish. What causes one person and not another to develop an allergy is not completely understood.

An allergic response occurs in the following manner. On first exposure to the allergen, the person becomes sensitized to it—that is, develops antibodies and specific T cells to the allergen. An allergic reaction does not usually accompany this initial event. When reexposure occurs, however, symptoms of the allergic response appear. These symptoms range from the mild response of sneezing and a runny nose to the sometimes life-threatening reaction of anaphylaxis, or anaphylactic shock, symptoms of which include vascular collapse and potentially fatal respiratory distress.

Allergic reactions exhibit different symptoms depending on which immune mechanisms are responsible. On the basis of this criterion, they can be categorized into four types, the first three of which involve antibodies and occur in a matter of minutes or hours. Type I hypersensitivity, which occurs immediately after the sensitized person comes in contact again with the allergen, is responsible for most common allergies. The allergen reacts with antibodies attached to the surface of either of two types of cells: mast cells, which are scattered throughout the supporting tissues of the body, and basophilic leukocytes (white blood cells that stain readily with basic dyes), which circulate in the blood. The cells release various substances such as histamine, which causes dilation of blood vessels and contraction of smooth muscles in the bronchial airways, characteristic symptoms of asthma and anaphylaxis. In type II, or cytotoxic, reactions, antibodies are not bound to cells, as in the type I reaction, but circulate freely and interact with cell-bound antigens in the same way that antibodies bind to cells containing infectious agents. Complement is usually activated, leading to cell destruction. A special class of type II hypersensitivity involves an immune response to certain "self" proteins (antigens that belong to the host) on the surface of cells, a mechanism that underlies autoimmune disorders such as autoimmune hemolytic anemia. Type III, or immune-complex, reactions are directed against soluble antigens. Circulating antibodies combine with antigens, usually not bound to the cell surface, to form an immune complex, which is deposited in tissues or the walls of blood vessels.

The complex attracts complement, to which polymorphonuclear leukocytes are drawn. These cells then release powerful enzymes that cause inflammation and vessel damage. Immune complexes also form in autoimmune disorders such as rheumatoid arthritis. Type IV hypersensitivity, unlike the other reactions, does not involve antibodies but instead is mediated by T cells. In these reactions, also called delayed-type because they arise in a matter of days rather than minutes or hours, T cells either activate a local inflammatory reaction, which can cause extensive tissue damage, or they kill tissue cells directly. Chronic inflammation characteristic of many autoimmune disorders, such as chronic thyroiditis, results from this reaction. With the exception of the type I response, all responses are seen in both allergies and autoimmune disorders.

Autoimmune Disorders

Immune responses can be mounted against proteins that belong to the host, giving rise to autoimmune diseases. Although the immune system naturally generates antibodies to its own cells, mechanisms exist to keep this activity in check. Two mechanisms that prevent the immune system from mounting an attack against the host's own tissues have been identified. The first involves the elimination of self-reactive lymphocytes during their development and maturation in the thymus, a lymphoid organ in the chest. Self-reactive lymphocytes present in these cell populations are destroyed when they encounter the self-antigen to which they react. Because this protective selection process is not highly efficient, some self-reactive lymphocytes survive, exit the thymus, and enter the blood and tissues. Outside the thymus a second line of defence against immune self-destruction is afforded in which self-reactive lymphocytes lose their ability to react to self-antigens when they are encountered in blood and tissues. This state is referred to as immunologic ignorance. Autoimmune diseases arise when this mechanism fails and self-reactive lymphocytes are activated by self-antigens in the host's own tissues, often with devastating effects. Systemic lupus erythematosus, thyroiditis, insulin-dependent diabetes mellitus, and rheumatoid arthritis are examples of this type of disorder.

Graft Rejection

Transplantation of organs and cells from one individual to another has become an important medical treatment. As are other forms of therapy, it is accompanied by certain risks. Each individual's cells have a spectrum of genetically determined cell surface protein antigens, the major histocompatibility complex (MHC) antigens, or human leukocyte antigens as they are referred to in humans. MHC antigens determine a person's tissue type just as red blood cell antigens determine blood type. There are two classes of MHC antigens: class I molecules, encoded by three genes, and class II molecules, encoded by four possible sets of genes. Each of these genes has many alternative forms, and thus the probability of any two individuals—aside from siblings, especially identical twins—having the same form of each gene is extremely small. Even parents will have different tissue antigens from their children.

These differences in tissue antigens pose an obstacle to transplantation because it is highly likely that foreign donor tissue will introduce antigens in the recipient that will trigger an immune response leading to tissue death and rejection. However, by careful matching of the MHC type of donor and recipient, rejection can be diminished or avoided. Because perfect matching is possible only between identical twins or very close relatives, many transplants occur between less closely matched tissue types, and success is achieved with the administration of powerful immunosuppressive drugs.

Diseases of Biotic Origin

Factors in Infection

Biotic agents include life-forms that range in size from the smallest virus, measuring approximately 20 nanometres (0.000 000 8 inch) in diameter, to tapeworms that achieve lengths of 10 metres (33 feet). These agents are commonly grouped as viruses, rickettsiae, bacteria, fungi, and parasites. The disease that these organisms cause is only incidental to their struggle for survival. Most of these agents do not require a human host for their life cycles. Many survive readily in soil, water, or lower animal species and are harmless to humans. Other living organisms, which require the temperature range of endothermic (warm-blooded) animals, may flourish on the skin or in the secretions of fluids of the mouth or intestinal tract but do not invade tissue or cause disease under normal conditions. Thus there is a distinction to be made between infection and disease.

All animals are infected with biotic agents. Those agents that do not cause disease are termed nonpathogenic, or commensal. Those that invade and cause disease are termed pathogenic. *Streptococcus viridans* bacteria, for example, are found in the throats of more than 90 percent of healthy persons. In this area they are not considered pathogenic. The same organism cultured from the bloodstream, however, is highly pathogenic and usually indicates the presence of the disease subacute bacterial endocarditis (chronic bacterial invasion of the valves of the heart). In order for such nonpathogenic agents to achieve pathogenicity, they obviously must overcome the defences of the host. Most biotic agents require a portal of entry through the intact skin or mucosal linings of the body. They must be present in sufficient number to escape the phagocytes. They must be capable of surviving the inflammatory and immune response. Ultimately, to induce disease, they must have sufficient virulence and invasiveness to cause significant tissue injury.

Invasiveness and Virulence

Invasiveness is the capability of penetrating and spreading throughout tissues. Remarkably, little is known of the factors that condition it. In a few instances enzymes produced by biotic agents have been identified that are capable of breaking down the integrity of the supporting tissues of the body, thereby preparing a pathway for the spread of the organism.

Only very few bacteria release such enzymes, however, and there are marked differences in invasiveness to be found among the various types of bacteria. The organism that causes diphtheria (*Corynebacterium diphtheriae*), for example, is capable of invading only the surface cells of the mouth and throat. The disease that results is caused by the production of a powerful exotoxin (a chemical substance produced by the organism and released into the surrounding tissues) that is absorbed into the bloodstream from the local infection within the throat. This exotoxin causes major damage in the heart and the nervous system. The diphtheria bacillus, therefore, is an example of a serious infection in which the organism has low invasiveness. In contrast, the bacterium that causes syphilis (*Treponema pallidum*) has a high degree of invasiveness. It is one of the rare biotic agents that are capable of penetrating intact skin and mucosal linings of the body.

The invasiveness of viruses undoubtedly is facilitated by their extremely small size, but, because of this size, the exact mechanism is difficult to study. In the case of fungi and parasites, the invasiveness is related to the life cycle of the organism. The formation of tiny spores by fungi and the smaller reproductive forms of the parasites provide vehicles by which infection may be drawn into the lungs or may pass through tiny defects in the skin or mucosal linings of the various openings and tracts of the body.

In general, virulence is the degree of toxicity or the injury-producing potential of a microorganism. The words virulence and pathogenicity are often used interchangeably. The virulence of bacteria usually relates to their capability of producing a powerful exotoxin or endotoxin. Invasiveness also adds to an organism's virulence by permitting it to spread.

Predisposition of the Host

Up to this point, diseases caused by biotic agents have been considered in terms of the role of the invader. Equally important is the role of the host, the individual who contracts the disease. Any infectious disease is a test between the invader and the defender. Virulent organisms may be capable of inducing serious illness even in the most robust. The converse is perhaps more important. The weak host is prey to many forms of biotic infection, even those of low virulence and invasiveness. Some of the more important of the many factors that condition the level of resistance to biotic infection in the individual are age, with infancy and old age being times of maximum vulnerability; poor nutrition; genetic disorders and immunosuppressive agents, such as the human immunodeficiency virus, that compromise the immunologic system; and metabolic disorders such as diabetes that increase vulnerability to infectious agents.

Therapeutic agents, paradoxically, also have become important factors in predisposing to disease of biotic origin and indeed in altering the incidence patterns of infectious disease. The drugs that are principally involved include those used to suppress the immune response, as well as the host of antimicrobial and antibiotic agents now employed in the treatment of infectious disease. Immunosuppressive drugs are used to block the immune response in patients about to receive an organ transplant and in the treatment of the autoimmune diseases, but such treatment renders the patient vulnerable to attack by biotic agents. Indeed, these immunologically compromised persons become susceptible to organisms of extremely low virulence.

Antimicrobial drugs also have drawbacks as well as benefits. A patient suffering from a streptococcal disease, for example, may appropriately be treated with penicillin. Certain strains of staphylococci, however, are resistant to penicillin. Although the streptococcal organisms, as well as other commensals, may be eradicated by the antibiotic, the resistant staphylococci begin to proliferate, possibly because the competition with other bacteria for nutrients and food supply has been removed. In this noncompetitive situation they may cause disease. More powerful antibiotics may destroy all bacteria, including staphylococci, but permit the unrestrained proliferation of fungi and other agents of low virulence that are nonetheless resistant to the antibiotic. Thus antibiotics have changed the entire frequency pattern of biotic disease. Organisms that have proved to be more resistant to antibiotics have become the more common causes of serious clinical infection. For this reason certain forms of drug-resistant bacteria that include *Escherichia coli*, *Aerobacter aerogenes*, *Pseudomonas aeruginosa*, and strains of *Proteus* as well as fungi have emerged as the important biotic causes of death.

Viral Diseases

Of the many existing viruses, a few are of great importance as causes of human sickness. They are responsible for such diseases as smallpox, poliomyelitis, encephalitis, influenza, yellow fever, measles, and mumps and such minor disorders as warts and the common cold.

Viruses may survive for some time in the soil, in water, or in milk, but they cannot multiply unless they invade or parasitize living cells. Certain viruses proliferate within the host cells and accumulate in sufficient number to cause rupture and death of the cells. Others multiply within the cell body and compete with the host for nutrition or vital constituents of the cell's metabolism. Both types of viruses are said to be cytotoxic.

Viral agents, particularly those capable of producing tumours in humans and lower animals, flourish within cells and stimulate the cells to active growth. These viruses are referred to as oncogenic (tumour-producing). The number of oncogenic viruses that cause tumours in lower animals is large. In humans, several DNA viruses and one RNA virus have been implicated strongly in the induction of a variety of tumours.

Most viral infections occur in childhood. This age distribution has been explained on immunologic grounds. Viruses usually induce a firm and enduring immunity. On first exposure to a virus, children may or may not contract the disease, depending on their resistance, the size of the infective dose of virus, and many other variables. Those who contract the disease, as well as those who resist the infection, develop a permanent immunity to any further exposure. By either pathway, as children grow older they progressively gather protection against viral infections. Consequently, the incidence of these infections falls in adulthood and later life. The frequency of common colds is explained on the grounds that a host of different viral agents all induce similar respiratory infections, and, while a single attack confers immunity against the specific causative agent, it provides no protection against the rest.

Viral diseases are resistant to antibiotics and other antimicrobial agents. This point is made because of a distressing tendency among individuals to take penicillin or another antibiotic for a common cold.

Rickettsial Diseases

Human rickettsial diseases are caused by microorganisms that fall between viruses and bacteria in size. These minute agents are barely visible under the ordinary light microscope. Like viruses, they multiply only within the cells of susceptible hosts. They are found in nature in a variety of ticks and lice and, when transmitted to humans by the bite of one of these arthropods, usually cause acute febrile (fever-producing) illnesses, most of which are characterized by skin rashes. Rocky Mountain spotted fever, a systemic rickettsial infection, invades and kills the cells lining blood vessels and causes hemorrhage, inflammation, blood clots, and extensive tissue death; if untreated, it is fatal in about 20 to 30 percent of cases.

Bacterial Diseases

The diseases produced by bacteria are the most common of infectious biotic diseases. They range from trivial skin infections to such devastating disorders as bubonic plague and tuberculosis. Various types of pneumonia; infections of the cerebrospinal fluid (meningitis), the liver, and the kidneys; and the sexually transmitted diseases syphilis and gonorrhea are all forms of bacterial infection.

All bacteria induce disease by one of three methods: (1) the production of an exotoxin, a harmful chemical substance that is secreted or excreted by the bacterium (as in food poisoning caused by *Clostridium botulinum*), (2) the elaboration of an endotoxin, a harmful chemical substance that is liberated only after disintegration of the micro-organism (as in typhoid, caused by *Salmonella typhi*), or (3) the induction of sensitivity within the host to antigenic properties of the bacterial organism (as in tuberculosis, after sensitization to *Mycobacterium tuberculosis*).

Fungi and Other Parasites

Diseases caused by fungi and parasites are relatively uncommon in developed countries. Fungal infections, also known as mycotic infections, may affect the skin surfaces or the internal organs of the body. The superficial mycotic infections are generally not serious and include such well-known disorders as athlete's foot (tinea pedis), caused by the dermatophyte *Trichophyton*. Deep mycotic infections such as histoplasmosis and candidiasis are potentially life-threatening.

Other parasites that attack humans range in size from unicellular organisms such as *Entamoeba histolytica* to such multicellular forms as tapeworms and roundworms. Most parasitic infestations are encountered in the less-developed areas of the world where sanitation is not optimal. Indeed, parasitic infestations constitute major causes of death in regions of Central and South America, Africa, India, and Asia.

Abnormal Growth of Cells

Normal and Abnormal Cell Growth

Cell Growth Inhibition: The growth of cells in the body is a closely controlled function, which, together with limited and regulated expression of various genes, gives rise to the many different tissues that constitute the whole organism. For the most part, control of cell growth persists throughout life except for episodic instances such as healing of an injured tissue. In this situation the growth of a localized group of cells is accelerated to reconstitute the tissue to its previous state of normal structure and function, following which tightly regulated growth resumes. Such areas of increased cell growth are referred to as hyperplasias; they consist of expanded numbers of normal-appearing cells and, depending on the duration of growth, can result in an enlargement of tissues and organs. In general, hyperplasias arise to meet special needs of the body and subside once these needs are met. Hyperplasias are the result of the sustained impact over time of stimulatory influences together with a loss of growth-inhibitory factors that are normally found within or around cells. As long as the loss of inhibition of cell growth is temporary, the capacity for enhanced cell proliferation when necessary has obvious advantages. However, if cells permanently lose their ability to respond to growth-inhibitory factors, their growth becomes irrepressible, and cancer may result.

Neoplasms: Malignant and Benign Tumours: Diseases arising from uncontrolled cell growth and behaviour collectively constitute the second most common cause of human death (the most common cause being heart disease). Cancers, the most important form of abnormal growth and behaviour, were responsible for approximately 538,000 deaths, or almost one-fourth of all deaths, in the United States in 1994. The significance of this incidence is placed in proper perspective by a consideration of the following facts. While cancer arises at all stages of life, its incidence (number of cases) increases with age, reaching a peak between 55 and 74 years. This fact, together with the increasing longevity of the general population and improved diagnostic modalities that enable clinicians to detect cancers with greater frequency, tempers the notion that the incidence of cancer is increasing.

In addition to cancers—malignant tumours that may eventually kill the host—there are benign tumours that rarely produce serious disease. The two types of tumours are collectively referred to as neoplasms (new growths), and their study is known as oncology. Tumours are referred to as malignant or benign based on the structural and functional properties of their component cells and their biological behaviour. The cells and tissues of malignant tumours differ from the tissues from which they arise. They exhibit more rapid growth and altered structure and function, including stimulation of new blood vessel growth (angiogenesis) and a capacity to invade adjacent normal tissues, enter the blood vascular system, and spread (metastasize) to distant sites. The properties of malignant tumour cells serve to enhance and support their proliferation and extension throughout the body tissues and organs, eventually leading to death of the host.

In contrast, the cells and tissues of benign tumours tend to grow more slowly and in general closely resemble their normal tissues of origin. When the structure and function of benign tumour cells are morphologically and functionally indistinguishable from those of normal cells, their growth as a tumour mass is the sole feature indicative of their neoplastic nature. It is hoped that a greater understanding of malignant cell growth and behaviour will lead to the development of novel cancer therapies based on tumour cell biology that will complement or replace the current treatments of surgical extirpation (complete excision), chemotherapy, and radiation.

Characteristics of Cancer

Epidemiology

Epidemiological studies of the worldwide incidence of cancers have identified striking differences among countries and population groups. For example, the incidence of and death rates for skin cancer are much higher in Australia and New Zealand than in the Scandinavian countries—presumably because of the marked differences between these two regions in total annual hours of exposure to sunlight. The importance of environmental influences is highlighted by comparing the incidence of and death rates for cancers among populations in different geographic regions. For example, prostate and colon cancer rates in Japanese persons living in Japan differ from the rates in Japanese persons who have emigrated to the United States, the rates of their offspring born in California, and the rates of long-term white residents of that state. These rates are much lower among Japanese living in Japan than they are in white Californians. However, the rates for each type of tumour among first-generation Japanese immigrants are intermediate between the rates in Japan and those in California, suggesting that environmental and cultural factors may play a more important role than genetic ones.

The Role of Genetics

The irreversibility of the structural and behavioural changes of cancer cells has long been recognised and has favoured the postulate that they are probably due to permanent genetic alterations. This postulate remained speculative until the discovery in 1979 that oncogenes (cancer-causing genes) are derived from proto-oncogenes (normal growth-regulatory cellular genes). When proto-oncogenes become mutated or deregulated, they are converted to oncogenes, which are capable of causing the malignant transformation of cells, including those of humans. Cellular proto-oncogenes code for proteins involved in cell regulation, such as growth factors, their receptors, and transmembrane signal transducers.

Thus, changes in the structure of proto-oncogenes and their conversion to oncogenes results in the synthesis of abnormal proteins that are incapable of carrying out their usual growth-regulatory functions. In identifying the genes involved in the development of cancer, researchers discovered a group of cellular genes—tumour-suppressor, or suppressor, genes—whose protein products normally negatively regulate cell growth by suppressing cell proliferation, thus counterbalancing the growth-stimulatory effects of proteins synthesized by proto-oncogenes. Genetic analyses of various animal and human cancers have demonstrated that, in the majority, alterations of oncogenes and suppressor genes were often simultaneously present. These analyses suggest that multiple genetic alterations involving growth-stimulatory and growth-inhibitory genes are required for the induction of malignancy. Such discoveries have ushered in a new era in cancer biology and may well lead to the eventual control, cure, and prevention of malignant diseases.

Heredity and Environment

The many causes of cancer include intrinsic factors, such as heredity, and extrinsic factors, such as environment and lifestyle. Hereditary causes of cancer are less common and are due to the inheritance of a single mutant gene that greatly increases the risk of developing a malignant tumour. Such cancers include

(1) a childhood tumour of the eye, retinoblastoma, and a bone tumour, osteosarcoma, both of which involve the loss of a tumour suppressor gene, and

(2) familial adenomatous polyposis, in which all patients develop colon cancer by age 50.

The most common types of cancer that occur sporadically, such as cancers of the breast, ovary, colon, and pancreas, also have been documented to occur in familial forms. The children in such families appear to have a two- to threefold increased risk of developing a particular tumour, but the transmission pattern is unclear. A still rarer hereditary cause of cancer is an inherited deficiency in the ability to repair DNA. Patients with this defect (known as xeroderma pigmentosum) are particularly sensitive to sunlight and develop skin cancer during early adolescence because of unrepaired mutations induced by ultraviolet (UV) light.

Although the environment contains many agents that can cause cancer in humans, the extent to which they contribute to the human disease is often difficult to assess. For example, the link between tobacco smoking and lung cancer is clear; however, little is known about the cause of cancer of the prostate, the most common form of cancer in males, despite the fact that many factors—including age, race, male hormone, increased consumption of dietary fat, and a genetic basis—have been implicated.

Three categories of carcinogens (chemical or physical agents that mutate DNA) that induce cancer in experimental animals and humans have been identified in the environment: (1) chemicals, (2) radiant energy, and (3) oncogenic viruses.

Carcinogenic Agents

Chemicals

Chemicals capable of causing cancer arise from a variety of sources. These include certain synthetic chemicals used in industry, some natural compounds formed during the curing and burning of tobacco, compounds formed during the cooking of meat, and chemicals present in certain plants and molds. Two categories have been identified, those capable of causing DNA damage and mutations directly (genotoxic, or direct-acting, carcinogens) and those that require prior metabolic activation by cells of the host to be converted to mutagens (epigenic, or indirect-acting, carcinogens). In the industrial countries much progress has been made in significantly decreasing and preventing exposure to chemical carcinogens in the workplace. However, exposure to carcinogens as a consequence of cultural practices, such as tobacco smoking and the cooking and consumption of meats, is difficult if not impossible to control or eradicate.

Radiant Energy

Sustained exposure to two forms of radiant energy—namely, UV light and ionizing radiation—is carcinogenic for humans. Repeated and sustained exposure to UV rays emanating from the Sun causes mutations of DNA that ultimately are capable of inducing three different types of skin cancer. As one would expect, the incidence of UV-induced skin cancer is high among farmers, sailors, and sunbathing enthusiasts. The degree of risk depends on the extent of exposure and the amount of melanin pigment in the skin, which absorbs UV rays. Dark-skinned individuals are protected by the high content of melanin in their skin; in contrast, fair-skinned persons and albinos have very little or no protective melanin pigment in their skin.

The carcinogenic effects of ionizing radiation first became apparent from the results of inappropriate exposure of early uranium ore miners and of physicians who first used X-ray machines for diagnostic purposes and were unaware of the health hazards. The devastating complications that resulted are rare today because of stricter indications for the use of radiation therapy, careful focusing of radiation beams, and effective shielding of adjacent normal tissues. However, the risks of exposure to ionizing radiation have been re-emphasized from time to time by the appearance of neoplastic disease following radiation therapy and following the release of enormous amounts of radiation into the environment, as occurred from atomic bombing of Hiroshima and Nagasaki in Japan and the accident at the Chernobyl nuclear power station in Ukraine.

Reactive forms of carcinogenic chemicals and, in the case of ionizing radiation, reactive forms of oxygen damage DNA directly. If repair of damaged DNA is slow, error-prone, or not accomplished at all and cell replication occurs, the damage is amplified and becomes a permanent (fixed) mutation.

Viruses

In recent years certain DNA viruses have been strongly implicated as causal agents for a variety of cancers in humans. These include human papillomavirus (HPV) as a cause of genital cancers in both sexes worldwide, the Epstein-Barr virus (EBV) for childhood lymphoma in Africa and cancer of the nose and throat in Asia and Africa, and the hepatitis viruses B and C that cause liver cancer worldwide with the highest incidence in Asia and Africa. However, at present only one type of human cancer, the rare adult T-cell leukemia, has been solidly linked to infection with an RNA virus, the human T-cell leukemia virus (HTLV-1). While much experimental and clinical evidence supports the carcinogenic role of the above-mentioned viruses in humans, additional research suggests that other factors also may be required.

Observations that support the multifactorial nature of viral carcinogenesis include the continuous but not neoplastic growth of human cells infected in culture with HPV, the restricted geographic distribution of cancers induced by EBV, and the lack of either an oncoprotein (protein product produced by an oncogene) for HBV or evidence of consistent integration of the virus near a proto-oncogene encoding for a growth-regulatory protein. Thus far, oncogenic viruses have not been shown to induce DNA mutations directly in human cells; rather, their contribution seems to lie in promoting and hastening the process of mutation.

Diseases of Metabolic-endocrine Origin

The term metabolism encompasses all the chemical reactions vital to the growth and maintenance of the body. Defects in metabolism are found in almost every disease condition. Most are secondary; i.e., they result from some other basic disorder (infection, kidney disease, or heart disease, for example). In a few primary metabolic disorders, small genetic mutations lead to structural alterations of specific proteins that disrupt protein function and are responsible for the disease state. At this point, another group of primary metabolic disorders—those associated with hormonal defects—will be touched on.

Hormones are large organic molecules secreted in small amounts by specific cells in the various endocrine (ductless) glands. These secretions are carried by the blood to distant sites (target organs), where they bind to specific receptors on target cells and act to regulate specific chemical reactions.

All endocrine disease stems from either an overproduction (hyperfunction) or underproduction (hypofunction) of some hormone-secreting endocrine gland. There are relatively few causes of hormone overproduction. In general, overproduction results from hyperplasia, an increase in the number of cells (in this case, hormone-secreting cells) in a specific endocrine gland. It can also be caused by neoplasia, the growth of a tumour in an endocrine gland. Although most endocrine tumours are benign, the resulting hypersecretion of hormone can have far-reaching effects. For example, the pituitary gland, tucked into the base of the skull, produces many hormones that have far-ranging effects, mostly controlling the function of the other endocrine glands, such as the thyroid, adrenals, ovaries, and testes.

Acromegaly, characterized by the enlargement of many skeletal parts, is a rare endocrine disease caused by excess secretion of pituitary growth hormone in the adult. An example of hormone overproduction because of hyperplasia is hyperthyroidism, the disease produced by an excess of thyroid hormone. It is characterized by a rapid pulse, increased sweating, weight loss, heat intolerance, and frequent disturbances in the heart rhythm. Cushing's syndrome, an exception to the generalization that hypersecretion of hormones is due to either neoplasia or hyperplasia, results from an overproduction of the adrenal steroid hormones (such as cortisol). Although the disease is occasionally caused by tumours or by hyperplasia of the adrenals, in most instances it is not. It has been suggested that the disease results from excessive adrenocorticotropic hormone (ACTH) from the pituitary; in rare cases when the level of ACTH is not elevated, it is thought that autoantibodies to ACTH receptors cause the hyperplasia.

Underproduction of hormone is most often the result of destruction of hormone-secreting cells. This destruction may be caused by infection, infarction (tissue death due to loss of blood supply), or obliteration of endocrine glands by cancer. Underproduction of hormone also may result from failure of the gland to undergo normal fetal development, or it may be a feature of an autoimmune disease (as in juvenile diabetes mellitus).

Treatment of endocrine disease involves either hormone supplementation, in the case of hypofunction, or, in cases of hyperfunction, destruction of endocrine gland tissue by surgery or radiation.

Diseases of Nutrition

Diseases of nutrition include the effects of undernutrition, prevalent in less-developed areas but present even in affluent societies, and the effects of nutritional excess.

Diseases of Nutritional Excess

Obesity, perhaps the most important nutritional disease in the United States and Europe, results usually from excessive caloric intake, although emotional, genetic, and endocrine factors may be present.

Obesity predisposes one towards several serious disorders, including a state of chronic oxygen deficiency called the hypoventilation syndrome; high blood pressure; and atherosclerosis, a degenerative condition of the blood vessels that is discussed further below.

Excessive intake of certain vitamins, especially vitamins A and D, can also produce disease. Vitamins A and D are both fat-soluble and tend to accumulate to toxic levels in the bodily tissues when taken in excessive quantities. Vitamin C and the B vitamins, soluble in water, are more easily metabolized or excreted and, therefore, rarely accumulate to toxic levels.

Diseases of Nutritional Deficiency

Nutritional deficiencies may take the form of inadequacies of (1) total caloric intake, (2) protein intake, or (3) certain essential nutrients such as the vitamins and, more rarely, specific amino acids (components of proteins) and fatty acids.

Protein-calorie malnutrition remains prevalent in certain areas. It has been estimated that about two-thirds of the world's population has less than enough food to eat. Not only is the quantity inadequate but the quality of the food is nutritionally deficient and usually lacks protein. In deprived areas malnutrition has its greatest impact on the young. Deaths from protein-calorie malnutrition result from the failure of the child to thrive, with progressive weight loss and weakness, which in turn can lead to infection and disease, usually some form of gastrointestinal bacterial or parasitic disorder. In other circumstances adequate calories may be available, but a deficiency of protein induces a disorder known as kwashiorkor.

Vitamin deficiencies, the most important forms of selective malnutrition, may arise in a variety of ways, the most common and the most important being an improper, inadequate diet. When the total caloric intake is inadequate, vitamin deficiencies may also occur, but in these circumstances the more profound lack of calories and proteins masks the lack of vitamins.

Vitamin deficiencies may also be encountered despite a diet that is apparently adequate nutritionally. One source of such a deficiency, called secondary, is interference with absorption of the vitamin. Pernicious anemia is a classic example of this phenomenon. This disorder results from an autoimmune response to intrinsic factor, a substance normally found in the stomach lining with which vitamin B_{12} must form a complex to be absorbed. (Vitamin B_{12} is necessary for red cells to form properly.) The basis of pernicious anemia, then, is a lack of absorption of vitamin B_{12}. The absence of certain digestive enzymes, as is found in pancreatic disease, can lead to the inability to digest and absorb fats and the fat-soluble vitamins (A, D, E, and K). Impaired uptake of vitamins may be encountered in gastrointestinal diseases. Some of these diseases reduce the absorptive function of the bowel. Similarly, diseases associated with severe, prolonged vomiting may interfere with adequate absorption.

Avitaminosis (vitamin lack) may be encountered when there are increased losses of vitamins such as occur with chronic severe diarrhea or excessive sweating or when there are increased requirements for vitamins during periods of rapid growth, especially during childhood and pregnancy. Fever and the endocrine disorder hyperthyroidism are two additional examples of conditions that require higher than the usual levels of vitamin intake. Unless the diet is adjusted to the increased requirements, deficiencies may develop. Lastly, artificial manipulation of the body and its natural metabolic pathways, as by certain surgical procedures or the administration of various drugs, can lead to avitaminoses. (Diseases involving deficiencies of particular vitamins are discussed in nutrition: Deficiency diseases: Vitamins.)

Diseases of Neuropsychiatric Origin

Diseases of neuropsychiatric origin afflict large segments of the population. For example, a total of about 2.8 million persons in the United States suffer from three major psychiatric diseases—schizophrenia, major depression, and mania—and three major neurological disorders—Alzheimer's disease, Huntington's chorea, and Parkinson's disease. These six conditions will be briefly reviewed here. More in-depth coverage is found in the articles mental disorder and nervous system disease.

The key function of the nervous system is to collect information about the body and its external environment, process the information, and coordinate the body's responses to that information. This complex function depends on each nerve cell (neuron) receiving signals from other neurons and transmitting this input to still other neurons. This critical input and output of communication (signalling) between neurons is mediated by chemical transmitter molecules (neurotransmitters). Neurotransmitters are synthesized by nerve cells and released from one cell to another across a narrow gap between the two neurons known as the synapse. Eight different major neurotransmitters and a large number of neuropeptide molecules (which serve to modulate the effects of neurotransmitters) have been identified. Different types of nerve cells respond to different neurotransmitters and neuropeptides. Chemical signalling between nerve cells is rapid and precise and can occur over long distances. The precision is due to receptor molecules, which are activated following their recognition and binding of specific neurotransmitters. In some types of nerves the synapses do not possess receptors, in which case interneuronal communication is achieved by electrical transmission. In many neuropsychiatric diseases alterations in the levels of transmitter substances appear to play a major role in pathogenesis.

Psychiatric Diseases

Mental illnesses affect the very fabric of human nature, robbing it of its various facets of personality, purposeful behaviour, abstract thinking, creativity, emotion, and mood. Those suffering from mental disorders exhibit a spectrum of symptoms depending on the severity of their disease. These diseases include obsessive-compulsive personality disorder, dementia, schizophrenia, major depression, and manic disorders.

Schizophrenia in its severe form is a catastrophic mental illness that begins in adolescence or early adult life. It is relatively common, occurring in about 1 percent of the general population worldwide. Because the incidence of schizophrenia among parents, children, and siblings of patients with the disease is increased to 15 percent, it is believed that heredity plays an important role in the genesis of the disease. However, other studies suggest that nongenetic factors are also influential. The biochemical basis of the disease may be an excess of the neurotransmitter substance dopamine, as high levels of dopamine and its metabolites, as well as increased dopamine receptors, are found in the brains of persons with schizophrenia. Further evidence for this hypothesis is that the drugs most effective in treating the disease are those that have a high capacity to block dopamine receptors.

Pathological disturbances of mood, ranging from severe depression to manic behaviour, are common forms of mental illnesses. Severe depression is characterized by despondency, diminished interest in most or all activities, weight fluctuation not due to dieting, disruption in sleep patterns, psychomotor agitation or retardation, feelings of worthlessness, excessive quiet, and recurrent thoughts of death or suicide. Manic behaviour involves a period in which an expansive, elevated, or irritable mood persists abnormally. During this episode symptoms such as increased talkativeness, distractibility, decreased need for sleep, inflated self-esteem, and excessive involvement in pleasurable yet risky activities may be present. Major depression is associated with decreased brain levels of the neurotransmitters norepinephrine and serotonin, and the most effective therapy consists of drugs that inhibit the breakdown of these compounds. The neurochemical alterations in mania are less clearly understood, but it is well established that drugs effective in the treatment of mania are those that antagonize dopamine and serotonin. The mechanism responsible for the therapeutic efficacy of lithium for the treatment of mania is not yet clear. Although mood disorders have a familial background, the evidence for a genetic component is not convincing.

Neurological Diseases

The three neurological diseases considered in this section—Alzheimer's disease, Huntington's chorea, and Parkinson's disease—are age-related, and to varying degrees they manifest as deterioration of mental function that involves the loss of memory and of acquired intellectual skills. This deterioration is referred to as dementia. Because dementia can result from many causes, other features of each disease must be present before a definitive diagnosis can be made.

Alzheimer's Disease

Alzheimer's disease is the most common form of dementia, being responsible for about two-thirds of the cases of dementia in patients over 60 years of age. Women are affected twice as often as men. More rarely there are familial forms of the disease that have an early onset affecting individuals in the fourth and fifth decades of life. Alzheimer's disease is insidious in onset. Early manifestations include memory loss, temporary confusion, restlessness, poor judgement, and lethargy. A failure to retain new information and a deterioration of social relationships often ensue. In some patients paranoia and delusions, which worsen during the night, are the first symptoms of the disease. Whatever the onset, the last stages are characterized by intellectual vacuity and loss of control over all body functions.

The brains of patients with Alzheimer's disease are characterized by the loss of neurons, which, as the disease progresses, becomes severe and leads to decreased brain size and weight. Because nerve cells synthesize the neurotransmitters necessary for interneuronal communication, it is not surprising that Alzheimer's disease is associated with diminished levels of neurotransmitters, including acetylcholine, norepinephrine, and serotonin, as well as modulatory neuropeptide molecules that transmit signals between nerve cells. Two other characteristic tissue lesions found in the cerebral cortex of patients with Alzheimer's disease are neuritic plaques and neurofibrillary tangles. Neuritic plaques are deposits of neuron fragments surrounding a core of amyloid β-protein. Neurofibrillary tangles are twisted fibres of the protein tau found within neurons.

A variety of genetic factors have been identified in the different forms of Alzheimer's disease. The rare cases of the early familial forms of the disease are linked to three different genetic defects found on three different chromosomes—chromosomes 1, 14, and 21. Another gene on chromosome 19 is believed to play a part in the more common late-onset cases. The gene on chromosome 21 was the first to be identified. (This finding is significant because an abnormality in chromosome 21—an extra copy—is found in patients with Down syndrome, virtually all of whom develop Alzheimer's disease if they live to age 35.) The defective gene on chromosome 21 normally codes for amyloid precursor protein. A defect in this gene is thought to result in abnormal cleavage of the protein that increases the production and deposition of amyloid β-protein. This gene, however, is linked to only 2 to 3 percent of all early familial cases of the disease. The majority of patients with early-onset disease—70 to 80 percent—have the genetic mutation on chromosome 14, and another group of patients have a defective gene on chromosome 1. The gene on chromosome 19 codes for apolipoprotein E, a protein involved in cholesterol transport and metabolism. Three forms, or alleles, of the gene exist. The presence of one form—ApoE4—in an individual's genome seems to increase the deposition of amyloid β-protein in the brain and may also increase the number of neurofibrillary tangles.

Huntington's Chorea

Huntington's chorea occurs at the rate of about 5 per 100,000 individuals. It affects both sexes equally and usually becomes manifest in the fourth decade of life. The disorder is characterized by uncontrolled movements (chorea), dementia, and death within 20 years after onset. The symptoms worsen until the patient becomes totally incapacitated and bedridden. Huntington's chorea is a hereditary disease passed on as an autosomal dominant trait. Because of its highly regular familial inheritance, the disease is often traceable to the original carriers who introduced the defective gene. For example, British immigrants to colonial America in the 17th century are believed to be responsible for almost all cases of Huntington's chorea in the eastern United States, and an English sailor is thought to have introduced the defective gene into Venezuela almost 200 years ago. The recent localization of the Huntington's chorea gene to chromosome 4 and its cloning will allow identification of the gene product, insight into the mechanism responsible for the disease, and perhaps effective treatment. It will also permit the disease to be diagnosed in fetuses as well as in children before the onset of symptoms.

Parkinson's Disease

Parkinson's disease is a motor disorder characterized by the onset of a "pill rolling" rhythmic tremor, muscle rigidity, difficulty and slowness in movement, and stooped posture. As the disease progresses, the face of the patient becomes expressionless, the rate of swallowing is reduced, leading to drooling, and depression and dementia increase. The prevalence of Parkinson's disease is estimated to be about 160 per 100,000 persons in the general population, with about 16 to 19 new cases per 100,000 appearing each year. Men are slightly more affected than women, and there are no apparent racial differences. The disease appears typically in the sixth and seventh decades, although occasionally it can begin as early as the third decade. Parkinson's disease has no known cause. A marked decrease in the level of dopamine, a major neurotransmitter, has been noted in the brains of patients with Parkinson's disease, and this change has been attributed to the loss of so-called dopaminergic neurons that normally synthesize and use dopamine to communicate with other neurons in parts of the brain that regulate motor function. This information has opened a new approach to the treatment of the disease—namely, administration of the metabolic precursor to dopamine (L-dopa) that can be converted by the body to dopamine. Although initially beneficial in causing a significant remission of symptoms, L-dopa frequently is effective for only 5 to 10 years, and serious side effects accompany treatment. Co-treatment with an inhibitor of the enzyme that breaks down L-dopa and thus allows the substance to remain in the brain longer has yielded an effective therapy, which allows many patients to live reasonably normal lives. Nevertheless, although treatment may slow the progress of the disease, it does not alter its course. This suggests that factors other than variation in neurotransmitter levels are responsible for the disease.

Diseases of Senescence

The process of aging begins at the time of conception. Throughout life the body undergoes a series of changes that can be considered as manifestations of aging. During the first half of life these changes are generally referred to as maturation, during the last half of life as progressive senescence. Visual acuity, sensitivity of hearing, and muscular vigour begin to deteriorate after the third decade of life. These changes, although they may begin at different ages and progress at differing rates, are universal among all individuals and must therefore be considered as the normal aging process. A critical question remains unanswered concerning the cause of the intrinsic retrogressive changes in cell and organ structure and function that occur throughout the aging process. Are these changes genetically determined, or are they a result of accumulated sublethal injuries that the cell sustains from exposure to noxious environmental factors over time? Or perhaps both elements act in concert to effect the changes that occur as life progresses. It is extremely difficult to draw a sharp line between the deleterious effects of normal aging and the deleterious effects of the diseases of aging. The diseases most commonly manifested in the elderly are disorders of the heart, blood vessels, and joints. The heart disease of the elderly is related to the generalized vascular disease known as arteriosclerosis, which frequently attacks the major coronary arteries of the heart. Arteriosclerosis and arthritis will therefore be briefly touched upon here. More extended discussions may be found in cardiovascular disease and in joint disease. These problems and other aspects of aging are also considered in human aging.

Arteriosclerosis is not a specific disease. The term is applied to all diseases that cause hardening of the arteries. Several minor processes can induce hardening of the arteries, but the overwhelming preponderance of cases of arteriosclerosis are caused by atherosclerosis. This disorder, which eventually affects all individuals to varying degrees, begins relatively early in life in most persons. There are great variations, however, in the severity of this disease among individuals and among racial, national, and ethnic populations. These differences depend on the presence or absence of risk factors such as diet, hypertension, tobacco smoking, diabetes, obesity, family history, and stress.

Atherosclerosis is characterized by the deposition of fats (cholesterol and other complex lipids) in the linings (intima) of the arteries. It is accompanied by cell injury, cell death, and scarring and sometimes produces total obstruction of an artery. Atherosclerosis has a predilection for the aorta, the major artery of the body, and the arteries of the heart, brain, and legs. Atherosclerosis of the arteries of the heart (the coronaries) causes myocardial infarction, otherwise known as heart attack.

When atherosclerosis narrows but does not totally block the coronary arteries, the heart also is injured by lack of adequate blood supply and nutrition and becomes progressively smaller and weaker; even though this disease is not as life-threatening as a heart attack, it nonetheless frequently causes heart failure, an inability of the heart to deliver an adequate supply of blood to the tissues. Atherosclerosis of the arteries of the brain is the usual cause of stroke. When the arteries to the legs become affected in this way, gangrene may develop.

Arthritis, probably the second most common and distressing disease among the elderly, is a disease of the joints. It causes considerable pain, discomfort, and lack of mobility and so makes life burdensome. Moreover, arthritic individuals are more subject to other illnesses. Degenerative arthritis (osteoarthritis) is common to all elderly people to a lesser or greater degree. Osteoarthritis usually begins in the fourth decade of life and slowly progresses with increasing age. Coinciding with the characteristic degeneration of the joints are changes involving the bone itself. The bone of elderly persons is known to be less dense and more brittle; it tends, therefore, to fracture more easily. It also heals with greater difficulty.

There are many subtle changes that occur with the normal aging process. These may include degenerative changes in the brain, leading to impaired mental ability and even senility. As this damage is usually accompanied by atherosclerosis of the arteries of the brain, it is difficult to know how much of the change is the result of impaired blood flow and how much is related to normal aging. Finally, but of no less significance, is the general decline in the body's ability to defend itself against disease. Thus elderly persons are more susceptible to infections, trauma, and a number of other bodily defects. Simple, uncomplicated pneumonia, which might be easily tolerated by the young, healthy adult, may be fatal for an elderly, weakened person.

Chapter 7

Emerging Infectious Disease

An emerging infectious disease (EID) is an infectious disease whose incidence has increased in the past 35 years and could increase in the near future. Emerging infections account for at least 12% of all human pathogens. EIDs are caused by newly identified species or strains (e.g. SARS, AIDS) that may have evolved from a known infection (e.g. influenza) or spread to a new population (e.g. West Nile virus) or area undergoing ecologic transformation (e.g. Lyme disease), or be *re-emerging* infections, like drug resistant tuberculosis. Nosocomial infections, such as MRSA are emerging in hospitals, and extremely problematic in that they are resistant to many antibiotics. Of growing concern are adverse synergistic interactions between emerging diseases and other infectious and non-infectious conditions leading to the development of novel syndemics.

An example of this is MRSA, a common nosocomial infection. MRSA, the pathogen that we know today, evolved from Methicillin-susceptible Staphylococcus aureus (MSSA) otherwise known as common S. Aureus. Many people are natural carriers of S. Aureus, without being affected in any way, shape, or form. MSSA was treatable with the antibiotic methicillin until it acquired the gene for antibiotic resistance. Though genetic mapping of various strains of MRSA, scientists have found that MSSA acquired the mecA gene in the 1960s, which accounts for its pathogenicity, before this it had a predominantly commensal relationship with humans. It is theorized that when this S. Aureus strain that had acquired the mecA gene was introduced into hospitals, it came into contact with other hospital bacteria that had already been exposed to high levels of antibiotics. When exposed to such high levels of antibiotics, the hospital bacteria suddenly found themselves in an environment that had a high level of selection for antibiotic resistance, and thus resistance to multiple antibiotics formed with in these hospital populations. When S. Aureus came into contact with these populations, the multiple genes that code for antibiotic resistance to different drugs were then acquired by MRSA, making it nearly impossible to control.

It is thought that MSSA acquired the resistance gene through the horizontal gene transfer, a method in which genetic information can be passed within a generation, and spread rapidly through its own population as was illustrated in multiple studies. Horizontal gene transfer speeds the process of genetic transfer since there is no need to wait an entire generation time for gene to be passed on. Since most antibiotics do not work on MRSA, physicians have to turn to alternative methods based in Darwinian medicine.

However prevention is the most preferred method of avoiding antibiotic resistance. By reducing unnecessary antibiotic use within society as a whole, antibiotics resistance can be slowed.

The U.S. Centres for Disease Control and Prevention (CDC) publishes a journal *Emerging Infectious Diseases* that identifies the following factors contributing to disease emergence:

- Microbial adaption; e.g. genetic drift and genetic shift in Influenza A
- Changing human susceptibility; e.g. mass immunocompromisation with HIV/AIDS
- Climate and weather; e.g. diseases with zoonotic vectors such as West Nile Disease (transmitted by mosquitoes) are moving further from the tropics as the climate warms
- Change in human demographics and trade; e.g. rapid travel enabled SARS to rapidly propagate around the globe
- Economic development; e.g. use of antibiotics to increase meat yield of farmed cows leads to antibiotic resistance
- Breakdown of public health; e.g. the current situation in Zimbabwe
- Poverty and social inequality; e.g. tuberculosis is primarily a problem in low-income areas
- War and famine
- Bioterrorism; e.g. 2001 Anthrax attacks
- Dam and irrigation system construction; e.g. malaria and other mosquito borne diseases

Diet, Nutrition and Chronic Diseases in Context

The diets people eat, in all their cultural variety, define to a large extent people's health, growth and development. Risk behaviours, such as tobacco use and physical inactivity, modify the result for better or worse. All this takes place in a social, cultural, political and economic environment that can aggravate the health of populations unless active measures are taken to make the environment a health-promoting one.

Although this report has taken a disease approach for convenience, the Expert Consultation was mindful in all its discussions that diet, nutrition and physical activity do not take place in a vacuum. Since the publication of the earlier report in 1990, there have been great advances in basic research, considerable expansion of knowledge, and much community and international experience in the prevention and control of chronic diseases. At the same time, the human genome has been mapped and must now enter any discussion of chronic disease.

Concurrently there has been a return to the concept of the basic life course, i.e. of the continuity of human lives from fetus to old age. The influences in the womb work differently from later influences, but clearly have a strong effect on the subsequent manifestation of chronic disease. The known risk factors are now recognised as being amenable to alleviation throughout life, even into old age. The continuity of the life course is seen in the way that both undernutrition and overnutrition (as well as a host of other factors) play a role in the development of chronic disease. The effects of man-made and natural environments (and the interaction between the two) on the development of chronic diseases are increasingly recognised. Such factors are also being recognised as happening further and further "upstream" in the chain of events predisposing humans to chronic disease. All these broadening perceptions not only give a clearer picture of what is happening in the current epidemic of chronic diseases, but also present many opportunities to address them. The identities of those affected are now better recognised: those most disadvantaged in more affluent countries, and - in numerical terms far greater - the populations of the developing and transitional worlds.

There is a continuity in the influences contributing to chronic disease development, and thus also to the opportunities for prevention. These influences include the life course; the microscopic environment of the gene to macroscopic urban and rural environments; the impact of social and political events in one sphere affecting the health and diet of populations far distant; and the way in which already stretched agriculture and oceanic systems will affect the choices available and the recommendations that can be made. For chronic diseases, risks occur at all ages; conversely, all ages are part of the continuum of opportunities for their prevention and control. Both undernutrition and overnutrition are negative influences in terms of disease development, and possibly a combination is even worse; consequently the developing world needs additional targeting. Those with least power need different preventive approaches from the more affluent. Work has to start with the individual risk factors, but, critically, attempts at prevention and health promotion must also take account of the wider social, political and economic environment. Economics, industry, consumer groups and advertising all must be included in the prevention equation.

Diet, Nutrition and the Prevention of Chronic Diseases Through the Life Course

The rapidly increasing burden of chronic diseases is a key determinant of global public health. Already 79% of deaths attributable to chronic diseases are occurring in developing countries, predominantly in middleaged men. There is increasing evidence that chronic disease risks begin in fetal life and continue into old age. Adult chronic disease, therefore, reflects cumulative differential lifetime exposures to damaging physical and social environments.

For these reasons a life-course approach that captures both the cumulative risk and the many opportunities to intervene that this affords, was adopted by the Expert Consultation. While accepting the imperceptible progression from one life stage to the next, five stages were identified for convenience. These are: fetal development and the maternal environment; infancy; childhood and adolescence; adulthood; and ageing and older people.

Fetal Development and the Maternal Environment

The four relevant factors in fetal life are: (i) intrauterine growth retardation (IUGR); (ii) premature delivery of a normal growth for gestational age fetus; (iii) overnutrition in utero; and (iv) intergenerational factors. There is considerable evidence, mostly from developed countries, that IUGR is associated with an increased risk of coronary heart disease, stroke, diabetes and raised blood pressure. It may rather be the pattern of growth, i.e. restricted fetal growth followed by very rapid postnatal catch-up growth, that is important in the underlying disease pathways. On the other hand, large size at birth (macrosomia) is also associated with an increased risk of diabetes and cardiovascular disease. Among the adult population in India, an association was found between impaired glucose tolerance and high ponderal index (i.e. fatness) at birth. In Pima Indians, a U-shaped relationship to birth weight was found, whereas no such relationship was found amongst Mexican Americans. Higher birth weight has also been related to an increased risk of breast and other cancers.

In sum, the evidence suggests that optimal birth weight and length distribution should be considered, not only in terms of immediate morbidity and mortality but also in regard to long-term outcomes such as susceptibility to diet-related chronic disease later in life.

Infancy

Retarded growth in infancy can be a reflected in a failure to gain weight and a failure to gain height. Both retarded growth and excessive weight or height gain ("crossing the centiles") can be factors in later incidence of chronic disease. An association between low growth in early infancy (low weight at 1 year) and an increased risk of coronary heart disease (CHD) has been described, irrespective of size at birth. Blood pressure has been found to be highest in those with retarded fetal growth and greater weight gain in infancy. Short stature, a reflection of socioeconomic deprivation in childhood, is also associated with an increased risk of CHD and stroke, and to some extent, diabetes. The risk of stroke, and also of cancer mortality at several sites, including breast, uterus and colon, is increased if shorter children display an accelerated growth in height.

Breastfeeding

There is increasing evidence that among term and pre-term infants, breastfeeding is associated with significantly lower blood pressure levels in childhood. Consumption of formula instead of breast milk in infancy has also been shown to increase diastolic and mean arterial blood pressure in later life. Nevertheless, studies with older cohorts (*22*) and the Dutch study of famine have not identified such associations. There is increasingly strong evidence suggesting that a lower risk of developing obesity may be directly related to length of exclusive breastfeeding although it may not become evident until later in childhood. Some of the discrepancy may be explained by socioeconomic and maternal education factors confounding the findings.

Data from most, but not all, observational studies of term infants have generally suggested adverse effects of formula consumption on the other risk factors for cardiovascular disease (as well as blood pressure), but little information to support this finding is available from controlled clinical trials. Nevertheless, the weight of current evidence indicates adverse effects of formula milk on cardiovascular disease risk factors; this is consistent with the observations of increased mortality among older adults who were fed formula as infants. The risk for several chronic diseases of childhood and adolescence (e.g. type 1 diabetes, coeliac disease, some childhood cancers, inflammatory bowel disease) have also been associated with infant feeding on breast-milk substitutes and short-term breastfeeding.

There has been great interest in the possible effect of high-cholesterol feeding in early life. Reiser et al. proposed the hypothesis that high cholesterol feeding in early life may serve to regulate cholesterol and lipoprotein metabolism in later life. Animal data in support of this hypothesis are limited, but the idea of a possible metabolic imprinting served to trigger several retrospective and prospective studies in which cholesterol and lipoprotein metabolism in infants fed human milk were compared with those fed formula. Studies in suckling rats have suggested that the presence of cholesterol in the early diet may serve to define a metabolic pattern for lipoproteins and plasma cholesterol that could be of benefit later in life. The study by Mott, Lewis & McGill on differential diets in infant baboons, however, provided evidence to the contrary in terms of benefit. Nevertheless, the observation of modified responses of adult cholesterol production rates, bile cholesterol saturation indices, and bile acid turnover, depending on whether the baboons were fed breast milk or formula, served to attract further interest. It was noted that increased atherosclerotic lesions associated with increased levels of plasma total cholesterol were related to increased dietary cholesterol in early life. No long-term human morbidity and mortality data supporting this notion have been reported.

Short-term human studies have been in part confounded by diversity in solid food weaning regimens, as well as by the varied composition of fatty acid components of the early diet. The latter are now known to have an impact on circulating lipoprotein cholesterol species. Mean plasma total cholesterol by age 4 months in infants fed breast milk reached 180 mg/dl or greater, while cholesterol values in infants fed formula tended to remain under 150 mg/dl. In a study by Carlson, DeVoe & Barness, infants receiving predominantly a linoleic acidenriched oil blend exhibited a mean cholesterol concentration of approximately 110 mg/dl. A separate group of infants in that study who received predominantly oleic acid had a mean cholesterol concentration of 133 mg/dl. Moreover, infants who were fed breast milk and oleic acid-enriched formula had higher high-density lipoprotein

(HDL) cholesterol and apoproteins A-I and A-II than the predominantly linoleic acid-enriched oil diet group. The ratio of low density lipoprotein (LDL) cholesterol plus very low-density lipoprotein (VLDL) cholesterol to HDL cholesterol was lowest for infants receiving the formula in which oleic acid was predominant. Using a similar oleic acid predominant formula, Darmady, Fosbrooke & Lloyd reported a mean value of 149 mg/dl at age 4 months, compared with 196 mg/dl in a parallel breast-fed group. Most of those infants then received an uncontrolled mixed diet and cow's milk, with no evident differences in plasma cholesterol levels by 12 months, independent of the type of early feeding they had received. A more recent controlled study suggests that the specific fatty acid intake plays a predominant role in determining total and LDL cholesterol. The significance of high dietary cholesterol associated with exclusive human milk feeding during the first 4 months of life has no demonstrated adverse effect. Measurements of serum lipoprotein concentrations and LDL receptor activity in infants suggests that it is the fatty acid content rather than the cholesterol in the diet which regulates cholesterol homeostasis. The regulation of endogenous cholesterol synthesis in infants appears to be regulated in a similar manner to that of adults.

Childhood and Adolescence

An association between low growth in childhood and an increased risk of CHD has been described, irrespective of size at birth. Although based only on developed country research at this point, this finding gives credence to the importance that is currently attached to the role of immediate postnatal factors in shaping disease risk. Growth rates in infants in Bangladesh, most of whom had chronic intrauterine undernourishment and were breastfed, were similar to growth rates of breastfed infants in industrialized countries, but catch-up growth was limited and weight at 12 months was largely a function of weight at birth.

In a study of 11-12 year-old Jamaican children, blood pressure levels were found to be highest in those with retarded fetal growth and greater weight gain between the ages of 7 and 11 years. Similar results were found in India. Low birth weight Indian babies have been described as having a characteristic poor muscle but high fat preservation, so-called "thin-fat" babies. This phenotype persists throughout the postnatal period and is associated with an increased central adiposity in childhood that is linked to the highest risk of raised blood pressure and disease. In most studies, the association between low birth weight and high blood pressure has been found to be particularly strong if adjusted to current body size - body mass index (BMI) - suggesting the importance of weight gain after birth.

Relative weight in adulthood and weight gain have been found to be associated with increased risk of cancer of the breast, colon, rectum, prostate and other sites. Whether there is an independent effect of childhood weight is difficult to determine, as childhood overweight is usually continued into adulthood. Relative weight in adolescence was significantly associated with colon cancer in one retrospective cohort study. Frankel, Gunnel & Peters, in the follow-up to an earlier survey by Boyd Orr in the late 1930s, found that for both sexes, after accounting for the confounding effects of social class, there was a significant positive relationship between childhood energy intake and adult cancer mortality. The recent review by the International Agency for Research on Cancer (IARC) in Lyon, France, concluded that there was clear evidence of a relationship between onset of obesity (both early and later) and cancer risk.

Short stature (including measures of childhood leg length), a reflection of socioeconomic deprivation in childhood, is associated with an increased risk of CHD and stroke, and to some extent diabetes. Given that short stature, and specifically short leg length, are particularly sensitive indicators of early socioeconomic deprivation, their association with later disease very likely reflects an association between early undernutrition and infectious disease load.

Height serves partly as an indicator of socioeconomic and nutritional status in childhood. As has been seen, poor fetal development and poor growth during childhood have been associated with increased cardiovascular disease risk in adulthood, as have indicators of unfavourable social circumstances in childhood. Conversely, a high calorie intake in childhood may be related to an increased risk of cancer in later life. Height is inversely associated with mortality among men and women from all causes, including coronary heart disease, stroke and respiratory disease.

Height has also been used as a proxy for usual childhood energy intake, which is particularly related to body mass and the child's level of activity. However, it is clearly an imperfect proxy because when protein intake is adequate (energy appears to be important in this regard only in the first 3 months of life), genetics will define adult height. Protein, particularly animal protein, has been shown to have a selective effect in promoting height growth. It has been suggested that childhood obesity is related to excess protein intake and, of course, overweight or obese children tend to be in the upper percentiles for height. Height has been shown to be related to cancer mortality at several sites, including breast, uterus and colon. The risk of stroke is increased by accelerated growth in height during childhood. As accelerated growth has been linked to development of hypertension in adult life, this may be the mechanism (plus an association with low socioeconomic status).

There is a higher prevalence of raised blood pressure not only in adults of low socioeconomic status, but also in children from low socioeconomic backgrounds, although the latter is not always associated with higher blood pressure later in life. Blood pressure has been found to track from childhood to predict hypertension in adulthood, but with stronger tracking seen in older ages of childhood and in adolescence.

Higher blood pressure in childhood (in combination with other risk factors) causes target organ and anatomical changes that are associated with cardiovascular risk, including reduction in artery elasticity, increased ventricular size and mass, haemodynamic increase in cardiac output and peripheral resistance. High blood pressure in children is strongly associated with obesity, in particular central obesity, and clusters and tracks with an adverse serum lipid profile (especially LDL cholesterol) and glucose intolerance.

There may be some ethnic differences, although these often seem to be explained by differences in body mass index. A retrospective mortality follow-up of a survey of family diet and health in the United Kingdom (1937-1939) identified significant associations between childhood energy intake and mortality from cancer. The presence and tracking of high blood pressure in children and adolescents occurs against a background of unhealthy lifestyles, including excessive intakes of total and saturated fats, cholesterol and salt, inadequate intakes of potassium, and reduced physical activity, often accompanied by high levels of television viewing. In adolescents, habitual alcohol and tobacco use contributes to raised blood pressure.

There are three critical aspects of adolescence that have an impact on chronic diseases:

(i) the development of risk factors during this period;

(ii) the tracking of risk factors throughout life; and, in terms of prevention,

(iii) the development of healthy or unhealthy habits that tend to stay throughout life, for example physical inactivity because of television viewing.

In older children and adolescents, habitual alcohol and tobacco use contribute to raised blood pressure and the development of other risk factors in early life, most of which track into adulthood.

The clustering of risk factor variables occurs as early as childhood and adolescence, and is associated with atherosclerosis in young adulthood and thus risk of later cardiovascular disease. This clustering has been described as the metabolic - or "syndrome X" - clustering of physiological disturbances associated with insulin resistance, including hyperinsulinaemia, impaired glucose tolerance, hypertension, elevated plasma triglyceride and low HDL cholesterol. Raised serum cholesterol both in middle age and in early life are known to be associated with an increased risk of disease later on. The Johns Hopkins Precursor Study showed that serum cholesterol levels in adolescents and young white males were strongly related to subsequent risk of cardiovascular disease mortality and morbidity.

Although the risk of obesity does not apparently increase in adults who were overweight at 1 and 3 years old, the risk rises steadily thereafter, regardless of parental weight. Tracking has also been reported in China, where overweight children were 2.8 times as likely to become overweight adolescents; conversely, underweight children were 3.6 times as likely to remain underweight as adolescents. The study found that parental obesity and underweight, and the child's initial body mass index, dietary fat intake and family income helped predict tracking and changes. However, in a prospective cohort study conducted in the United Kingdom, little tracking from childhood overweight to adulthood obesity was found when using a measure of fatness (percentage body fat for age) that was independent of build. The authors also found that only children obese at 13 years of age had an increased risk of obesity as adults, and that there was no excess adult health risk from childhood or adolescent overweight. Interestingly, they found that in the thinnest children, the more obese they became as adults, the greater was their subsequent risk of developing chronic diseases.

The real concern about these early manifestations of chronic disease, besides the fact that they are occurring earlier and earlier, is that once they have developed they tend to track in that individual throughout life. On the more positive side, there is evidence that they can be corrected. Overweight and obesity are, however, notoriously difficult to correct after becoming established, and there is an established risk of overweight during childhood persisting into adolescence and adulthood. Recent analyses have shown that the later the weight gain in childhood and adolescence, the greater the persistence. More than 60% of overweight children have at least one additional risk factor for cardiovascular disease, such as raised blood pressure, hyperlipidaemia or hyperinsulinaemia, and more than 20% have two or more risk factors.

Habits Leading to Noncommunicable Disease Development During Adolescence

It seems increasingly likely that there are widespread effects of early diet on later body composition, physiology and cognition. Such observations "provide strong support for the recent shift away from defining nutritional needs for prevention of acute deficiency symptoms towards long-term prevention of morbidity and mortality".

Increased birth weight increases the risk of obesity later, but children with low birth weight tend to remain small into adulthood. In industrialized countries there have been only modest increases in birth weight so the increased levels of obesity described earlier must reflect environmental changes.

The "obesogenic" environment appears to be largely directed at the adolescent market, making healthy choices that much more difficult. At the same time, exercise patterns have changed and considerable parts of the day are spent sitting at school, in a factory, or in front of a television or computer. Raised blood pressure, impaired glucose tolerance and dyslipidaemia are associated in children and adolescents with unhealthy lifestyles, such as diets containing excessive intakes of fats (especially saturated), cholesterol and salt, an inadequate intake of fibre and potassium, a lack of exercise, and increased television viewing. Physical inactivity and smoking have been found independently to predict CHD and stroke in later life.

It is increasingly recognised that unhealthy lifestyles do not just appear in adulthood but drive the early development of obesity, dyslipidaemia, high blood pressure, impaired glucose tolerance and associated disease risk. In many countries, perhaps most typified by the United States, changes in family eating patterns, including the increased consumption of fast foods, pre-prepared meals and carbonated drinks, have taken place over the past 30 years. At the same time, the amount of physical activity has been greatly reduced both at home and in school, as well as by increasing use of mechanized transport.

Adulthood

The three critical questions relating to adulthood were identified as:

(i) to what extent do risk factors continue to be important in the development of chronic diseases;

(ii) to what extent will modifying such risk factors make a difference to the emergence of disease; and

(iii) what is the role of risk factor reduction and modification in secondary prevention and the treatment of those with disease?

Reviewing the evidence within the framework of a life-course approach highlights the importance of the adult phase of life, it being both the period during which most chronic diseases are expressed, as well as a critical time for the preventive reduction of risk factors and for increasing effective treatment.

The most firmly established associations between cardiovascular disease or diabetes and factors in the lifespan are the ones between those diseases and the major known "adult" risk factors, such as tobacco use, obesity, physical inactivity, cholesterol, high blood pressure and alcohol consumption. The factors that have been confirmed to lead to an increased risk of CHD, stroke and diabetes are: high blood pressure for CHD or stroke; high cholesterol (diet) for CHD, and tobacco use for CHD. Other associations are robust and consistent, although they have not necessarily been shown to be reversible: obesity and physical inactivity for CHD, diabetes and stroke; and heavy or binge drinking for CHD and stroke. Most of the studies are from developed countries, but supporting evidence from developing countries is beginning to emerge, for example, from India.

In developed countries, low socioeconomic status is associated with higher risk of cardiovascular disease and diabetes. As in the affluent industrialized countries, there appears to be an initial preponderance of cardiovascular disease among the higher socioeconomic groups, for example, as has been found in China. It is presumed that the disease will progressively shift to the more disadvantaged sectors of society. There is some evidence that this is already happening, especially among women in low-income groups, for example in Brazil and South Africa, as well as in countries in economic transition such as Morocco.

Other risk factors are continually being recognised or proposed. These include the role of high levels of homocysteine, the related factor of low folate, and the role of iron. From a social sciences perspective, Losier has suggested that socioeconomic level is less important than a certain stability in the physical and social environment. In other words, an individual's sense of understanding of his or her environment, coupled with control over the course and setting of his or her own life appears to be the most important determinant of health. Marmot, among others, has demonstrated the impact of the wider environment and societal and individual stress on the development of chronic disease.

Ageing and Older People

There are three critical aspects relating to chronic diseases in the later part of the life-cycle:

(i) most chronic diseases will be manifested in this later stage of life;

(ii) there is an absolute benefit for ageing individuals and populations in changing risk factors and adopting health-promoting behaviours such as exercise and healthy diets; and

(iii) the need to maximize health by avoiding or delaying preventable disability.

Along with the societal and disease transitions, there has been a major demographic shift. Although older people are currently defined as those aged 60 years and above, this definition of older people has a very different meaning from the middle of the last century, when 60 years of age and above often exceeded the average life expectancy, especially in industrialized countries. It is worth remembering, however, that the majority of elderly people will, in fact, be living in the developing world.

Most chronic diseases are present at this period of life - the result of interactions between multiple disease processes as well as more general losses in physiological functions. Cardiovascular disease peaks at this period, as does type 2 diabetes and some cancers. The main burden of chronic diseases is observed at this stage of life and, therefore, needs to be addressed.

Changing Behaviours in Older People

In the 1970s, it was thought that risks were not significantly increased after certain late ages and that there would be no benefit in changing habits, such as dietary habits, after 80 years old as there was no epidemiological evidence that changing habits would affect mortality or even health conditions among older people. There was also a feeling that people "earned" some unhealthy behaviours simply because of reaching "old age". Then there was a more active intervention phase, when older people were encouraged to change their diets in ways that were probably overly rigorous for the expected benefit. More recently, older people have been encouraged to eat a healthy diet - as large and as varied as possible while maintaining their weight - and particularly to continue exercise. Liu et al. have reported an observed risk of atherosclerotic disease among older women that was approximately 30% less in women who ate 5-10 servings of fruits and vegetables per day than in those who ate 2-5 servings per day. It seems that, as elderly patients have a higher cardiovascular risk, they are more likely to gain from risk factor modification.

Although this age group has received relatively little attention as regards primary prevention, the acceleration in decline caused by external factors is generally believed to be reversible at any age. Interventions aimed at supporting the individual and promoting healthier environments will often lead to increased independence in older age.

Interactions between Early and Later Factors Throughout the Life Course

Low birth weight, followed by subsequent adult obesity, has been shown to impart a particularly high risk of CHD, as well as diabetes. Risk of impaired glucose tolerance has been found to be highest in those who had low birth weight, but who subsequently became obese as adults. A number of recent studies have demonstrated that there is an increased risk of adult disease when IUGR is followed by rapid catch-up growth in weight and height. Conversely, there is also fairly consistent evidence of higher risk of CHD, stroke, and probably adult onset diabetes with shorter stature. Further research is needed to define optimal growth in infancy in terms of prevention of chronic disease. A WHO multicentre growth reference study currently under way may serve to generate much needed information on this matter.

Clustering of Risk Factors

Impaired glucose tolerance and an adverse lipid profile are seen as early as childhood and adolescence, where they typically appear clustered together with higher blood pressure and relate strongly to obesity, in particular central obesity. Raised blood pressure, impaired glucose tolerance and dyslipidaemia also tend to be clustered in children and adolescents with unhealthy lifestyles and diets, such as those with excessive intakes of saturated fats, cholesterol and salt, and inadequate intake of fibre. Lack of exercise and increased television viewing add to the risk. In older children and adolescents, habitual alcohol and tobacco use also contribute to raised blood pressure and to the development of other risk factors in early adulthood. Many of the same factors continue to act throughout the life course. Such clustering represents an opportunity to address more than one risk at a time.

The clustering of health-related behaviours is also a well described phenomenon.

Intergenerational Effects

Young girls who grow poorly become stunted women and are more likely to give birth to low-birth-weight babies who are then likely to continue the cycle by being stunted in adulthood, and so on. Maternal birth size is a significant predictor of a child's birth size after controlling for gestational age, sex of the child, socioeconomic status, and maternal age, height and pre-pregnant weight. There are clear indications of intergenerational factors in obesity, such as parental obesity, maternal gestational diabetes and maternal birth weight. Low maternal birth weight is associated with higher blood pressure levels in the offspring, independent of the relation between the offspring's own birth weight and blood pressure. Unhealthy lifestyles can also have a direct effect on the health of the next generation, for example, smoking during pregnancy.

Gene-nutrient Interactions and Genetic Susceptibility

There is good evidence that nutrients and physical activity influence gene expression and have shaped the genome over several million years of human evolution. Genes define opportunities for health and susceptibility to disease, while environmental factors determine which susceptible individuals will develop illness. In view of changing socioeconomic conditions in developing countries, such added stress may result in exposure of underlying genetic predisposition to chronic diseases. Gene-nutrient interactions also involve the environment.

The dynamics of the relationships are becoming better understood but there is still a long way to go in this area, and also in other aspects, such as disease prevention and control. Studies continue on the role of nutrients in gene expression; for example, researchers are currently trying to understand why omega-3 fatty acids suppress or decrease the mRNA of interleukin, which is elevated in atherosclerosis, arthritis and other autoimmune diseases, whereas the omega-6 fatty acids do not. Studies on genetic variability to dietary response indicate that specific genotypes raise cholesterol levels more than others. The need for targeted diets for individuals and subgroups to prevent chronic diseases was acknowledged as being part of an overall approach to prevention at the population level. However, the practical implications of this issue for public health policy have only begun to be addressed. For example, a recent study of the relationship between folate and cardiovascular disease revealed that a common single gene mutation that reduces the activity of an enzyme involved in folate metabolism (MTHFR) is associated with a moderate (20%) increase in serum homocysteine and higher risk of both ischaemic heart disease and deep vein thrombosis.

Although humans have evolved being able to feed on a variety of foods and to adapt to them, certain genetic adaptations and limitations have occurred in relation to diet. Understanding the evolutionary aspects of diet and its composition might suggest a diet that would be consistent with the diet to which our genes were programmed to respond. However, the early diet was presumably one which gave evolutionary advantage to reproduction in the early part of life, and so may be less indicative of guidance for healthy eating, in terms of lifelong health and prevention of chronic disease after reproduction has been achieved. Because there are genetic variations among individuals, changes in dietary patterns have a differential impact on a genetically heterogeneous population, although populations with a similar evolutionary background have more similar genotypes. While targeted dietary advice for susceptible populations, subgroups or individuals is desirable, it is not feasible at present for the important chronic diseases considered in this report. Most are polygenic in nature and rapidly escalating rates suggest the importance of environmental change rather than change in genetic susceptibility.

Intervening Throughout Life

There is a vast volume of scientific evidence highlighting the importance of applying a life-course approach to the prevention and control of chronic disease. The picture is, however, still not complete, and the evidence sometimes contradictory. From the available evidence, it is possible to state the following:

- Unhealthy diets, physical inactivity and smoking are confirmed risk behaviours for chronic diseases.
- The biological risk factors of hypertension, obesity and lipidaemia are firmly established as risk factors for coronary heart disease, stroke and diabetes.
- Nutrients and physical activity influence gene expression and may define susceptibility.
- The major biological and behavioural risk factors emerge and act in early life, and continue to have a negative impact throughout the life course.
- The major biological risk factors can continue to affect the health of the next generation.

- An adequate and appropriate postnatal nutritional environment is important.
- Globally, trends in the prevalence of many risk factors are upwards, especially those for obesity, physical inactivity and, in the developing world particularly, smoking.
- Selected interventions are effective but must extend beyond individual risk factors and continue throughout the life course.
- Some preventive interventions early in the life course offer lifelong benefits.
- Improving diets and increasing levels of physical activity in adults and older people will reduce chronic disease risks for death and disability.
- Secondary prevention through diet and physical activity is a complementary strategy in retarding the progression of existing chronic diseases and decreasing mortality and the disease burden from such diseases.

From the above, it is clear that risk factors must be addressed throughout the life course. As well as preventing chronic diseases, there are clearly many other reasons to improve the quality of life of people throughout their lifespan. The intention of primary prevention interventions is to move the profile of the whole population in a healthier direction. Small changes in risk factors in the majority who are at moderate risk can have an enormous impact in terms of population-attributable risk of death and disability. By preventing disease in large populations, small reductions in blood pressure, blood cholesterol and so on can dramatically reduce health costs. For example, it has been demonstrated that improved lifestyles can reduce the risk of progression to diabetes by a striking 58% over 4 years. Other population studies have shown that up to 80% of cases of coronary heart disease, and up to 90% of cases of type 2 diabetes, could potentially be avoided through changing lifestyle factors, and about one-third of cancers could be avoided by eating healthily, maintaining normal weight and exercising throughout life.

For interventions to have a lasting effect on the risk factor prevalence and the health of societies, it is also essential to change or modify the environment in which these diseases develop. Changes in dietary patterns, the influence of advertising and the globalization of diets, and widespread reduction in physical activity have generally had negative impacts in terms of risk factors, and presumably also in terms of subsequent disease. Reversing current trends will require a multifaceted public health policy approach.

While it is important to avoid inappropriately applying nutritional guidelines to populations that may differ genetically from those for whom the dietary and risk data were originally determined, to date the information regarding genes or gene combinations is insufficient to define specific dietary recommendations based on a population distribution of specific genetic polymorphisms. Guidelines should try to ensure that the overall benefit of recommendations to the majority of the population substantially outweighs any potential adverse effects on selected subgroups of the population. For example, population-wide efforts to prevent weight gain may trigger a fear of fatness and, therefore, undernutrition in adolescent girls.

The population nutrient goals recommended by the Joint WHO/FAO Expert Consultation at the present meeting are based on current scientific knowledge and evidence, and are intended to be further adapted and tailored to local or national diets and populations, where diet has evolved to be appropriate for the culture and local environment.

The goals are intended to reverse or reduce the impact of unfavourable dietary changes that have occurred over the past century in the industrialized world and more recently in many developing countries. Present nutrient intake goals also need to take into account the effects of long-term environmental changes, i.e. those that have occurred over time-scales of hundreds of years. For example, the metabolic response to periodic famine and chronic food shortage may no longer represent a selective advantage but instead may increase susceptibility to chronic diseases. An abundant stable food supply is a recent phenomenon; it was not a factor until the advent of the industrial revolution (or the equivalent process in more recently industrialized countries).

A combination of physical activity, food variety and extensive social interaction is the most likely lifestyle profile to optimize health, as reflected in increased longevity and healthy ageing. Some available evidence suggests that, within the time frame of a week, at least 20 and probably as many as 30 biologically distinct types of foods, with the emphasis on plant foods, are required for healthy diets.

The recommendations given in this report consider the wider environment, of which the food supply is a major part. The implications of the recommendations would be to increase the consumption of fruits and vegetables, to increase the consumption of fish, and to alter the types of fats and oils, as well as the amount of sugars and starch consumed, especially in developed countries. The current move towards increasing animal protein in diets in countries in economic transition is unlikely to be reversed in those countries where there are increased consumer resources, but is unlikely to be conducive to adult health, at least in terms of preventing chronic diseases.

Finally, what success can be expected by developing and updating the scientific basis for national guidelines? The percentage of British adults complying with national dietary guidelines is discouraging; for example, only 2-4% of the population are currently consuming the recommended level of saturated fat, and 5-25% are achieving the recommended levels of fibre. The figures would not be dissimilar in many other developed countries, where the majority of people are not aware of what exactly the dietary guidelines suggest.

In using the updated and evidence-based recommendations in this report, national governments should aim to produce dietary guidelines that are simple, realistic and food-based. There is an increasing need, recognised at all levels, for the wider implications to be specifically addressed; these include the implications for agriculture and fisheries, the role of international trade in a globalized world, the impact on countries dependent on primary produce, the effect of macroeconomic policies, and the need for sustainability. The greatest burden of disease will be in the developing world and, in the transitional and industrialized world, amongst the most disadvantaged socioeconomically.

In conclusion, it may be necessary to have three mutually reinforcing strategies that will have different magnitudes of impact over differing time frames. First, with the greatest and most immediate impact, there is the need to address risk factors in adulthood and, increasingly, among older people. Risk-factor behaviours can be modified in these groups and benefits seen within 3-5 years. With all populations ageing, the sheer numbers and potential cost savings are enormous and realisable. Secondly, societal changes towards health-promoting environments need to be greatly expanded as an integral part of any intervention.

Ways to reduce the intake of sugars-sweetened drinks (particularly by children) and of high-energy density foods that are micronutrient poor, as well as efforts to curb cigarette smoking and to increase physical activity will have an impact throughout society. Such changes need the active participation of communities, politicians, health systems, town planners and municipalities, as well as the food and leisure industries. Thirdly, the health environment, in which those who are most at risk grow up, needs to change. This is a more targeted and potentially costly approach, but one that has the potential for cost-effective returns even though they are longer term.

Inequality in Disease

While rates of incidence for many diseases vary based on biological factors and inheritable characteristics, a larger disparity, which cannot be explained by biological factors, exists in disease rates among varying racial and socioeconomic groups in the United States (for example, lower-income African-Americans and upper-class Caucasians). This suggests that social and economic factors play a role in determining who acquires certain diseases in the United States. For example, heart disease is the most dangerous disease in America, followed closely by cancer, with the fifth most deadly being diabetes. The general risk factors associated with these three diseases include obesity and poor diet, tobacco and alcohol use, physical inactivity, and access to medical care and health information.

While some of these risk factors are individual health choices, all of them are also correlated with socioeconomic factors, such as gender, race, income, environment, and education, and consequently, a person's likelihood for developing heart disease, cancer, or diabetes is in part correlated with these social factors. Men are more likely than women to die from heart disease. Likewise, African-Americans and other racial minorities have higher mortality rates from heart disease, cancer, and diabetes than their white counterparts. Among all racial groups, individuals who are impoverished or low income, have lower levels of educational attainment, and live in lower-income neighbourhoods are all more likely to develop heart disease, cancer, and diabetes.

Gender

Gender as a defining characteristic of a social group has different effects for the different diseases. Men are 30% more likely to suffer a stroke than women. Women generally have a healthier diet, and tend to consume fewer fats and carbohydrates. Women are also more likely to engage in regular exercise and follow their doctor's orders concerning healthy habits. Men are more inclined to hot tempers and emotional outbursts that can increase blood pressure. Men are also more likely to be smokers than women. Both men and women battle cancer, but different forms of cancer pertain more or less to the different sexes. Breast cancer affects women more than men, and prostate cancer affects only men. Lung cancer, however, is the number one cancer-related killer for both men and women, but men are more likely to develop and die from it. Diabetes, on the other hand, is more deadly for women. In recent years, the mortality rate for diabetes is higher for women than it is for men.

Race

Race is a strong determinant of disease rates, mostly because racial minorities make up a large portion of the lowest social level. More African Americans are obese or overweight and are smokers. Similarly, African Americans have the highest death rate and shortest survival rate of any racial and ethnic group for most cancers. African Americans are more likely to smoke mentholated cigarettes with higher carbon monoxide concentrations, which put them at greater risk for developing lung cancer. Obesity is more common in African Americans in part because they are less likely to engage in leisure-time physical activity. The prevalence of Type 2 diabetes is four times higher among African Americans and other racial minorities due to both poorer diets and less physical activity.

Income

Income is highly correlated with the prevalence of heart disease because it is correlated with many other social factors, such as one's neighbourhood, education level, occupation, and overall social status. Income itself, as well as the distribution of income, affect the occurrence of heart disease. Populations with high levels of income inequality display higher rates of heart disease than populations with more evenly distributed income. People living in poverty are less able to afford healthy food, spend time participating in physical activity, and pay for medical care that can reduce the risk of heart disease. The lack of insurance for those in poverty is another cause of health disparities relating to heart disease. Low-income individuals tend to face greater stress, and with low funds, many people turn to high levels of food consumption, smoking, and alcohol use as a way to cope. People living in poverty are also more likely to die from cancer than their more affluent peers because they do not have access to high quality cancer prevention, early detection, and treatment services. There is a close correlation between increased poverty and increased diabetes, as well. The reasons for the diabetes discrepancy are probably the same as those for heart disease and cancer; low-income individuals cannot afford healthy food or medication, and tend to have more stress in their day-to-day lives.

Environment

The neighbourhoods and areas people live in, as well as their occupation, make up the environment in which they exist. People living in poverty stricken neighbourhoods are at a greater risk for heart disease, possibly because the supermarkets in their area do not sell healthy foods and there is increased availability of stores selling alcohol and tobacco than in more affluent parts of town. People living in rural areas are also more susceptible to heart disease, as well. An agriculturally based diet rich in fat and cholesterol, combined with an isolated environment in which there is limited access to health care and ways to distribute information probably creates a pattern in which people living in rural environments have higher levels of heart disease. Occupational cancer is one way in which the environment one works in can increase their rate of disease. Employees exposed to smoke, asbestos, diesel fumes, paint, and chemicals in factories can develop cancer from their workplace. All of these jobs tend to be low-paying and typically held by low-status individuals. The decreased amount of healthy food in stores located in low-income areas also contributes to the increased rates of diabetes for persons living in those neighbourhoods.

Education

The lower a person's level of education, the higher their chance of being diagnosed with heart disease. People who have not graduated from high school have a 2.4% greater risk of dying than those who did graduate high school. Education level is also related to smoking, overeating, and not exercising; thus, education also affects rates of cancer and diabetes by influencing health behaviours. A lack of knowledge about the risk factors of these diseases, as well as the understanding of symptoms and when to go to the doctor, greatly affects both the development of disease as well as the prognosis of it.

Health Equity

Health equity refers to the study of differences in the quality of health and healthcare across different populations. Health equity is different from health equality, as it refers only to the absence of disparities in controllable or remediable aspects of health. It is not possible to work towards complete equality in health, as there are some factors of health that are beyond human influence. Equity implies some kind of social injustice. Thus, if one population dies younger than another because of genetic differences, a non-remediable/controllable factor, we tend to say that there is a health inequality. On the other hand, if a population has a lower life expectancy due to lack of access to medications, the situation would be classified as a health inequity. These inequities may include differences in the "presence of disease, health outcomes, or access to health care" between populations with a different race, ethnicity, sexual orientation or socioeconomic status.

Health equity falls into two major categories: horizontal equity, the equal treatment of individuals or groups in the same circumstances; and vertical equity, the principle that individuals who are unequal should be treated differently according to their level of need. Disparities in the quality of health across populations are well-documented globally in both developed and developing nations. The importance of equitable access to healthcare has been cited as crucial to achieving many of the Millennium Development Goals.

Socioeconomic Status

Socioeconomic status is both a strong predictor of health, and a key factor underlying health inequities across populations. Poor socioeconomic status has the capacity to profoundly limit the capabilities of an individual or population, manifesting itself through deficiencies in both financial and social capital. It is clear how a lack of financial capital can compromise the capacity to maintain good health. In the UK, prior to the institution of the NHS reforms in the early 2000s, it was shown that income was an important determinant of access to healthcare resources. Maintenance of good health through the utilisation of proper healthcare resources can be quite costly and therefore unaffordable to certain populations.

In China, for instance, the collapse of the Cooperative Medical System left many of the rural poor uninsured and unable to access the resources necessary to maintain good health. Increases in the cost of medical treatment made healthcare increasingly unaffordable for these populations. This issue was further perpetuated by the rising income inequality in the Chinese population. Poor Chinese were often unable to undergo necessary hospitalization and failed to complete treatment regimens, resulting in poorer health outcomes.

Similarly, in Tanzania, it was demonstrated that wealthier families were far more likely to bring their children to a healthcare provider: a significant step towards stronger healthcare. Some scholars have noted that unequal income distribution itself can be a cause of poorer health for a society as a result of "underinvestment in social goods, such as public education and health care; disruption of social cohesion and the erosion of social capital".

The role of socioeconomic status in health equity extends beyond simple monetary restrictions on an individual's purchasing power. In fact, social capital plays a significant role in the health of individuals and their communities. It has been shown that those who are better connected to the resources provided by the individuals and communities around them (those with more social capital) live longer lives. The segregation of communities on the basis of income occurs in nations worldwide and has a significant impact on quality of health as a result of a decrease in social capital for those trapped in poor neighbourhoods. Social interventions, which seek to improve healthcare by enhancing the social resources of a community, are therefore an effective component of campaigns to improve a community's health. A 1998 epidemiological study showed that community healthcare approaches fared far better than individual approaches in the prevention of heart disease mortality.

Education

Education is an important factor in healthcare utilisation, though it is closely intertwined with economic status. An individual may not go to a medical professional or seek care if they don't know the ills of their failure to do so, or the value of proper treatment. In Tajikistan, since the nation gained its independence, the likelihood of giving birth at home has increased rapidly among women with lower educational status. Education also has a significant impact on the quality of prenatal and maternal healthcare. Mothers with primary educations consulted a doctor during pregnancy at significantly lower rates (72%) when compared to those with a secondary education (77%), technical training (88%) or a higher education (100%). There is also evidence for a correlation between socioeconomic status and health literacy; one study showed that wealthier Tanzanian families were more likely to recognise disease in their children than those that were poorer.

Spatial Disparities in Health

For some populations, access to healthcare and health resources is physically limited, resulting in health inequities. For instance, an individual might be physically incapable of travelling the distances required to reach healthcare services, or such distances might make seeking regular care unappealing despite the potential benefits.

Costa Rica, for example, has demonstrable health spatial inequities with 12-14% of the population living in areas where healthcare is inaccessible. Inequity has decreased in some areas of the nation as a result of the work of healthcare reform programmes, however those regions not served by the programmes have experienced a slight increase in inequity.

China experienced a serious decrease in spatial health equity following the Chinese economic revolution in the 1980s as a result of the degradation of the Cooperative Medical System (CMS). The CMS provided an infrastructure for the delivery of healthcare to rural locations, as well as a framework to provide funding based upon communal contributions and government subsidies. In its absence, there was a significant decrease in the quantity of healthcare professionals (35.9%), as well as functioning clinics (from 71% to 55% of villages over 14 years) in rural areas, resulting in inequitable healthcare for rural populations. The significant poverty experienced by rural workers (some earning less than 1 USD per day) further limits access to healthcare, and results in malnutrition and poor general hygiene, compounding the loss of healthcare resources. The loss of the CMS has had noticeable impacts on life expectancy, with rural regions such as areas of Western China experiencing significantly lower life expectancies.

Similarly, populations in rural Tajikistan experience spatial health inequities. A study by Jane Falkingham noted that physical access to healthcare was one of the primary factors influencing quality of maternal healthcare. Further, many women in rural areas of the country did not have adequate access to healthcare resources, resulting in poor maternal and neonatal care. These rural women were, for instance, far more likely to give birth in their homes without medical oversight.

Ethnic and Racial Disparities

The United States historically had large disparities in health and access to adequate healthcare between races, and current evidence supports the notion that these racially centred disparities continue to exist and are a significant social health issue. The disparities in access to adequate healthcare include differences in the quality of care based on race and overall insurance coverage based on race. The Journal of the American Medical Association identifies race as a significant determinant in the level of quality of care, with ethnic minority groups receiving less intensive and lower quality care. Ethnic minorities also receive less preventative care, are seen less by specialists, and have fewer expensive and technical procedures than non-ethnic minorities. In 2009, Hispanic children were almost three times less likely to receive routine health care as white children, and only 16% of white patients lacked routine health care, as compared to about 20% of African Americans and 30% of Hispanic patients. There are also considerable racial disparities in access to insurance coverage, with ethnic minorities generally having less insurance coverage than non-ethnic minorities. For example, Hispanic Americans tend to have less insurance coverage than white Americans and as a result receive less regular medical care.

The level of insurance coverage is directly correlated with access to healthcare including preventative and ambulatory care. A 2010 study on racial and ethnic disparities in health done by the Institute of Medicine has shown that the aforementioned disparities cannot solely be accounted for in terms of certain demographic characteristics like: insurance status, household income, education, age, geographic location and quality of living conditions. Even when the researchers corrected for these factors, the disparities persist.

Ethnic health inequities also appear in nations across the African continent. A survey of the child mortality of major ethnic groups across 11 African nations (Central African Republic, Côte d'Ivoire, Ghana, Kenya, Mali, Namibia, Niger, Rwanda, Senegal, Uganda, and Zambia) was published in 2000 by the WHO. The study described the presence of significant ethnic parities in the child mortality rates among children younger than 5 years old, as well as in education and vaccine use. In South Africa, the legacy of apartheid still manifests itself as a differential access to social services, including healthcare based upon race and social class, and the resultant health inequities. Further, evidence suggests systematic disregard of indigenous populations in a number of countries. The Pygmys of Congo, for instance, are excluded from government health programmes, discriminated against during public health campaigns, and receive poorer overall healthcare.

In a survey of five European countries (Sweden, Switzerland, the UK, Italy, and France), a 1995 survey noted that only Sweden provided access to translators for 100% of those who needed it, while the other countries lacked this service potentially compromising healthcare to non-native populations. Given that non-natives composed a considerable section of these nations (6%, 17%, 3%, 1%, and 6% respectively), this could have significant detrimental effects on the health equity of the nation. In France, an older study noted significant differences in access to healthcare between native French populations, and non-French/ migrant populations based upon health expenditure; however this was not fully independent of poorer economic and working conditions experienced by these populations.

A 1996 study of race-based health inequity in Australia revealed that Aborigines experienced higher rates of mortality than non-Aborigine populations. Aborigine populations experienced 10 times greater mortality in the 30-40 age range; 2.5 times greater infant mortality rate, and 3 times greater age standardized mortality rate. Rates of diarrheal diseases and tuberculosis are also significantly greater in this population (16 and 15 times greater respectively), which is indicative of the poor healthcare of this ethnic group. At this point in time, the parities in life expectancy at birth between indigenous and non-indigenous peoples were highest in Australia, when compared to the US, Canada and New Zealand. In South America, indigenous populations faced similarly poor health outcomes with maternal and infant mortality rates that were significantly higher (up to 3 to 4 times greater) than the national average. The same pattern of poor indigenous healthcare continues in India, where indigenous groups were shown to experience greater mortality at most stages of life, even when corrected for environmental effects.

LGBT Minority Group Health Disparities

Sexuality has become a major source of discrimination and inequity in health. Homosexual, bisexual, and transgender populations experience a wide range of health problems related to their sexuality and gender identity. One of the egregious inequities that faces LGBT individuals is discrimination from healthcare workers or institutions. In a study of the quality of healthcare for South African MSM (Men who have Sex with Men), a cohort of individuals were interviewed about their health experiences. The researchers found that homosexually identified MSM felt that their access to healthcare was limited by their inability to find clinics that employed healthcare workers who did not discriminate based upon their sexuality. They often faced "homophobic verbal harassment from healthcare workers when presenting for STI treatment." Further, those MSM who did not identify as homosexuals did not feel comfortable discussing - and did not disclose - their sexual activity with healthcare workers, limiting the quality of their sexual healthcare. Similarly, a survey of the United States revealed that transgender individuals faced a significant level of discrimination with 19% of individuals having experienced a healthcare worker refuse care because of their gender, 28% having faced harassment from a healthcare worker, 2% having faced violence, and 50% having a doctor who was not able or qualified to provide transgender care.

Furthermore, healthcare for LGBT populations is hindered by a lack of medical research on such groups. Without the appropriate studies, it is difficult to assess what the proper strategies are for treatment of these groups. For instance, a review of medical literature regarding LGBT patients revealed that there is a significant gap in our understanding of breast cancer, which is more prevalent among lesbian and bisexual women. It is unclear whether this is a result of probability or another preventable cause. Similarly, the review notes that it is generally assumed that these groups of women have a lower incidence of cervical cancer than their heterosexual counterparts, and as a result they have low rates of screening, despite the fact that it is unclear whether they are actually at a decreased risk for the disease. In addition, it is difficult to conduct retrospective epidemiological studies on LGBT populations as a result of the practice that sexual orientation is not noted on death certificates.

Healthcare Equity and Sex

In the United States, women have better access to healthcare than many other places in the world, in part because they have higher rates of health insurance. In one study of a population group in Harlem, 86% of women reported having health insurance (privatized or publicly assisted), while only 74% of men reported having any health insurance. This trend in women reporting higher rates of insurance coverage is not unique to this population and is representative of the general population of the US. In China, gender is a significant determining factor in health, though disparities have lessened in recent years as females start receiving higher quality care.

In India, gender inequities in health start in early childhood, as many families provide better nutrition for boys than girls in the interest of maximizing future productivity (as boys are generally seen as breadwinners). In addition, boys receive better care, and are hospitalized when seriously ill at a greater rate than girls. The magnitude of these disparities increased with the severity of poverty in a given population. In general the 2012 WDR noted that women in developing nations experienced greater mortality rates than men when comparing developing nations to more developed nations. That said, men do face greater mortality than females in a number of countries as a result of behaviour or violence.

Health Inequality and Environmental Influence

Minority populations have increase exposure to environmental hazards that include lack of neighbourhood resources, structural and community factors as well as residential segregation that result in a cycle of disease and stress. The environment that surrounds us can influence individual behaviours and lead to poor health choices and therefore outcomes. Minority neighbourhoods have been continuously noted to have more fast food chains and fewer grocery stores than predominantly white neighbourhoods. These food deserts affect a family's ability to have easy access to nutritious food for their children. This lack of nutritious food extends beyond the household into the schools that have a variety of vending machines and deliver over processed foods. These environmental condition have social ramifications and in the first time in US history is it projected that the current generation will live shorter lives than their predecessors will.

In addition, minority neighbourhoods have various health hazards that result from living close to highways and toxic waste factories or general dilapidated structures and streets. These environmental conditions create varying degrees of health risk from noise pollution, to carcinogenic toxic exposures from asbestos and radon that result in increase chronic disease, morbidity, and mortality. The quality of residential environment such as damaged housing has been shown to increase the risk of adverse birth outcomes, which is reflective of a communities health. Housing conditions can create varying degrees of health risk that lead to complications of birth and long-term consequences in the aging population. In addition, occupational hazards can add to the detrimental effects of poor housing conditions. It has been reported that a greater number of minorities work in jobs that have higher rates of exposure to toxic chemical, dust and fumes.

Racial segregation is another environmental factor that occurs through the discriminatory action of those organisations and working individuals within the real estate industry, whether in the housing markets or rentals. Even though residential segregation is noted in all minority groups, blacks tend to be segregated regardless of income level when compared to Latinos and Asians. Thus, segregation results in minorities clustering in poor neighbourhoods that have limited employment, medical care, and educational resources, which is associated with high rates of criminal behaviour. In addition, segregation affects the health of individual residents because the environment is not conducive to physical exercise due to unsafe neighbourhoods that lack recreational facilities and have nonexistent park space. Racial and ethnic discrimination adds an additional element to the environment that individuals have to interact with daily. Individuals that reported discrimination have been shown to have an increase risk of hypertension in addition to other physiological stress related affects. The high magnitude of environmental, structural, socioeconomic stressors leads to further compromise on the psychological and physical being, which leads to poor health and disease.

Individuals living in rural areas, especially poor rural areas, have access to fewer health care resources. Although 20 percent of the U.S. population lives in rural areas, only 9 percent of physicians practice in rural settings. Individuals in rural areas typically must travel longer distances for care, experience long waiting times at clinics, or are unable to obtain the necessary health care they need in a timely manner. Rural areas characterized by a largely Hispanic population average 5.3 physicians per 10,000 residents compared with 8.7 physicians per 10,000 residents in nonrural areas. Financial barriers to access, including lack of health insurance, are also common among the urban poor.

Disparities in Access to Health Care

Reasons for disparities in access to health care are many, but can include the following:

- Lack of universal health care or health insurance coverage. Without health insurance, patients are more likely to postpone medical care, more likely to go without needed medical care, and more likely to go without prescription medicines. Minority groups in the United States lack insurance coverage at higher rates than whites. This problem does not exist in countries with fully funded public health systems, such as the examplar of the NHS.
- Lack of a regular source of care. Without access to a regular source of care, patients have greater difficulty obtaining care, fewer doctor visits, and more difficulty obtaining prescription drugs. Compared to whites, minority groups in the United States are less likely to have a doctor they go to on a regular basis and are more likely to use emergency rooms and clinics as their regular source of care. In the United Kingdom, which is much more racially harmonious, this issue arises for a different reason; since 2004, NHS GPs have not been responsible for care out of normal GP surgery opening hours, leading to significantly higher attendances in A+E
- Lack of financial resources. Although the lack of financial resources is a barrier to health care access for many Americans, the impact on access appears to be greater for minority populations.
- Legal barriers. Access to medical care by low-income immigrant minorities can be hindered by legal barriers to public insurance programmes. For example, in the United States federal law bars states from providing Medicaid coverage to immigrants who have been in the country fewer than five years.
- Structural barriers. These barriers include poor transportation, an inability to schedule appointments quickly or during convenient hours, and excessive time spent in the waiting room, all of which affect a person's ability and willingness to obtain needed care.

- The health care financing system. The Institute of Medicine in the United States says fragmentation of the U.S. health care delivery and financing system is a barrier to accessing care. Racial and ethnic minorities are more likely to be enrolled in health insurance plans which place limits on covered services and offer a limited number of health care providers.
- Scarcity of providers. In inner cities, rural areas, and communities with high concentrations of minority populations, access to medical care can be limited due to the scarcity of primary care practitioners, specialists, and diagnostic facilities. In the UK, Monitor (a quango) has a legal obligation to ensure that sufficient provision exists in all parts of the nation.
- Linguistic barriers. Language differences restrict access to medical care for minorities in the United States who are not English-proficient.
- Health literacy. This is where patients have problems obtaining, processing, and understanding basic health information. For example, patients with a poor understanding of good health may not know when it is necessary to seek care for certain symptoms. While problems with health literacy are not limited to minority groups, the problem can be more pronounced in these groups than in whites due to socioeconomic and educational factors.
- Lack of diversity in the health care workforce. A major reason for disparities in access to care are the cultural differences between predominantly white health care providers and minority patients. Only 4% of physicians in the United States are African American, and Hispanics represent just 5%, even though these percentages are much less than their groups' proportion of the United States population.
- Age. Age can also be a factor in health disparities for a number of reasons. As many older Americans exist on fixed incomes which may make paying for health care expenses difficult. Additionally, they may face other barriers such as impaired mobility or lack of transportation which make accessing health care services challenging for them physically. Also, they may not have the opportunity to access health information via the internet as less than 15% of Americans over the age of 65 have access to the internet. This could put older individuals at a disadvantage in terms of accessing valuable information about their health and how to protect it. On the other hand, older

individuals in the US (65 or above) are provided with medical care via Medicare.

Disparities in Quality of Health Care

Health disparities in the quality of care exist and are based on language and ethnicity/race which includes:

Problems with Patient-provider Communication

Communication is critical for the delivery of appropriate and effective treatment and care, regardless of a patient's race, and miscommunication can lead to incorrect diagnosis, improper use of medications, and failure to receive follow-up care. The patient provider relationship is dependent on the ability of both individuals to effectively communicate. Language and culture both play a significant role in communication during a medical visit. Among the patient population, minorities face greater difficulty in communicating with their physicians. Patients when surveyed responded that 19% of the time they have problems communicating with their providers which included understanding doctor, feeling doctor listened, and had questions but did not ask. In contrast, the Hispanic population had the largest problem communicating with their provider, 33% of the time. Communication has been linked to health outcomes, as communication improves so does patient satisfaction which leads to improved compliance and then to improved health outcomes. Quality of care is impacted as a result of an inability to communicate with health care providers. Language plays a pivotal role in communication and efforts need to be taken to ensure excellent communication between patient and provider. Among limited English proficient patients in the United States, the linguistic barrier is even greater.

Less than half of non-English speakers who say they need an interpreter during clinical visits report having one. The absence of interpreters during a clinical visit adds to the communication barrier. Furthermore, inability of providers to communicate with limited English proficient patients leads to more diagnostic procedures, more invasive procedures, and over prescribing of medications. Poor communication contributes to poor medical compliance and health outcomes. Many health-related settings provide interpreter services for their limited English proficient patients. This has been helpful when providers do not speak the same language as the patient. However, there is mounting evidence that patients need to communicate with a language concordant physician (not simply an interpreter) to receive the best medical care, bond with the physician, and be satisfied with the care experience. Having patient-physician language discordant pairs (i.e. Spanish-speaking patient with an English-speaking physician) may also lead to greater medical expenditures and thus higher costs to the organisation. Additional communication problems result from a decrease or lack of cultural competence by providers. It is important for providers to be cognizant of patients' health beliefs and practices without being judgemental or reacting. Understanding a patients' view of health and disease is important for diagnosis and treatment. So providers need to assess patients' health beliefs and practices to improve quality of care. Patient health decisions can be influenced by religious beliefs, mistrust of Western medicine, and familial and hierarchical roles, all of which a white provider may not be familiar with. Other type of communication problems are seen in LGBT health care with the spoken heterosexist (conscious or unconscious) attitude on LGBT patients, lack of understanding on issues like having no sex with men (lesbians, gynecologic examinations) and other issues.

Provider Discrimination

Provider discrimination occurs when health care providers either unconsciously or consciously treat certain racial and ethnic patients differently from other patients. This may be due to stereotypes that providers may have towards ethnic/racial groups. Doctors are more likely to ascribe negative racial stereotypes to their minority patients. This may occur regardless of consideration for education, income, and personality characteristics. Two types of stereotypes may be involved, automatic stereotypes or goal modified stereotypes. Automated stereotyping is when stereotypes are automatically activated and influence judgements/behaviours outside of consciousness. Goal modified stereotype is a more conscious process, done when specific needs of clinician arise (time constraints, filling in gaps in information needed) to make a complex decisions. Physicians are unaware of their implicit biases. Some research suggests that ethnic minorities are less likely than whites to receive a kidney transplant once on dialysis or to receive pain medication for bone fractures. Critics question this research and say further studies are needed to determine how doctors and patients make their treatment decisions. Others argue that certain diseases cluster by ethnicity and that clinical decision making does not always reflect these differences.

Lack of Preventive Care

According to the 2009 National Healthcare Disparities Report, uninsured Americans are less likely to receive preventive services in health care. For example, minorities are not regularly screened for colon cancer and the death rate for colon cancer has increased among African Americans and Hispanic populations.

Furthermore, limited English proficient patients are also less likely to receive preventive health services such as mammograms. Studies have shown that use of professional interpreters have significantly reduced disparities in the rates of fecal occult testing, flu immunizations and pap smears.

In the UK, Public Health England, a universal service free at the point of use, which forms part of the NHS, offers regular screening to any member of the population considered to be in an at-risk group (such as individuals over 45) for major disease (such as colon cancer, or diabetic-retinopathy).

Plans for Achieving Health Equity

There are a multitude of strategies for achieving health equity and reducing disparities outlined in scholarly texts, some examples include:

- Provider based incentives to improve healthcare for ethnic populations. One source of health inequity stems from unequal treatment of non-white patients in comparison with white patients. Creating provider based incentives to create greater parity between treatment of white and non-white patients is one proposed solution to eliminate provider bias. These incentives typically are monetary because of its effectiveness in influencing physician behaviour.
- Using Evidence Based Medicine (EBM). Evidence Based Medicine (EBM) shows promise in reducing healthcare provider bias in turn promoting health equity. In theory EBM can reduce disparities however other research suggests that it might exacerbate them instead. Some cited shortcomings include EBM's injection of clinical inflexibility in decision making and its origins as a purely cost driven measure.
- Increasing awareness. The most cited measure to improving health equity relates to increasing public awareness. A lack of public awareness is a key reason why there has not been significant gains in reducing health disparities in ethnic and minority populations. Increased public awareness would lead to increased congressional awareness, greater availability of disparity data, and further research into the issue of health disparities.

Health Inequalities

Health inequality is the term used in a number of countries to refer to those instances whereby the health of two demographic groups (not necessarily ethnic or racial groups) differs despite comparative access to health care services. Such examples include higher rates of morbidity and mortality for those in lower occupational classes than those in higher occupational classes, and the increased likelihood of those from ethnic minorities being diagnosed with a mental health disorder. In Canada, the issue was brought to public attention by the LaLonde report. In UK, the Black Report was produced in 1980 to highlight inequalities. On 11 February 2010, Sir Michael Marmot, an epidemiologist at University College London, published the *Fair Society, Healthy Lives* report on the relationship between health and poverty. Marmot described his findings as illustrating a "social gradient in health": the life expectancy for the poorest is seven years shorter than for the most wealthy, and the poor are more likely to have a disability. In its report on this study, *The Economist* argued that the material causes of this contextual health inequality include unhealthful lifestyles - smoking remains more common, and obesity is increasing fastest, amongst the poor in Britain.

Poor Health and Economic Inequality

Poor health outcomes appear to be an effect of economic inequality across a population. Nations and regions with greater economic inequality show poorer outcomes in life expectancy, mental health, drug abuse, obesity, educational performance, teenage birthrates, and ill health due to violence. On an international level, there is a positive correlation between developed countries with high economic equality and longevity. This is unrelated to average income per capita in wealthy nations. Economic gain only impacts life expectancy to a great degree in countries in which the mean per capita annual income is less than approximately $25,000. The United States shows exceptionally low health outcomes for a developed country, despite having the highest national healthcare expenditure in the world. The US ranks 31st in life expectancy. Americans have a lower life expectancy than their European counterparts, even when factors such as race, income, diet, smoking, and education are controlled for.

Relative inequality negatively affects health on an international, national, and institutional levels. The patterns seen internationally hold true between more and less economically equal states in the United States. The patterns seen internationally hold true between more and less economically equal states in the United States, that is, more equal states show more desirable health outcomes. Importantly, inequality can have a negative health impact on members of lower echelons of institutions. The Whitehall I and II studies looked at the rates of cardiovascular disease and other health risks in British civil servants and found that, even when lifestyle factors were controlled for, members of lower status in the institution showed increased mortality and morbidity on a sliding downward scale from their higher status counterparts. The negative aspects of inequality are spread across the population. For example, when comparing the United States (a more unequal nation) to England (a less unequal nation), the US shows higher rates of diabetes, hypertension, cancer, lung disease, and heart disease across all income levels. This is also true of the difference between mortality across all occupational classes in highly equal Sweden as compared to less-equal England

Chapter 8

Social Determinants of Health

The social determinants of health are the economic and social conditions – and their distribution among the population – that influence individual and group differences in health status. They are risk factors found in one's living and working conditions (such as the distribution of income, wealth, influence, and power), rather than individual factors (such as behavioural risk factors or genetics) that influence the risk for a disease, or vulnerability to disease or injury. According to some viewpoints, these distributions of social determinants are shaped by public policies that reflect the influence of prevailing political ideologies of those governing a jurisdiction. The World Health Organisation says that "This unequal distribution of health-damaging experiences is not in any sense a 'natural' phenomenon but is the result of a toxic combination of poor social policies, unfair economic arrangements [where the already well-off and healthy become even richer and the poor who are already more likely to be ill become even poorer], and bad politics."

Commonly Accepted Social Determinants of Health

There is no single definition of the social determinants of health, but there are commonalities, and many governmental and non-governmental organisations recognise that there are social factors which impact the health of individuals.

In 2003, the World Health Organisation (WHO) Europe suggested that the social determinants of health included:

- Social gradients (life expectancy is shorter and disease is more common further down the social ladder)
- Stress (including stress in the workplace)

- Early childhood development
- Social exclusion
- Unemployment
- Social support networks
- Addiction
- Availability of healthy food
- Availability of healthy transportation / active travel

In Canada these social determinants of health have gained wide usage.

1. Income and Income Distribution
2. Education
3. Unemployment and Job Security
4. Employment and Working Conditions
5. Early Childhood Development
6. Food Insecurity
7. Housing
8. Social Exclusion
9. Social Safety Network
10. Health Services
11. Aboriginal Status
12. Gender
13. Race
14. Disability

These SDOH are clearly related to health outcomes, are closely tied to public policy, and are clearly understandable by the public. Sadly, they tend to cluster together such that those living in poverty, for example, also experience numerous other adverse social determinants. The quality and equitable distribution of these social determinants in Canada and the USA are clearly well below the standards seen in other developed nations.

The WHO later developed a Commission on Social Determinants of Health, which in 2008 published a report entitled "Closing the Gap in a Generation". This report identified two broad areas of social determinants of health that needed to be addressed. The first area was daily living conditions, which included healthy physical environments, fair employment and decent work, social protection across the lifespan, and access to health care. The second major area was distribution of power, money, and resources, including equity in health programmes, public financing of action on the social determinants, economic inequalities, resource depletion, healthy working conditions, gender equity, political empowerment, and a balance of power and prosperity of nations.

The 2011 World Conference on Social Determinants of Health brought together delegations from 125 member states and resulted in the Rio Political Declaration on Social Determinants of Health. This declaration involved an affirmation that health inequities are unacceptable, and noted that these inequities arise from the societal conditions in which people are born, grow, live, work, and age, including early childhood development, education, economic status, employment and decent work, housing environment, and effective prevention and treatment of health problems. The United States Centres for Disease Control defines social determinants of health as "life-enhancing resources, such as food supply, housing, economic and social relationships, transportation, education, and health care, whose distribution across populations effectively determines length and quality of life". These include access to care and resources such as food, insurance coverage, income, housing, and transportation. Social determinants of health influence health-promoting behaviours, and health equity among the population is not possible without equitable distribution of social determinants among groups.

Woolf states, "The degree to which social conditions affect health is illustrated by the association between education and mortality rates". Reports in 2005 revealed the mortality rate was 206.3 per 100,000 for adults aged 25 to 64 years with little education beyond high school, but was twice as great (477.6 per 100,000) for those with only a high school education and 3 times as great (650.4 per 100,000) for those less educated. Based on the data collected, the social conditions such as education, income, and race were very much dependent on one another, but these social conditions also apply independent health influences.

Marmot and Bell found that in wealthy countries, income and mortality are correlated as a marker of relative position within society, and this relative position is related to social conditions that are important for health including good early childhood development, access to good quality education, rewarding work with some degree of autonomy, decent housing, and a clean and safe living environment. The social condition of autonomy, control, and empowerment turns are important influences on health and disease, and individuals who lack social participation and control over their lives are at a greater risk for heart disease and mental illness.

International Health Disparities

Even in the wealthiest countries, there are disparities in health between the rich and the poor. Canadian authors Labonte and Schrecker from the University of Ottawa note that globalization is a key context for the study of the social determinants of health, and the impacts of globalization are asymmetric.

As a result, there is an uneven distribution of wealth and influence both within and across national borders, leading to negative impacts on the social determinants of health. The Organisation for Economic Cooperation and Development found significant differences among developed nations in health status indicators such as life expectancy, infant mortality, incidence of disease, and death from injuries.

These disparities may exist in the context of the health care system, or in broader social approaches. According to the WHO's Commission on Social Determinants of Health, access to health care is essential for equitable health, and it argued that health care should be a common good rather than a market commodity. However, there is substantial variation in health care systems and coverage from country to country.

The Commission also calls for government action on such things as access to clean water and safe, equitable working conditions, and it notes that dangerous working conditions exist even in some wealthy countries. In the Rio Political Declaration on Social Determinants of Health, several key areas of action were identified to address disparities, including promotion of participatory policy-making processes, strengthening global governance and collaboration, and encouraged developed countries to reach a target of 0.7% of gross national product (GNP) for official development assistance.

Theoretical Approaches

The UK *Black* and *The Health Divide* reports considered two primary mechanisms for understanding the process by which the social determinants influence health: cultural/ behavioural and materialist/ structuralist. The cultural/behavioural explanation was that individuals' behavioural choices (e.g., tobacco and alcohol use, diet, physical activity, etc.) were responsible for their developing and dying from a variety of diseases. However, both the Black and Health divide reports found that behavioural choices are heavily structured by one's material conditions of life, and these behavioural risk factors account for a relatively small proportion of variation in the incidence and death from various diseases.

The materialist/structuralist explanation emphasizes the material conditions under which people live. These conditions include availability of resources to access the amenities of life, working conditions, and quality of available food and housing among others. Within this view, three frameworks have been developed to explain how social determinants influence health. These frameworks are: (a) materialist; (b) neo-materialist; and (c) psychosocial comparison. The materialist explanation is about how living conditions – and the social determinants of health that constitute these living conditions—shape health. The neo-materialist explanation extends the materialist analysis by asking how these living conditions come about. The psychosocial comparison explanation considers whether people compare themselves to others and how these comparisons affect health and wellbeing.

The wealth of nations is a strong indicator of population health. But within nations, socio-economic position is a powerful predictor of health as it is an indicator of material advantage or disadvantage over the lifespan. Material conditions of life determine health by influencing the quality of individual development, family life and interaction, and community environments. Material conditions of life lead to differing likelihood of physical (infections, malnutrition, chronic disease, and injuries), developmental (delayed or impaired cognitive, personality, and social development), educational (learning disabilities, poor learning, early school leaving), and social (socialization, preparation for work, and family life) problems. Overall wealth of nations is a strong indicator of population health. But within nations, socio-economic position is a powerful predictor of health as it is an indicator of material advantage or disadvantage over the lifespan. Material conditions of life also lead to differences in psychosocial stress The fight-or-flight reaction—chronically elicited in response to threats such as income, housing, and food insecurity, among others—weakens the immune system, leads to increased insulin resistance, greater incidence of lipid and clotting disorders, and other biomedical insults that are precursors to adult disease.

Adoption of health-threatening behaviours is also influenced by material deprivation and stress. Environments influence whether individuals take up tobacco, use alcohol, experience poor diets, and have low levels of physical activity. Tobacco and excessive alcohol use, and carbohydrate-dense diets are also means of coping with difficult circumstances. The materialist approach offers insight into the sources of health inequalities among individuals and nations and the role played by the social determinants of health.

The neo-materialist approach is concerned with how nations, regions, and cities differ on how economic and other resources are distributed among the population. This distribution of resources can vary widely from country to country. The neo-materialist view therefore, directs attention to both the effects of living conditions – the social determinants of health—on individuals' health and the societal factors that determine the quality of the distribution of these social determinants of health. How a society decides to distribute resources among citizens is especially important.

The social comparison approach holds that the social determinants of health play their role through citizens' interpretations of their standings in the social hierarchy. There are two mechanisms by which this occurs. At the individual level, the perception and experience of one's status in unequal societies lead to stress and poor health. Feelings of shame, worthlessness, and envy can lead to harmful effects upon neuro-endocrine, autonomic and metabolic, and immune systems. Comparisons to those of a higher social class can also lead to attempts to alleviate such feelings by overspending, taking on additional employment that threaten health, and adopting health-threatening coping behaviours such as overeating and using alcohol and tobacco. At the communal level, widening and strengthening of hierarchy weakens social cohesion, which is a determinant of health. The social comparison approach directs attention to the psychosocial effects of public policies that weaken the social determinants of health. However, these effects may be secondary to how societies distribute material resources and provide security to its citizens, which are described in the materialist and neo-materialist approaches.

Life-course Perspective

Life-course approaches emphasize the accumulated effects of experience across the life span in understanding the maintenance of health and the onset of disease. The economic and social conditions—the social determinants of health—under which individuals live their lives have a cumulative effect upon the probability of developing any number of diseases, including heart disease and stroke Studies into the childhood and adulthood antecedents of adult-onset diabetes show that adverse economic and social conditions across the life span predispose individuals to this disorder.

Hertzman outlines three health effects that have relevance for a life-course perspective. Latent effects are biological or developmental early life experiences that influence health later in life. Low birth weight, for instance, is a reliable predictor of incidence of cardiovascular disease and adult-onset diabetes in later life. Experience of nutritional deprivation during childhood has lasting health effects.

Pathway effects are experiences that set individuals onto trajectories that influence health, well-being, and competence over the life course. As one example, children who enter school with delayed vocabulary are set upon a path that leads to lower educational expectations, poor employment prospects, and greater likelihood of illness and disease across the lifespan. Deprivation associated with poor-quality neighbourhoods, schools, and housing sets children off on paths that are not conducive to health and well-being.

Cumulative effects are the accumulation of advantage or disadvantage over time that manifests itself in poor health. These involve the combination of latent and pathways effects. Adopting a life-course perspective directs attention to how social determinants of health operate at every level of development—early childhood, childhood, adolescence, and adulthood—to both immediately influence health and provide the basis for health or illness later in life.

Steps to Improve Conditions of Health Worldwide

Reducing the health gap in a generation requires that governments build systems that allow a healthy standard of living where no one should fall below due to circumstances beyond his or her control. Social protection schemes can be instrumental in realising developmental goals rather than being dependent on achieving those goals. They can be effective ways to reduce poverty and local economies can benefit.

Policies to reduce child poverty are particularly important, as elevated stress hormones in children interfere with the development of brain circuitry and connections, causing long term chemical damage. Studies showed that the immune system of participants were stronger if their parents had the security of home ownership while the participants were growing up. In most wealthy countries, the relative child poverty rate is 10 percent or less; in the United States, it is 21.9 percent. The lowest poverty rates are more common in smaller well-developed and high-spending welfare states like Sweden and Finland, with about 5 or 6 percent . Middle-level rates are found in major European countries where unemployment compensation is more generous and social policies provide more generous support to single mothers and working women (through paid family leave, for example), and where social assistance minimums are high. For instance, the Netherlands, Austria, Belgium and Germany have poverty rates that are in the 7 to 8 percent range.

The Commission on Social Determinants of Health (CSDH) in 2005 made recommendations for action to promote health equity based on 3 principles of action: "improve the circumstances in which people are born, grow, live, work, and age; tackle the inequitable distribution of power, money, and resources, the structural drivers of conditions of daily life, globally, nationally, and locally; and measure the problem, evaluate action, and expand the knowledge base."

These recommendations would involve providing resources such as quality education, decent housing, access to affordable health care, access to healthy food, and safe places to exercise for everyone despite gaps in affluence. Expansion of knowledge of the social determinants of health, including among healthcare workers, can improve the quality and standard of care for people who are marginalized, poor or living in developing nations by preventing early death and disability while working to improve quality of life.

Public Policy

The Rio Political Declaration on Social Determinants of Health embraces a transparent, participatory model of policy development that, among other things, addresses the social determinants of health leading to persistent health inequalities for indigenous peoples.

The United States Department of Health and Human Services includes social determinants in its model of population health, and one of its missions is to strengthen policies which are backed by the best available evidence and knowledge in the field Social determinants of health do not exist in a vacuum. Their quality and availability to the population are usually a result of public policy decisions made by governing authorities. For example, early life is shaped by availability of sufficient material resources that assure adequate educational opportunities, food and housing among others. Much of this has to do with the employment security and the quality of working conditions and wages. The availability of quality, regulated childcare is an especially important policy option in support of early life. These are not issues that usually come under individual control. A policy-oriented approach places such findings within a broader policy context. In this context, Health in All Policies has seen as a response to incorporate health and health equity into all public policies as means to foster synergy between sectors and ultimately promote health.

Yet it is not uncommon to see governmental and other authorities individualize these issues. Governments may view early life as being primarily about parental behaviours towards their children. They then focus upon promoting better parenting, assist in having parents read to their children, or urge schools to foster exercise among children rather than raising the amount of financial or housing resources available to families. Indeed, for every social determinant of health, an individualized manifestation of each is available. There is little evidence to suggest the efficacy of such approaches in improving the health status of those most vulnerable to illness in the absence of efforts to modify their adverse living conditions. One of the recommendations by the CSDH is expanding knowledge - particularly to health care workers.

Health Literacy

Health literacy is the ability to obtain, read, understand and use healthcare information to make appropriate health decisions and follow instructions for treatment. There are multiple definitions of health literacy, in part, because health literacy involves both the context (or setting) in which health literacy demands are made (e.g., health care, media, internet or fitness facility) and the skills that people bring to that situation (Rudd, Moeykens, & Colton, 1999). Studies reveal that up to half of patients cannot understand basic healthcare information. Low health literacy reduces the success of treatment and increases the risk of medical error.

Various interventions, such as simplified information and illustrations, avoiding jargon, "teach back" methods and encouraging patients questions, have improved health behaviours in persons with low health literacy. Health literacy is of continued and increasing concern for health professionals, as it is a primary factor behind health disparities. The Healthy People 2020 initiative of the United States Department of Health and Human Services has included it as a pressing new topic, with objectives for addressing it in the decade to come.

Characteristics

Many factors determine the health literacy level of health education materials or other health interventions: Reading level, numeracy level, language barriers, cultural appropriateness, format and style, sentence structure, use of illustrations, interactiveness of intervention, and numerous other factors will affect how easily health information is understood and followed.

A study of 2,600 patients conducted in 1995 by two US hospitals found that between 26% and 60% of patients could not understand medication directions, a standard informed consent or basic health care materials.

History

The young and multidisciplinary field of health literacy emerged from two expert groups; physicians, other health providers, and health educators, and Adult Basic Education (ABE) and English as a Second Language (ESL) practitioners. Physicians are a source of groundbreaking patient comprehension and compliance studies. Adult Basic Education / English for Speakers of Languages Other Than English (ABE/ESOL) specialists study and design interventions to help people develop reading, writing, and conversation skills and increasingly infuse curricula with health information to promote better health literacy. A range of approaches to adult education brings health literacy skills to people in traditional classroom settings, as well as where they work and live.

Biomedical Approach

The biomedical approach to health literacy that became dominant (in the U.S.) during the 1980s and 1990s often depicted individuals as lacking, or "suffering" from, low health literacy, assumed that recipients are passive in their possession and reception of health literacy, and believed that models of literacy and health literacy are politically neutral and universally applicable. This approach is found lacking when placed in the context of broader ecological, critical, and cultural approaches to health. This approach has produced, and continues to reproduce, numerous correlational studies.

Where there are adequate levels of health literacy, that is where the population has sufficient knowledge and skills and where members of a community have the confidence to guide their own health, people are able to stay healthy, recover from illness and live with disease or disability.

McMurray states that health literacy is important in a community as it addresses health inequities, as those at the lower levels of health literacy are often the ones who live in lower socio-economic communities. Being aware of information relevant to improving their health, or how to access health resources creates higher levels of disadvantage. For some people, a lack of education and health literacy that would flow from education prevents them from becoming empowered at any time in their lives.

A more robust view of health literacy includes the ability to understand scientific concepts, content, and health research; skills in spoken, written, and online communication; critical interpretation of mass media messages; navigating complex systems of health care and governance; and knowledge and use of community capital and resources, as well as using cultural and indigenous knowledge in health decision making (Nutbeam, 2000; Ratzan, 2001; Zarcadoolas, Pleasant, & Greer, 2002). This view sees health literacy as a social determinant of health that offers a powerful opportunity to reduce inequities in health.

This perspective defines health literacy as the wide range of skills, and competencies that people develop over their lifetimes to seek out, comprehend, evaluate, and use health information and concepts to make informed choices, reduce health risks, and increase quality of life (Zarcadoolas, Pleasant, & Greer, 2006). While definitions vary in wording, they all fall within the conceptual framework offered in this definition.

Defining health literacy in that manner builds the foundation for a multi-dimensional model of health literacy built around four central domains:

- fundamental literacy,
- scientific literacy,
- civic literacy, and
- cultural literacy.

Patient Safety and Outcomes

According to an Institute of Medicine (2004) report, low health literacy negatively affects the treatment outcome and safety of care delivery. These patients have a higher risk of hospitalization and longer hospital stays, are less likely to comply with treatment, are more likely to make errors with medication, and are more ill when they seek medical care.

The mismatch between a clinician's level of communication and a patient's ability to understand can lead to medication errors and adverse medical outcomes. The lack of health literacy affects all segments of the population, although it is disproportionate in certain demographic groups, such as the elderly, ethnic minorities, recent immigrants and persons with low general literacy. Health literacy skills are not only a problem in the public. Health care professionals (doctors, nurses, public health workers) can also have poor health literacy skills, such as a reduced ability to clearly explain health issues to patients and the public. A well arranged layout, pertinent illustrations, and intuitive format can improve the usability of health care literature. This in turn can help in effective communication between health care providers and patients and their families.

Risk Identification

Identifying patients at risk due to low health literacy is productive. Health behaviours such as correct medication use, taking advantage of health screening and effective preventive measures such as exercise and smoking cessation improved when low literacy patients were given visual aids, easy readability brochures or videotapes. Several tests of health literacy have been developed to validate research studies, but a practical, three-minute assessment can be completed in a doctor's office. A recent review on health literacy in the Journal of the American Medical Association's "Rational Clinical Examination Series" showed that single-item questions can be useful. The simple enquiry, "How confident are you in filling out medical forms by yourself?" gives a likelihood ratio (LR) for limited literacy of 5.0 (95% confidence interval [CI], 3.8-6.4) for an answer of "a little confident" or "not at all confident"; an LR of 2.2 (95% CI, 1.5-3.3) for "somewhat confident"; and an LR of 0.44 (95% CI, 0.24-0.82) for "quite a bit" or "extremely confident."

Intervention

Once identified, low health literacy patients benefit from providing limited but clear information at each visit, avoidance of medical jargon, using illustrations of important concepts and confirming information by a "teach back" method. A programme called "Ask Me 3" is designed to bring public and physician attention to this issue, by letting patients know that they should ask three questions each time they talk to a doctor, nurse, or pharmacist:

- What is my main problem?
- What do I need to do?
- Why is it important for me to do this?

A public information programme by the US Department of Health and Human Services encourages patients to improve healthcare quality and avoid errors by asking questions about health conditions and treatment.

Health Illiterate-related Diabetes Prevalence in Vietnamese-American Populations

Diabetes is a rapidly growing health problem among immigrants—affecting approximately 10 percent of Asian-Americans. It is the fifth-leading cause of death in Asian-Americans between the ages of 45 and 64. In addition, type 2 diabetes is the most common form of the disease. Those who are diagnosed with type 2 diabetes have high levels of blood glucose because the body does not effectively respond to insulin. It is a lifelong disease with no known cure. Diabetes is a chronic, debilitating, and costly social burden—costing healthcare systems about $100 billion annually.

Diabetes disproportionately affects underserved and ethnically diverse populations, such as Vietnamese-American communities. The relationship between the disease and health literacy level is in part because of an individual's ability to read English, evaluate blood glucose levels, and communicate with medical professionals. Other studies also suggest lack in knowledge of diabetes symptoms and complications. According to an observational cross-sectional study conducted, many Vietnamese-American diabetic patients show signs of poor blood glucose control and adherence due to inadequate self-management knowledge and experience. Diabetes health literacy research is needed to fully understand the burden of the chronic disease in Vietnamese-American communities, with respect to language and culture, health literacy, and immigrant status. Ethnic minority groups and immigrant communities have less knowledge of health promoting behaviour, face considerable obstacles to health services, and experience poor communication with medical professionals. According to a recent review, studies has supported an independent relationship between literacy and knowledge of diabetes management and glucose control, but its impact on patients has not been sufficiently described. With the demand of chronic disease self-management (e.g., diabetic diet, glucose monitoring, etc.), a call for cultural-specific patient education is needed to achieve the control of diabetes and its adverse health outcomes in low- to middle-income Vietnamese-American immigrant communities.

EHealth Literacy

E-Health literacy is a term that describes the relatively modern concept of an individual's ability to search for, successfully access, comprehend, and appraise desired health information from electronic sources and to then use such information to attempt to address a particular health problem. Due to the increasing influence of the internet for information-seeking and health information distribution purposes, eHealth literacy has become an important topic of research in recent years. Stellefson (2011) states, "8 out of 10 Internet users report that they have at least once looked online for health information, making it the third most popular Web activity next to checking email and using search engines in terms of activities that almost everybody has done." Though in recent years, individuals may have gained access to a multitude of health information via the Internet, access alone does not ensure that proper search skills and techniques are being used to find the most relevant online and electronic resources. The lines between a reputable medical source and an amateur opinion from a so-called expert can often be blurred; however the ability to differentiate between the two is becoming increasing important.

Health literacy requires a combination of several different literacy skills in order to facilitate eHealth promotion and care. Six core skills are delineated by an eHealth literacy model referred to as the Lily model. The Lily Model's six literacies are organised into two central types: analytic and context-specific. Analytic type literacies are those skills that can be applied to a broad range of sources, regardless of topic or content (i.e., skills that can also be applied to shopping or researching a term paper in addition to health) whereas context-specific skills arc those that are contextualized within a specific problem domain (can solely be applied to health). The six literacies are listed below, the first three of the analytic type and the latter three of the context-specific:

- Traditional literacy
- Media literacy
- Information literacy
- Computer literacy
- Scientific literacy
- Health literacy

According to Norman (2006), both analytical and context-specific literacy skills are "required to fully engage with electronic health resources." As the World Wide Web and technological innovations are more and more becoming a part of the health care environment, it is important for information technology to be properly utilised to promote health and deliver health care effectively.

Health Care

Health care (or healthcare) is the diagnosis, treatment, and prevention of disease, illness, injury, and other physical and mental impairments in human beings. Health care is delivered by practitioners in allied health, dentistry, midwifery (obstetrics), medicine, nursing, optometry, pharmacy, psychology and other health professions. It refers to the work done in providing primary care, secondary care, and tertiary care, as well as in public health.

Access to health care varies across countries, groups, and individuals, largely influenced by social and economic conditions as well as the health policies in place. Countries and jurisdictions have different policies and plans in relation to the personal and population-based health care goals within their societies. Health care systems are organisations established to meet the health needs of target populations. Their exact configuration varies between national and subnational entities. In some countries and jurisdictions, health care planning is distributed among market participants, whereas in others, planning occurs more centrally among governments or other coordinating bodies. In all cases, according to the World Health Organisation (WHO), a well-functioning health care system requires a robust financing mechanism; a well-trained and adequately-paid workforce; reliable information on which to base decisions and policies; and well maintained health facilities and logistics to deliver quality medicines and technologies.

Health care can contribute to a significant part of a country's economy. In 2011, the health care industry consumed an average of 9.3 percent of the GDP or US$ 3,322 (PPP-adjusted) per capita across the 34 members of OECD countries. The USA (17.7%, or US$ PPP 8,508), the Netherlands (11.9%, 5,099), France (11.6%, 4,118), Germany (11.3%, 4,495), Canada (11.2%, 5669), and Switzerland (11%, 5,634) were the top spenders, however life expectancy in total population at birth was highest in Switzerland (82.8 years), Japan and Italy (82.7), Spain and Iceland (82.4), France (82.2) and Australia (82.0), while OECD's average exceeds 80 years for the first time ever in 2011: 80.1 years, a gain of 10 years since 1970. The USA (78.7 years) ranges only on place 26 among the 34 OECD member countries, but has the highest costs by far. All OECD countries have achieved universal (or almost universal) health coverage, except Mexico and the USA.

Health care is conventionally regarded as an important determinant in promoting the general physical and mental health and well-being of people around the world. An example of this was the worldwide eradication of smallpox in 1980, declared by the WHO as the first disease in human history to be completely eliminated by deliberate health care interventions.

Health Care Delivery

The delivery of modern health care depends on groups of trained professionals and paraprofessionals coming together as interdisciplinary teams. This includes professionals in medicine, psychology, physiotherapy, nursing, dentistry, midwifery (obstetrics) and allied health, plus many others such as public health practitioners, community health workers and assistive personnel, who systematically provide personal and population-based preventive, curative and rehabilitative care services. While the definitions of the various types of health care vary depending on the different cultural, political, organisational and disciplinary perspectives, there appears to be some consensus that primary care constitutes the first element of a continuing health care process, that may also include the provision of secondary and tertiary levels of care. Healthcare can be defined as either public or private.

Primary Care

Primary care refers to the work of health professionals who act as a first point of consultation for all patients within the health care system. Such a professional would usually be a primary care physician, such as a general practitioner or family physician, a licensed independent practitioner such as a physiotherapist, or a non-physician primary care provider (mid-level provider) such as a physician assistant or nurse practitioner. Depending on the locality, health system organisation, and sometimes at the patient's discretion, they may see another health care professional first, such as a pharmacist, a nurse (such as in the United Kingdom), a clinical officer (such as in parts of Africa), or an Ayurvedic or other traditional medicine professional (such as in parts of Asia). Depending on the nature of the health condition, patients may then be referred for secondary or tertiary care.

Primary care is often used as the term for the health care services which play a role in the local community. It can be provided in different settings, such as Urgent care centres which provide services to patients same day with appointment or walk-in bases.

Primary care involves the widest scope of health care, including all ages of patients, patients of all socioeconomic and geographic origins, patients seeking to maintain optimal health, and patients with all manner of acute and chronic physical, mental and social health issues, including multiple chronic diseases. Consequently, a primary care practitioner must possess a wide breadth of knowledge in many areas. Continuity is a key characteristic of primary care, as patients usually prefer to consult the same practitioner for routine check-ups and preventive care, health education, and every time they require an initial consultation about a new health problem. The International Classification of Primary Care (ICPC) is a standardized tool for understanding and analyzing information on interventions in primary care by the reason for the patient visit.

Common chronic illnesses usually treated in primary care may include, for example: hypertension, diabetes, asthma, COPD, depression and anxiety, back pain, arthritis or thyroid dysfunction. Primary care also includes many basic maternal and child health care services, such as family planning services and vaccinations.

In the United States, the 2013 National Health Interview Survey found that skin disorders (42.7%), osteoarthritis and joint disorders (33.6%), back problems (23.9%), disorders of lipid metabolism (22.4%), and upper respiratory tract disease (22.1%, excluding asthma) were the most common reasons for accessing a physician.

In context of global population aging, with increasing numbers of older adults at greater risk of chronic non-communicable diseases, rapidly increasing demand for primary care services is expected in both developed and developing countries. The World Health Organisation attributes the provision of essential primary care as an integral component of an inclusive primary health care strategy.

Secondary Care

Secondary care is the health care services provided by medical specialists and other health professionals who generally do not have first contact with patients, for example, cardiologists, urologists and dermatologists.

It includes acute care: necessary treatment for a short period of time for a brief but serious illness, injury or other health condition, such as in a hospital emergency department. It also includes skilled attendance during childbirth, intensive care, and medical imaging services.

The "secondary care" is sometimes used synonymously with "hospital care". However many secondary care providers do not necessarily work in hospitals, such as psychiatrists, clinical psychologists, occupational therapists or physiotherapists, and some primary care services are delivered within hospitals. Depending on the organisation and policies of the national health system, patients may be required to see a primary care provider for a referral before they can access secondary care.

For example in the United States, which operates under a mixed market health care system, some physicians might voluntarily limit their practice to secondary care by requiring patients to see a primary care provider first, or this restriction may be imposed under the terms of the payment agreements in private or group health insurance plans. In other cases medical specialists may see patients without a referral, and patients may decide whether self-referral is preferred.

In the United Kingdom and Canada, patient self-referral to a medical specialist for secondary care is rare as prior referral from another physician (either a primary care physician or another specialist) is considered necessary, regardless of whether the funding is from private insurance schemes or national health insurance.

Allied health professionals, such as physical therapists, respiratory therapists, occupational therapists, speech therapists, and dietitians, also generally work in secondary care, accessed through either patient self-referral or through physician referral.

Tertiary Care

Tertiary care is specialised consultative health care, usually for inpatients and on referral from a primary or secondary health professional, in a facility that has personnel and facilities for advanced medical investigation and treatment, such as a tertiary referral hospital. Examples of tertiary care services are cancer management, neurosurgery, cardiac surgery, plastic surgery, treatment for severe burns, advanced neonatology services, palliative, and other complex medical and surgical interventions.

Quaternary Care

The term quaternary care is sometimes used as an extension of tertiary care in reference to advanced levels of medicine which are highly specialised and not widely accessed. Experimental medicine and some types of uncommon diagnostic or surgical procedures are considered quaternary care. These services are usually only offered in a limited number of regional or national health care centres. This term is more prevalent in the United Kingdom, but just as applicable in the United States. A quaternary care hospital may have virtually any procedure available, whereas a tertiary care facility may not offer a sub-specialist with that training.

Home and Community Care

Many types of health care interventions are delivered outside of health facilities. They include many interventions of public health interest, such as food safety surveillance, distribution of condoms and needle-exchange programmes for the prevention of transmissible diseases.

They also include the services of professionals in residential and community settings in support of self care, home care, long-term care, assisted living, treatment for substance use disorders and other types of health and social care services.

Community rehabilitation services can assist with mobility and independence after loss of limbs or loss of function. This can include prosthesis, orthotics or wheelchairs.

Many countries, especially in the west are dealing with aging populations, and one of the priorities of the health care system is to help seniors live full, independent lives in the comfort of their own homes. There is an entire section of health care geared to providing seniors with help in day-to-day activities at home, transporting them to doctor's appointments, and many other activities that are so essential for their health and well-being.

Although they provide home care for older adults in cooperation, family members and care workers may harbor diverging attitudes and values towards their joint efforts. This state of affairs presents a challenge for the design of ICT for home care.

With obesity in children rapidly becoming a major concern, health services often set up programmes in schools aimed at educating children in good eating habits; making physical education compulsory in school; and teaching young adolescents to have positive self-image.

Ratings

Health care ratings are ratings or evaluations of health care used to evaluate process of care, healthcare structures and/or outcomes of a healthcare services. This information is translated into report cards that are generated by quality organisations, nonprofit, consumer groups and media. This evaluation of quality can be based on:

- Measures of Hospital quality
- Measures of Health Plan Quality
- Measures of Physician Quality
- Measures of Quality for Other Health Professionals
- Measures of Patient Experience

Related Sectors

Health care extends beyond the delivery of services to patients, encompassing many related sectors, and set within a bigger picture of financing and governance structures.

Health System

A health system, also sometimes referred to as health care system or healthcare system is the organisation of people, institutions, and resources to deliver health care services to meet the health needs of target populations.

Health Care Industry

The health care industry incorporates several sectors that are dedicated to providing health care services and products. As a basic framework for defining the sector, the United Nations' International Standard Industrial Classification categorizes health care as generally consisting of hospital activities, medical and dental practice activities, and "other human health activities". The last class involves activities of, or under the supervision of, nurses, midwives, physiotherapists, scientific or diagnostic laboratories, pathology clinics, residential health facilities, or other allied health professions, e.g. in the field of optometry, hydrotherapy, medical massage, yoga therapy, music therapy, occupational therapy, speech therapy, chiropody, homeopathy, chiropractics, acupuncture, etc.

In addition, according to industry and market classifications, such as the Global Industry Classification Standard and the Industry Classification Benchmark, health care includes many categories of medical equipment, instruments and services as well as biotechnology, diagnostic laboratories and substances, and drug manufacturing and delivery.

For example, pharmaceuticals and other medical devices are the leading high technology exports of Europe and the United States. The United States dominates the biopharmaceutical field, accounting for three-quarters of the world's biotechnology revenues.

Health Care Research

The quantity and quality of many health care interventions are improved through the results of science, such as advanced through the medical model of health which focuses on the eradication of illness through diagnosis and effective treatment. Many important advances have been made through health research, including biomedical research and pharmaceutical research, which form the basis for evidence-based medicine and evidence-based practice in health care delivery.

For example, in terms of pharmaceutical research and development spending, Europe spends a little less than the United States (€22.50bn compared to €27.05bn in 2006). The United States accounts for 80% of the world's research and development spending in biotechnology.

In addition, the results of health services research can lead to greater efficiency and equitable delivery of health care interventions, as advanced through the social model of health and disability, which emphasizes the societal changes that can be made to make population healthier. Results from health services research often form the basis of evidence-based policy in health care systems. Health services research is also aided by initiatives in the field of AI for the development of systems of health assessment that are clinically useful, timely, sensitive to change, culturally sensitive, low burden, low cost, involving for the patient and built into standard procedures.

Health Care Financing

There are generally five primary methods of funding health care systems:

1. general taxation to the state, county or municipality
2. social health insurance
3. voluntary or private health insurance
4. out-of-pocket payments
5. donations to health charities

In most countries, the financing of health care services features a mix of all five models, but the exact distribution varies across countries and over time within countries. In all countries and jurisdictions, there are many topics in the politics and evidence that can influence the decision of a government, private sector business or other group to adopt a specific health policy regarding the financing structure.

For example, social health insurance is where a nation's entire population is eligible for health care coverage, and this coverage and the services provided are regulated. In almost every jurisdiction with a government-funded health care system, a parallel private, and usually for-profit, system is allowed to operate. This is sometimes referred to as two-tier health care or universal health care.

E.g. in Poland (former communist country) the costs of health services borne by the National Health Fund (financed by all that pay health insurance contributions) in 2012 amounted to 60.8 billion PLN (appr. 20 billion USD). The right to health services in Poland has about 99,9% of population (also registered unemployed persons and their spouses).

Health Care Administration and Regulation

The management and administration of health care is another sector vital to the delivery of health care services. In particular, the practice of health professionals and operation of health care institutions is typically regulated by national or state/provincial authorities through appropriate regulatory bodies for purposes of quality assurance. Most countries have credentialing staff in regulatory boards or health departments who document the certification or licensing of health workers and their work history.

Health Information Technology

Health information technology (HIT) is "the application of information processing involving both computer hardware and software that deals with the storage, retrieval, sharing, and use of health care information, data, and knowledge for communication and decision making." Technology is a broad concept that deals with a species' usage and knowledge of tools and crafts, and how it affects a species' ability to control and adapt to its environment. However, a strict definition is elusive; "technology" can refer to material objects of use to humanity, such as machines, hardware or utensils, but can also encompass broader themes, including systems, methods of organisation, and techniques. For HIT, technology represents computers and communications attributes that can be networked to build systems for moving health information. Informatics is yet another integral aspect of HIT.

Disease Surveillance

Disease surveillance is an epidemiological practice by which the spread of disease is monitored in order to establish patterns of progression. The main role of disease surveillance is to predict, observe, and minimize the harm caused by outbreak, epidemic, and pandemic situations, as well as increase knowledge about which factors contribute to such circumstances. A key part of modern disease surveillance is the practice of disease case reporting.

In modern times, reporting incidences of disease outbreaks has been transformed from manual record keeping to instant world wide internet communication.

The number of cases could be gathered from hospitals - which would be expected to see most of the occurrences - collated, and eventually made public. With the advent of modern communication technology, this has changed dramatically. Organisations like the World Health Organisation (WHO) and the Centres for Disease Control now can report cases and deaths from significant diseases within days - sometimes within hours - of the occurrence. Further, there is considerable public pressure to make this information available quickly and accurately.

Mandatory Reporting

Formal reporting of notifiable infectious diseases is a requirement placed upon health care providers by many regional and national governments, and upon national governments by the World Health Organisation. Since 1969, WHO has required that all cases of the following diseases be reported to the organisation: cholera, plague, yellow fever, smallpox, relapsing fever and typhus. In 2005, the list was extended to include polio and SARS. Regional and national governments typically monitor a larger set of (around 80 in the U.S.) communicable diseases that can potentially threaten the general population. Tuberculosis, HIV, botulism, hantavirus, anthrax, and rabies are examples of such diseases. The incidence counts of diseases are often used as health indicators to describe the overall health of a population.

World Health Organisation

The World Health Organisation is the lead agency for coordinating global response to major diseases. The WHO maintains Web sites for a number of diseases, and has active teams in many countries where these diseases occur. During the SARS outbreak in early 2004, for example, the Beijing staff of the WHO produced updates every few days for the duration of the outbreak. Beginning in January 2004, the WHO has produced similar updates for H5N1. These results are widely reported and closely watched.

WHO's Epidemic and Pandemic Alert and Response (EPR) to detect, verify rapidly and respond appropriately to epidemic-prone and emerging disease threats covers the following diseases:

- Anthrax
- Avian influenza
- Crimean-Congo hemorrhagic fever
- Dengue hemorrhagic fever
- Ebola virus disease
- Hepatitis
- Influenza
- Lassa fever
- Marburg hemorrhagic fever
- Meningococcal disease
- Plague
- Rift Valley fever
- Severe Acute Respiratory Syndrome
- Smallpox
- Tularaemia
- Yellow fever

Political Challenges

As the lead organisation in global public health, the WHO occupies a delicate role in global politics. It must maintain good relationships with each of the many countries in which it is active.

As a result, it may only report results within a particular country with the agreement of the country's government. Because some governments regard the release of *any* information on disease outbreaks as a state secret, this can place the WHO in a difficult position.

The WHO coordinated *International Outbreak Alert and Response* is designed to ensure "outbreaks of potential international importance are rapidly verified and information is quickly shared within the Network" but not necessarily by the public; integrate and coordinate "activities to support national efforts" rather than challenge national authority within that nation in order to "respect the independence and objectivity of all partners".

The commitment that "All Network responses will proceed with full respect for ethical standards, human rights, national and local laws, cultural sensitivities and tradition" ensures each nation that its security, financial, and other interests will be given full weight.

Technical Challenges

Testing for a disease can be expensive, and distinguishing between two diseases can be prohibitively difficult in many countries. One standard means of determining if a person has had a particular disease is to test for the presence of antibodies that are particular to this disease. In the case of H5N1, for example, there is a low pathogenic H5N1 strain in wild birds in North America that a human could conceivably have antibodies against.

It would be extremely difficult to distinguish between antibodies produced by this strain, and antibodies produced by Asian lineage HPAI A(H5N1). Similar difficulties are common, and make it difficult to determine how widely a disease may have spread.

There is currently little available data on the spread of H5N1 in wild birds in Africa and Asia. Without such data, predicting how the disease might spread in the future is difficult. Information that scientists and decision makers need to make useful medical products and informed decisions for health care, but currently lack include:

- Surveillance of wild bird populations
- Cell cultures of particular strains of diseases

H5N1

Surveillance of H5N1 in humans, poultry, wild birds, cats and other animals remains very weak in many parts of Asia and Africa. Much remains unknown about the exact extent of its spread.

H5N1 in China is less than fully reported. Blogs have described many discrepancies between official China government announcements concerning H5N1 and what people in China see with their own eyes. Many reports of total H5N1 cases have excluded China due to widespread disbelief in China's official numbers.

> *"Only half the world's human bird flu cases are being reported to the World Health Organisation within two weeks of being detected, a response time that must be improved to avert a pandemic, a senior WHO official said Saturday. Shigeru Omi, WHO's regional director for the Western Pacific, said it is estimated that countries would have only two to three weeks to stamp out, or at least slow, a pandemic flu strain after it began spreading in humans."*

David Nabarro, chief avian flu coordinator for the United Nations, says avian flu has too many unanswered questions.

CIDRAP reported on August 25, 2006 on a new US government Web site that allows the public to view current information about testing of wild birds for H5N1 avian influenza which is part of a national wild-bird surveillance plan that "includes five strategies for early detection of highly pathogenic avian influenza. Sample numbers from three of these will be available on HEDDS: live wild birds, subsistence hunter-killed birds, and investigations of sick and dead wild birds. The other two strategies involve domestic bird testing and environmental sampling of water and wild-bird droppings. A map on the new USGS site shows that 9,327 birds from Alaska have been tested so far this year, with only a few from most other states. Last year officials tested just 721 birds from Alaska and none from most other states, another map shows. The goal of the surveillance programme for 2006 is to collect 75,000 to 100,000 samples from wild birds and 50,000 environmental samples, officials have said."

Outbreak

In epidemiology, an outbreak is an occurrence of disease greater than expected at a particular time and place. It may affect a small and localized group or impact upon thousands of people across an entire continent. Two linked cases of a rare infectious disease may be sufficient to constitute an outbreak. Outbreaks may also refer to epidemics, which affect a region in a country or a group of countries, or pandemics, which describe global disease outbreaks.

Outbreak Investigation

When investigating disease outbreaks, the epidemiology profession has developed a number of widely accepted steps. As described by the Centres for Disease Control and Prevention, these include the following:

- Verify the diagnosis related to the outbreak
- Identify the existence of the outbreak (Is the group of ill persons normal for the time of year, geographic area, etc.?)
- Create a case definition to define who/what is included as a case
- Map the spread of the outbreak using Information technology as diagnosis is reported to insurance
- Develop a hypothesis (What appears to be causing the outbreak?)
- Study hypothesis (collect data and perform analysis)
- Refine hypothesis and carry out further study
- Develop and implement control and prevention systems
- Release findings to greater communities

Outbreak debriefing and review has also been recognised as an additional final step and iterative process by the Public Health Agency of Canada.

Types

There are several outbreak patterns, which can be useful in identifying the transmission method or source, and predicting the future rate of infection. Each has a distinctive epidemic curve, or histogram of case infections and deaths.

- Common source – All victims acquire the infection from the same source (e.g. a contaminated water supply).
    - o Continuous source – Common source outbreak where the exposure occurs over multiple incubation periods
    - o Point source – Common source outbreak where the exposure occurs in less than one incubation period
- Propagated – Transmission occurs from person to person.

Outbreaks can also be:

- Behavioural risk related (e.g., sexually transmitted diseases, increased risk due to malnutrition)
- Zoonotic – The infectious agent is endemic to an animal population.

Patterns of occurrence are:

- Endemic – a communicable disease, such as influenza, measles, mumps, pneumonia, colds, smallpox, which is characteristic of a particular place, or among a particular group, or area of interest or activity.
- Epidemic – when this disease is found to infect a significantly larger number of people at the same time than is common at that time, and among that population, and may spread through one or several communities.
- Pandemic – occurs when an epidemic spreads worldwide.

Outbreak Legislation

Outbreak legislation is still in its infancy and not many countries have had a direct and complete set of the provisions. However, some countries do manage the outbreaks using relevant acts, such as public health law.

Pandemic

A pandemic is an epidemic of infectious disease that has spread through human populations across a large region; for instance multiple continents, or even worldwide. A widespread endemic disease that is stable in terms of how many people are getting sick from it is not a pandemic. Further, flu pandemics generally exclude recurrences of seasonal flu. Throughout history there have been a number of pandemics, such as smallpox and tuberculosis. More recent pandemics include the HIV pandemic as well as the 1918 and 2009 H1N1 pandemics.

Definition and Stages

A pandemic is an epidemic occurring on a scale which crosses international boundaries, usually affecting a large number of people.

The World Health Organisation (WHO) has a six-stage classification that describes the process by which a novel influenza virus moves from the first few infections in humans through to a pandemic. This starts with the virus mostly infecting animals, with a few cases where animals infect people, then moves through the stage where the virus begins to spread directly between people, and ends with a pandemic when infections from the new virus have spread worldwide and it will be out of control until we stop it.

A disease or condition is not a pandemic merely because it is widespread or kills many people; it must also be infectious. For instance, cancer is responsible for many deaths but is not considered a pandemic because the disease is not infectious or contagious.

In a virtual press conference in May 2009 on the influenza pandemic, Dr Keiji Fukuda, Assistant Director-General *ad interim* for Health Security and Environment, WHO said "An easy way to think about pandemic ... is to say: a pandemic is a global outbreak. Then you might ask yourself: "What is a global outbreak"? Global outbreak means that we see both spread of the agent... and then we see disease activities in addition to the spread of the virus."

In planning for a possible influenza pandemic, the WHO published a document on pandemic preparedness guidance in 1999, revised in 2005 and in February 2009, defining phases and appropriate actions for each phase in an aide memoir entitled *WHO pandemic phase descriptions and main actions by phase*. The 2009 revision, including definitions of a pandemic and the phases leading to its declaration, were finalized in February 2009. The pandemic H1N1 2009 virus, was neither on the horizon at that time nor mentioned in the document All versions of this document refer to influenza. The phases are defined by the spread of the disease; virulence and mortality are not mentioned in the current WHO definition, although these factors have previously been included.

Current Pandemics

HIV and AIDS

HIV originated in Africa, and spread to the United States via Haiti between 1966 and 1972. AIDS is currently a pandemic, with infection rates as high as 25% in southern and eastern Africa. In 2006 the HIV prevalence rate among pregnant women in South Africa was 29.1%. Effective education about safer sexual practices and bloodborne infection precautions training have helped to slow down infection rates in several African countries sponsoring national education programmes. Infection rates are rising again in Asia and the Americas. AIDS death toll in Africa may reach 90–100 million by 2025.

Pandemics and Notable Epidemics Through History

There have been a number of significant pandemics recorded in human history, generally zoonoses which came about with domestication of animals, such as influenza and tuberculosis. There have been a number of particularly significant epidemics that deserve mention above the "mere" destruction of cities:

- Plague of Athens, 430 BC. Possibly typhoid fever killed a quarter of the Athenian troops, and a quarter of the population over four years. This disease fatally weakened the dominance of Athens, but the sheer virulence of the disease prevented its wider spread; i.e. it killed off its hosts at a rate faster than they could spread it. The exact cause of the plague was unknown for many years. In January 2006, researchers from the University of Athens analyzed teeth recovered from a mass grave underneath the city, and confirmed the presence of bacteria responsible for typhoid.
- Antonine Plague, 165–180. Possibly smallpox brought to the Italian peninsula by soldiers returning from the Near East; it killed a quarter of those infected, and up to five million in all. At the height of a second outbreak, the Plague of Cyprian (251–266), which may have been the same disease, 5,000 people a day were said to be dying in Rome.
- Plague of Justinian, from 541 to 750, was the first recorded outbreak of the bubonic plague. It started in Egypt, and reached Constantinople the following spring, killing (according to the Byzantine chronicler Procopius) 10,000 a day at its height, and perhaps 40% of the city's inhabitants. The plague went on to eliminate a quarter to a half of the human population that it struck throughout the known world. It caused Europe's population to drop by around 50% between 550 and 700.
- Black Death, from 1347 to 1453. The total number of deaths worldwide is estimated at 75 million people. Eight hundred years after the last outbreak, the plague returned to Europe. Starting in Asia, the disease reached Mediterranean and western Europe in 1348 (possibly from Italian merchants fleeing fighting in Crimea), and killed an estimated 20 to 30 million Europeans in six years; a third of the total population, and up to a half in the worst-affected urban areas. It was the first of a cycle of European plague epidemics that continued until the 18th century. There were more than 100 plague epidemics in Europe in this period. The disease recurred in England every two to five years from 1361 to 1480. By the 1370s, England's population was reduced by 50%. The Great Plague of London of 1665–66 was the last major outbreak of the plague in England.

The disease killed approximately 100,000 people, 20% of London's population.

- The third plague pandemic started in China in 1855, and spread to India, where 10 million people died. During this pandemic, the United States saw its first outbreak: the San Francisco plague of 1900–1904. Today, isolated cases of plague are still found in the western United States.

Encounters between European explorers and populations in the rest of the world often introduced local epidemics of extraordinary virulence. Disease killed part of the native population of the Canary Islands in the 16th century (Guanches). Half the native population of Hispaniola in 1518 was killed by smallpox. Smallpox also ravaged Mexico in the 1520s, killing 150,000 in Tenochtitlán alone, including the emperor, and Peru in the 1530s, aiding the European conquerors. Measles killed a further two million Mexican natives in the 17th century. In 1618–1619, smallpox wiped out 90% of the Massachusetts Bay Native Americans. During the 1770s, smallpox killed at least 30% of the Pacific Northwest Native Americans. Smallpox epidemics in 1780–1782 and 1837–1838 brought devastation and drastic depopulation among the Plains Indians. Some believe that the death of up to 95% of the Native American population of the New World was caused by Old World diseases such as smallpox, measles, and influenza. Over the centuries, the Europeans had developed high degrees of immunity to these diseases, while the indigenous peoples had no such immunity.

Smallpox devastated the native population of Australia, killing around 50% of Indigenous Australians in the early years of British colonisation. It also killed many New Zealand Mβori. As late as 1848–49, as many as 40,000 out of 150,000 Hawaiians are estimated to have died of measles, whooping cough and influenza. Introduced diseases, notably smallpox, nearly wiped out the native population of Easter Island. In 1875, measles killed over 40,000 Fijians, approximately one-third of the population. The disease devastated the Andamanese population. Ainu population decreased drastically in the 19th century, due in large part to infectious diseases brought by Japanese settlers pouring into Hokkaido.

Researchers concluded that syphilis was carried from the New World to Europe after Columbus' voyages. The findings suggested Europeans could have carried the nonvenereal tropical bacteria home, where the organisms may have mutated into a more deadly form in the different conditions of Europe. The disease was more frequently fatal than it is today. Syphilis was a major killer in Europe during the

Renaissance. Between 1602 and 1796, the Dutch East India Company sent almost a million Europeans to work in Asia. Ultimately, only less than one-third made their way back to Europe. The majority died of diseases. Disease killed more British soldiers in India than war.

As early as 1803, the Spanish Crown organised a mission (the Balmis expedition) to transport the smallpox vaccine to the Spanish colonies, and establish mass vaccination programmes there. By 1832, the federal government of the United States established a smallpox vaccination programme for Native Americans. From the beginning of the 20th century onwards, the elimination or control of disease in tropical countries became a driving force for all colonial powers. The sleeping sickness epidemic in Africa was arrested due to mobile teams systematically screening millions of people at risk. In the 20th century, the world saw the biggest increase in its population in human history due to lessening of the mortality rate in many countries due to medical advances. The world population has grown from 1.6 billion in 1900 to an estimated 7 billion today.

Cholera

Since it became widespread in the 19th century, cholera has killed tens of millions of people.

- First cholera pandemic 1816–1826. Previously restricted to the Indian subcontinent, the pandemic began in Bengal, then spread across India by 1820. 10,000 British troops and countless Indians died during this pandemic. It extended as far as China, Indonesia (where more than 100,000 people succumbed on the island of Java alone) and the Caspian Sea before receding. Deaths in India between 1817 and 1860 are estimated to have exceeded 15 million persons. Another 23 million died between 1865 and 1917. Russian deaths during a similar period exceeded 2 million.
- Second cholera pandemic 1829–1851. Reached Russia, Hungary (about 100,000 deaths) and Germany in 1831, London in 1832 (more than 55,000 persons died in the United Kingdom), France, Canada (Ontario), and United States (New York) in the same year, and the Pacific coast of North America by 1834. A two-year outbreak began in England and Wales in 1848 and claimed 52,000 lives. It is believed that over 150,000 Americans died of cholera between 1832 and 1849.
- Third pandemic 1852–1860. Mainly affected Russia, with over a million deaths. Throughout Spain, cholera caused more than 236,000 deaths in 1854–55. It claimed 200,000 lives in Mexico.

- Fourth pandemic 1863–1875. Spread mostly in Europe and Africa. At least 30,000 of the 90,000 Mecca pilgrims fell victim to the disease. Cholera claimed 90,000 lives in Russia in 1866.
- In 1866, there was an outbreak in North America. It killed some 50,000 Americans.
- Fifth pandemic 1881–1896. The 1883–1887 epidemic cost 250,000 lives in Europe and at least 50,000 in Americas. Cholera claimed 267,890 lives in Russia (1892); 120,000 in Spain; 90,000 in Japan and 60,000 in Persia.
- In 1892, cholera contaminated the water supply of Hamburg, and caused 8,606 deaths.
- Sixth pandemic 1899–1923. Had little effect in Europe because of advances in public health, but Russia was badly affected again (more than 500,000 people dying of cholera during the first quarter of the 20th century). The sixth pandemic killed more than 800,000 in India. The 1902–1904 cholera epidemic claimed over 200,000 lives in the Philippines.
- Seventh pandemic 1962–66. Began in Indonesia, called El Tor after the strain, and reached Bangladesh in 1963, India in 1964, and the USSR in 1966.

Influenza

- The Greek physician Hippocrates, the "Father of Medicine", first described influenza in 412 BC.
- The first influenza pandemic was recorded in 1580 and since then influenza pandemics occurred every 10 to 30 years.
- The 1889–1890 flu pandemic, also known as Russian Flu, was first reported in May 1889 in Bukhara, Uzbekistan. By October, it had reached Tomsk and the Caucasus. It rapidly spread west and hit North America in December 1889, South America in February–April 1890, India in February–March 1890, and Australia in March–April 1890. The H3N8 and H2N2 subtypes of the Influenza A virus have each been identified as possible causes. It had a very high attack and mortality rate, causing around a million fatalities.
- The "Spanish flu", 1918–1919. First identified early in March 1918 in US troops training at Camp Funston, Kansas. By October 1918, it had spread to become a worldwide pandemic on all continents, and eventually infected about one-third of the world's population (or $\approx$500 million persons). Unusually deadly and virulent, it ended nearly as quickly as it began,

vanishing completely within 18 months. In six months, some 50 million were dead; some estimates put the total of those killed worldwide at over twice that number. About 17 million died in India, 675,000 in the United States and 200,000 in the UK. The virus was recently reconstructed by scientists at the CDC studying remains preserved by the Alaskan permafrost. The H1N1 virus has a small, but crucial structure that is similar to the Spanish Flu.

- The "Asian Flu", 1957–58. An H2N2 virus caused about 70,000 deaths in the United States. First identified in China in late February 1957, the Asian flu spread to the United States by June 1957. It caused about 2 million deaths globally.
- The "Hong Kong Flu", 1968–69. An H3N2 caused about 34,000 deaths in the United States. This virus was first detected in Hong Kong in early 1968, and spread to the United States later that year. This pandemic of 1968 and 1969 killed approximately one million people worldwide. Influenza A (H3N2) viruses still circulate today.

Typhus

Typhus is sometimes called "camp fever" because of its pattern of flaring up in times of strife. (It is also known as "gaol fever" and "ship fever", for its habits of spreading wildly in cramped quarters, such as jails and ships.) Emerging during the Crusades, it had its first impact in Europe in 1489, in Spain. During fighting between the Christian Spaniards and the Muslims in Granada, the Spanish lost 3,000 to war casualties, and 20,000 to typhus. In 1528, the French lost 18,000 troops in Italy, and lost supremacy in Italy to the Spanish. In 1542, 30,000 soldiers died of typhus while fighting the Ottomans in the Balkans.

During the Thirty Years' War (1618–1648), about 8 million Germans were killed by bubonic plague and typhus. The disease also played a major role in the destruction of Napoleon's *Grande Armée* in Russia in 1812. During the retreat from Moscow, more French military personnel died of typhus than were killed by the Russians. Of the 450,000 soldiers who crossed the Neman on 25 June 1812, less than 40,000 returned. More military personnel were killed from 1500–1914 by typhus than from military action. In early 1813 Napoleon raised a new army of 500,000 to replace his Russian losses. In the campaign of that year, over 219,000 of Napoleon's soldiers died of typhus. Typhus played a major factor in the Irish Potato Famine. During World War I, typhus epidemics killed over 150,000 in Serbia. There were about 25 million infections and 3 million deaths from epidemic typhus in Russia from 1918 to 1922. Typhus also killed numerous prisoners in the Nazi concentration camps and Soviet prisoner of war camps during World War II. More than 3.5 million Soviet POWs died in the Nazi custody out of 5.7 million.

Smallpox

Smallpox is a highly contagious disease caused by the Variola virus. The disease killed an estimated 400,000 Europeans per year during the closing years of the 18th century. During the 20th century, it is estimated that smallpox was responsible for 300–500 million deaths. As recently as early 1950s an estimated 50 million cases of smallpox occurred in the world each year. After successful vaccination campaigns throughout the 19th and 20th centuries, the WHO certified the eradication of smallpox in December 1979. To this day, smallpox is the only human infectious disease to have been completely eradicated, and one of two infectious viruses ever to be eradicated.

Measles

Historically, measles was prevalent throughout the world, as it is highly contagious. According to the National Immunization Programme, 90% of people were infected with measles by age 15. Before the vaccine was introduced in 1963, there were an estimated 3–4 million cases in the U.S. each year. Measles killed around 200 million people worldwide over the last 150 years. In 2000 alone, measles killed some 777,000 worldwide out of 40 million cases globally.

Measles is an endemic disease, meaning that it has been continually present in a community, and many people develop resistance. In populations that have not been exposed to measles, exposure to a new disease can be devastating. In 1529, a measles outbreak in Cuba killed two-thirds of the natives who had previously survived smallpox. The disease had ravaged Mexico, Central America, and the Inca civilization.

Tuberculosis

One–third of the world's current population has been infected with *Mycobacterium tuberculosis*, and new infections occur at a rate of one per second. About 5–10% of these latent infections will eventually progress to active disease, which, if left untreated, kills more than half of its victims. Annually, 8 million people become ill with tuberculosis, and 2 million people die from the disease worldwide. In the 19th century, tuberculosis killed an estimated one-quarter of the adult population of Europe; by 1918 one in six deaths in France were still caused by TB.

During the 20th century, tuberculosis killed approximately 100 million people. TB is still one of the most important health problems in the developing world.

Leprosy

Leprosy, also known as Wopat's or Hansen's Disease, is caused by a bacillus, *Mycobacterium leprae.* It is a chronic disease with an incubation period of up to five years. Since 1985, 15 million people worldwide have been cured of leprosy.

Historically, leprosy has affected people since at least 600 BC. Leprosy outbreaks began to occur in Western Europe around 1000 AD. Numerous *leprosaria*, or leper hospitals, sprang up in the Middle Ages; Matthew Paris estimated that in the early 13th century there were 19,000 across Europe.

Malaria

Malaria is widespread in tropical and subtropical regions, including parts of the Americas, Asia, and Africa. Each year, there are approximately 350–500 million cases of malaria. Drug resistance poses a growing problem in the treatment of malaria in the 21st century, since resistance is now common against all classes of antimalarial drugs, except for the artemisinins.

Malaria was once common in most of Europe and North America, where it is now for all purposes non-existent. Malaria may have contributed to the decline of the Roman Empire. The disease became known as "Roman fever". *Plasmodium falciparum* became a real threat to colonists and indigenous people alike when it was introduced into the Americas along with the slave trade. Malaria devastated the Jamestown colony and regularly ravaged the South and Midwest. By 1830 it had reached the Pacific Northwest. During the American Civil War, there were over 1.2 million cases of malaria among soldiers of both sides. The southern U.S. continued to be afflicted with millions of cases of malaria into the 1930s.

Yellow Fever

Yellow fever has been a source of several devastating epidemics. Cities as far north as New York, Philadelphia, and Boston were hit with epidemics. In 1793, one of the largest yellow fever epidemics in U.S. history killed as many as 5,000 people in Philadelphia—roughly 10% of the population. About half of the residents had fled the city, including President George Washington. In colonial times, West Africa became known as "the white man's grave" because of malaria and yellow fever.

Concern About Possible Future Pandemics

Viral Hemorrhagic Fevers

Viruses causing viral hemorrhagic fever such as Lassa fever virus, Rift Valley fever, Marburg virus, Ebola virus and Bolivian hemorrhagic fever are highly contagious and deadly diseases, with the theoretical potential to become pandemics.

Their ability to spread efficiently enough to cause a pandemic is limited, however, as transmission of these viruses requires close contact with the infected vector, and the vector only has a short time before death or serious illness.

Furthermore, the short time between a vector becoming infectious and the onset of symptoms allows medical professionals to quickly quarantine vectors, and prevent them from carrying the pathogen elsewhere. Genetic mutations could occur, which could elevate their potential for causing widespread harm; thus close observation by contagious disease specialists is merited.

Antibiotic Resistance

Antibiotic-resistant microorganisms, sometimes referred to as "superbugs", may contribute to the re-emergence of diseases which are currently well controlled. For example, cases of tuberculosis that are resistant to traditionally effective treatments remain a cause of great concern to health professionals. Every year, nearly half a million new cases of multidrug-resistant tuberculosis (MDR-TB) are estimated to occur worldwide. China and India have the highest rate of multidrug-resistant TB.

The World Health Organisation (WHO) reports that approximately 50 million people worldwide are infected with MDR TB, with 79 percent of those cases resistant to three or more antibiotics. In 2005, 124 cases of MDR TB were reported in the United States. Extensively drug-resistant tuberculosis (XDR TB) was identified in Africa in 2006, and subsequently discovered to exist in 49 countries, including the United States. There are about 40,000 new cases of XDR-TB per year, the WHO estimates.

In the past 20 years, common bacteria including *Staphylococcus aureus*, *Serratia marcescens* and Enterococcus, have developed resistance to various antibiotics such as vancomycin, as well as whole classes of antibiotics, such as the aminoglycosides and cephalosporins. Antibiotic-resistant organisms have become an important cause of healthcare-associated (nosocomial) infections (HAI).

In addition, infections caused by community-acquired strains of methicillin-resistant *Staphylococcus aureus* (MRSA) in otherwise healthy individuals have become more frequent in recent years.

SARS

In 2003 the Italian physician Carlo Urbani (1956-2003) was to the first to identify severe acute respiratory syndrome (SARS) as a new and dangerously contagious disease although he became infected and died. It is caused by a coronavirus dubbed SARS-CoV.

Rapid action by national and international health authorities such as the World Health Organisation helped to slow transmission and eventually broke the chain of transmission, which ended the localized epidemics before they could become a pandemic. However, the disease has not been eradicated. It could re-emerge. This warrants monitoring and reporting of suspicious cases of atypical pneumonia.

H5N1 (Avian Flu)

In February 2004, avian influenza virus was detected in birds in Vietnam, increasing fears of the emergence of new variant strains. It is feared that if the avian influenza virus combines with a human influenza virus (in a bird or a human), the new subtype created could be both highly contagious and highly lethal in humans. Such a subtype could cause a global influenza pandemic, similar to the Spanish Flu, or the lower mortality pandemics such as the Asian Flu and the Hong Kong Flu.

From October 2004 to February 2005, some 3,700 test kits of the 1957 Asian Flu virus were accidentally spread around the world from a lab in the US.

In May 2005, scientists urgently called upon nations to prepare for a global influenza pandemic that could strike as much as 20% of the world's population.

In October 2005, cases of the avian flu (the deadly strain H5N1) were identified in Turkey. EU Health Commissioner Markos Kyprianou said: "We have received now confirmation that the virus found in Turkey is an avian flu H5N1 virus.

There is a direct relationship with viruses found in Russia, Mongolia and China." Cases of bird flu were also identified shortly thereafter in Romania, and then Greece. Possible cases of the virus have also been found in Croatia, Bulgaria and the United Kingdom.

By November 2007, numerous confirmed cases of the H5N1 strain had been identified across Europe. However, by the end of October only 59 people had died as a result of H5N1 which was atypical of previous influenza pandemics.

Avian flu cannot yet be categorized as a "pandemic", because the virus cannot yet cause sustained and efficient human-to-human transmission. Cases so far are recognised to have been transmitted from bird to human, but as of December 2006 there have been very few (if any) cases of proven human-to-human transmission.

Regular influenza viruses establish infection by attaching to receptors in the throat and lungs, but the avian influenza virus can only attach to receptors located deep in the lungs of humans, requiring close, prolonged contact with infected patients, and thus limiting person-to-person transmission.

Ebola Virus

Biological Warfare: In 1346, the bodies of Mongol warriors who had died of plague were thrown over the walls of the besieged Crimean city of Kaffa (now Theodosia). After a protracted siege, during which the Mongol army under Jani Beg was suffering the disease, they catapulted the infected corpses over the city walls to infect the inhabitants. It has been speculated that this operation may have been responsible for the arrival of the Black Death in Europe.

The Native American population was devastated after contact with the Old World by introduction of many fatal diseases.

There is, however, only one documented case of germ warfare, involving British commander Jeffrey Amherst and Swiss-British officer Colonel Henry Bouquet, whose correspondence included a reference to the idea of giving smallpox-infected blankets to Indians as part of an incident known as Pontiac's Rebellion, which occurred during the Siege of Fort Pitt (1763) late in the French and Indian War.

It is unclear whether or not this attempt succeeded. Smallpox after Pontiac's Rebellion killed 400,000–500,000 (possibly even up to 1.5 million) Native Americans.

During the Sino-Japanese War (1937–1945), Unit 731 of the Imperial Japanese Army conducted human experimentation on thousands, mostly Chinese. In military campaigns, the Japanese army used biological weapons on Chinese soldiers and civilians. Plague fleas, infected clothing, and infected supplies encased in bombs were dropped on various targets.

The resulting cholera, anthrax, and plague were estimated to have killed around 400,000 Chinese civilians.

Diseases considered for or known to be used as a weapon include anthrax, ebola, Marburg virus, plague, cholera, typhus, Rocky Mountain spotted fever, tularemia, brucellosis, Q fever, machupo, Coccidioides mycosis, Glanders, Melioidosis, Shigella, Psittacosis, Japanese B encephalitis, Rift Valley fever, yellow fever, and smallpox.

Spores of weaponized anthrax were accidentally released from a military facility near the Soviet closed city of Sverdlovsk in 1979. The Sverdlovsk anthrax leak is sometimes called "biological Chernobyl". In January 2009, an Al-Qaeda training camp in Algeria was reportedly wiped out by the plague, killing approximately 40 Islamic extremists. Some experts said that the group was developing biological weapons, however, a couple of days later the Algerian Health Ministry flatly denied this rumour stating "No case of plague of any type has been recorded in any region of Algeria since 2003".

Bibliography

Amanda J. Thomas: *The Lambeth cholera outbreak of 1848-1849: the setting, causes, course and aftermath of an epidemic in London*, McFarland, United States, 2010.

Anderson, Barbara A; Härm, Erna: *Human Fertility in Russia since the Nineteenth Century*, NJ: Princeton University Press, Princeton, 1979.

Bartley, M.: *Understanding Health Inequalities*, Polity Press, Oxford UK, 2003.

Begon, M.; Townsend, C. R.; Harper, J. L.: *Ecology: From Individuals to Ecosystems*, Blackwell Publishing, Oxford, UK, 2006.

Breslow, Lester, ed. (2002). Encyclopedia of Public Health. New York: Macmillan Reference USA.

Chesnais, Jean-Claude: *The Demographic Transition: Stages, Patterns, and Economic Implications*, Oxford Univercity Press, London. 1990.

Clayton, David and Michael Hills: *Statistical Models in Epidemiology, Oxford University Press*, London, 1993.

Darnell, Regna: *Histories of anthropology annual*, University of Nebraska Press, United States, 2008.

Esping-Andersen, G.: *A child-centred social investment strategy*, Oxford University Press, Oxford UK, 2002.

Garrett, Laurie: *Betrayal of Trust: the Collapse of Global Public Health*, Hyperion, New York, 2000.

Gillam Stephen; Yates, Jan; Badrinath, Padmanabhan: *Essential Public Health : theory and practice*, Cambridge University Press, 2007.

Graham, H.: *Unequal Lives: Health and Socioeconomic Inequalities*, Open University Press, New York, 2007.

Hanski, I.; Gaggiotti, O. E.: *Ecology, genetics and evolution of metapopulations*, Elsevier Academic Press, Burlington, MA, 2004.

Heggenhougen, Kris; Stella R Quah: *International Encyclopedia of Public Health*, Elsevier/Academic Press, Amsterdam Boston, 2008.

Khoury, M.J.; Beaty, T.H.; Cohen, B.H.: Fundamentals of genetic epidemiology, Oxford University Press, New York, 1993.

Khoury, Muin J.; Little, Julian; Burke, Wylie, *Human Genome Epidemiology: A scientific foundation for using genetic information to improve health and prevent disease*, Oxford University Press, 2003.

Marmot & R. G. Wilkinson: *Social Determinants of Health,* Oxford University Press, Oxford, UK, 1970.

Morabia, Alfredo: *A History of Epidemiologic Methods and Concepts*, Birkhauser Verlag, Basel, 2004.

Morton, Newton E; Chung, Chin Sik: *Genetic Epidemiology*, Academic Press, New York, 1978.

Notestein, Frank W.: *Population — The Long View* in Theodore W. Schultz, University of Chicago Press, Chicago, 1945.

Novick, Lloyd F; Cynthia B Morrow; Glen P Mays: *Public Health Administration: Principles for Population-Based Management,* Jones and Bartlett Pub., Sudbury, MA, 2008.

Odum, Eugene P.: *Fundamentals of Ecology,* W. B. Saunders Co., Philadelphia and London, 1959.

Patel, Kant; Rushefsky, Mark E.; McFarlane, Deborah R.: *The Politics of Public Health in the United States*, M.E. Sharpe, Armonk, New York, 2005.

Pencheon, David; Guest, Charles; Melzer, David; Gray, JA Muir: *Oxford Handbook of Public Health Practice*, Oxford University Press, 2006.

Ray M. Merrill: *Introduction to Epidemiology*, Jones & Bartlett Learning, United States, 2010.

Sanderson, Colin J.; Gruen, Reinhold: *Analytical Models for Decision Making*, Open University Press, United Kingdom, 2006

Schneider, Dona; David E Lilienfeld: *Public Health: the Development of a Discipline*, Rutgers University Press, New Brunswick, NJ, 2008.

Thomas, D.C.: *Statistical Methods in Genetic Epidemiology*, Oxford University Press, 2004.

Turnock, Bernard: *Public Health: What It Is and How It Works,* Jones and Bartlett Publishers, Sudbury, MA, 2009.

Vandermeer, J. H.; Goldberg, D. E.: *Population ecology: First principles. Woodstock,* Princeton University Press, Oxfordshire, 2003.

Vinten-Johansen, Peter, *Cholera, Chloroform, and the Science of Medicine: A Life of John Snow*, Oxford University Press, 2003.

White, Franklin; Stallones, Lorann; Last, John M.: *Global Public Health: Ecological Foundations*, Oxford University Press, 2013.

White, Kerr L.: *Healing the schism: Epidemiology, medicine, and the public's health*, Springer-Verlag, New York, 1991.

Wilkinson, R. G.: *Unhealthy Societies: The Afflictions of Inequality*, Routledge, New York, 1996.

Index

I

L

M

N

O

P

R

S

T

V

W

Y

❑❑❑